COMPARATIVE APPROACHES TO MEDICAL REASONING

ADVANCES IN FUZZY SYSTEMS – APPLICATIONS AND THEORY

Vol. 1: Between Mind and Computer: Fuzzy Science and Engineering
(*Eds. P.-Z. Wang and K.-F. Loe*)

Vol. 3: Comparative Approaches to Medical Reasoning
(*Eds. M. E. Cohen and D. L. Hudson*)

Forthcoming volumes:

Vol. 2: Industrial Applications of Fuzzy Technology in the World
(*Eds. K. Hirota and M. Sugeno*)

Vol. 4: Fuzzy Logic and Soft Computing
(*Eds. B. Bouchon-Meunier, R. R. Yager and L. A. Zadeh*)

Advances in Fuzzy Systems – Applications and Theory Vol. 3

COMPARATIVE APPROACHES TO MEDICAL REASONING

Editors

M. E. Cohen
California State University, Fresno
University of California, San Francisco

D. L. Hudson
University of California, San Francisco

World Scientific
Singapore • New Jersey • London • Hong Kong

Published by

World Scientific Publishing Co. Pte. Ltd.

P O Box 128, Farrer Road, Singapore 9128

USA office: Suite 1B, 1060 Main Street, River Edge, NJ 07661

UK office: 57 Shelton Street, Covent Garden, London WC2H 9HE

Library of Congress Cataloging-in-Publication Data

Comparative approaches to medical reasoning / editors, M. E. Cohen,
D. L. Hudson.
p. cm -- (Advances in fuzzy systems ; vol. 3)
Includes bibliographical references.
ISBN 9810221622
1. Clinical medicine -- Decision making -- Data processing.
2. Decision support systems. 3. Heart -- Diseases -- Treatment -
- Decision making -- Case studies. I. Cohen, M. E. (Maurice E.)
II. Hudson, D. L. (Donna L.) III. Series.
[DNLM: 1. Decision Making, Computer-Assisted. 2. Fuzzy Logic.
W26.55.D2 C737 1995]
R859.7.D42C66 1995
616'.001'1 -- dc20
DNLM/DLC
for Library of Congress

94-48854
CIP

Printed in Singapore.

PREFACE

In the last four decades, since the advent of the digital computer, numerous approaches have been tried to establish the computer as a tool to assist in medical decision making. Medical decision making is a good model for all types of decision making under uncertainty, in which some principles are known and others are not known or are only partially understood. This volume is a collection of papers which use unique approaches to deal with medical decision making. In order to facilitate comparison of methods, all papers deal with the same medical application: heart disease. The reader should be aware, however, that the contents of this book are in no way restricted to this area. In fact, each paper explains theoretical techniques which are applicable to any field in medicine, indeed to any field in which computer decision support tools are required. The use of a common problem makes it easier for readers to compare and contrast different approaches and see in practice the strengths and weaknesses of each approach.

The book is divided into five sections. The first section contains two chapters which deal with knowledge-based systems. These papers address some of the major issues confronting this approach, including handling of uncertain information and combination of diverse data types. The first paper by Kohout et al. focuses on interval-based fuzzy logic for decision making involving risk and uncertainty. The paper by Muscari addresses the role of varying data types, including temporal data, in the diagnostic process.

Section 2 focuses on neural network models, and contains four chapters. Proliferation of neural network systems in the last decade has led to considerable confusion. The four papers in this section contrast various approaches as well as represent the broad range of variables present in medical decision making. The first paper by Akay et al. uses three-layer back propagation to combine analysis of diastolic heart sounds with physical examination results. Paper two by Ding and Gupta addresses the use of fuzzy neural networks based on fuzzy min-max neurons. The paper by Kostis et al. uses a data base of 49,000 patients, some with five-year follow-up data, to predict long-term mortality in myocardial infarction. The concluding paper in this section by Sabbatini et al. uses a complex mixture of predictor variables for prognosis of one-year mortality for patients with congestive heart failure.

Section 3 addresses statistical approaches. The two papers in this section illustrate important extensions to traditional statistically-based systems. The paper by Patrick uses the CONSULT^R software developed by the author which includes a novel approach encompassing categories and subcategories of disease in which each subcategory uses a priori knowledge. The second paper by Römer and Kandel develops a generalized Bayes' Theorem for fuzzy evidences by means of Dempster-Shafer theory.

Section 4 presents two contributions using modeling techniques. The papers in this section illustrate the importance of physiologic modeling and its contribution to medical decision making when such models are available. The paper by Akay et al. uses multiresolution representations of heart fluctuations to characterize the autonomic nervous system regulation of cardiovascular activity before and after carotid surgery. The paper by Bachárová introduces a new concept for noninvasive diagnosis of left ventricular hypertrophy.

Finally, Section 5 contains three chapters on hybrid systems which use two or more of the techniques described in Sections 1 through 4 which have been integrated into a single comprehensive system. Assanelli et al. combine automatic electrocardiogram interpretation and measurement, questionnaire data, clinical observations, and epidemiological risk estimation. The contribution by Barschdorff et al. uses interpretation of filtered phonocardiographic signals by means of a neural network model. The final paper by Hudson, Cohen, and Deedwania combines a knowledge-based system, neural network model, and analysis of chaotic data to produce a comprehensive decision aid for chest pain.

Each approach in this book provides flexibility in application, and should be of interest to anyone working in the field of automated decision making. The contributions represent state-of-the-art work in medical decision making, and as such are also of interest to medical researchers in all areas, but especially in cardiology.

CONTENTS

CLINAID: MEDICAL KNOWLEDGE-BASED SYSTEM BASED ON FUZZY RELATIONAL STRUCTURES

LADISLAV J. KOHOUT

Department of Computer Science and the Institute for Cognitive Sciences, Florida State University, Tallahassee, Florida 32306-4019, USA

ISABEL STABILE

Academic Unit of Obstetrics and Gynaecology, The Royal London Hospital College, University of London, UK

WYLLIS BANDLER

Department of Computer Science and the Institute for Cognitive Sciences, Florida State University, Tallahassee, Florida 32306-4019, USA

JOHN ANDERSON, FRSM

King's College School of Medicine and Dentistry, University of London, UK

1. Introduction

In a series of papers and a monograph [1], we have described the conceptual structures as well as the basic architecture of the knowledge-based system CLINAID. Its architecture is aimed at supporting not only diagnosis but also other types of clinical activity and decision making in diverse clinical and/or hospital environments. In this chapter, we shall show the ways in which the cardiac body system fits within the overall scheme of the multiple body systems structure of medicine. The diagnostic structure of multiple body systems is in turn well-integrated into the overall context of other essential types of medical activities. The conceptual and formal framework of this paradigm is supported by the methodology of Activity Structures and of many-valued logic based (fuzzy) relational structures. A prominent mathematical and computational role in both knowledge representation & retrieval and approximate inference is played by triangle and square fuzzy relational products.

In general, CLINAID generic architecture is aimed at support of knowledge-based decision making with risk and under uncertainty. Such a system has to operate in a multi-environmental situation [2] and make decisions within a multiplicity of contexts [1]. Outstanding features of the context-dependent inference that do not fit conventional logic and Artificial Intelligence paradigms will be stressed, as these play an essential role in preserving the correctness of medical inference and judgement.

2. Challenges of Clinical Decision Making

2.1. Successes and Limitations of Conventional Expert System Shells

There were initially a substantial number of successful expert systems outside the medical field the majority of which were motivated by AI research in medicine. A typical example of the latter is PROSPECTOR that was heavily influenced by MYCIN. Most early successes in the medical field were expert systems operating within a narrow subdomain of some medical specialty, the problems of which were relatively easy to handle by means of rule-based expert systems technology.

To improve performance, rules were embedded into a frame structure in some systems, thus introducing explicit control over the dynamics of activation of the rules. Pioneering in this respect was the work of Aikins, who in her Ph.D. dissertation presented the design of CENTAUR in which frame-based control structures had access to clusters of rules, thus having the capability to control their activation. The knowledge and control structures of CENTAUR were a reworking of the knowledge representation structures of PUFFS, a purely rule-based system for the diagnosis of pulmonary diseases, implemented within the E-MYCIN shell. Clancey's NEO-MYCIN on the other hand resolved the problem of better structuring by grouping rules into partitions determined by the structure of concepts that these rules handled, and activating these by appropriate meta-rules. These developments were later transferred into very successful knowledge engineering tools and implementation shells. This technology allowed one to combine rule, frame and list structures in the expert system that were designed and implemented with help of these tools.

This early influence of medical expert systems on the development of new technology led to a rather paradoxical view within the non-medical part of the AI community and in some quarters of the industry. Namely, that everything in the mechanism of clinical decision making process is well understood, simple, almost trivial and hence of no interest to those outside Medicine. This opinion was also conditioned by the following incorrect and simplistic view: clinical decision making = making a diagnosis (sic!). As we shall see later, clinical decision making involves much more in addition to the diagnostic process. But it has been documented that even making diagnoses involves *multiple contexts, non-monotonicity of reasoning* and the need to handle *incomplete information.* These are the problems that the currently available routine knowledge engineering technologies cannot handle well, however good they are otherwise.

2.2. Context-Dependence of Diagnostic Inference

Problems remain not only in the context of global medical decision making, but also the diagnostic reasoning process. Extensive empirical enquiries conducted in response to the question "what are the basic features of clinical diagnostic inference", lead us to conclude that accomplished medical experts employ the reasoning process that can: [3]:

1. Handle successfully incompleteness of data.
2. Deal with locality of inference, where the validity of conclusions is limited to specific contexts.
3. Provide for directed complexity reduction of the inference that avoids pitfalls of combinatorial explosion.

Indeed, empirical evidence shows that, at its extremes, the path of diagnostic inference performed by an experienced clinician is qualitatively different from that of medical students (despite all their textbook knowledge). It transpires that an experienced clinician introduces new elements into the process of clinical judgement. These are the concepts of *a hierarchy of diagnostic levels* and *syndromes.* A syndrome is defined as a cluster of signs and symptoms that appear together and characterise a specific group of diseases. Syndromes perform an important function at a specific level of the diagnostic hierarchy. Indeed, the superior performance of an accomplished expert over that of a junior doctor (who due to clinical training has become familiar with syndromes and hierarchies) is primarily due to the fact that an experienced clinician utilizes this additional knowledge in a more efficient manner than a novice. These additional elements of knowledge are instrumental in vastly reducing the complexity of the inferential task as well as increasing its reliability. This is despite the fact that during the early stages of clinical training these additional elements appear to increase the possible difficulties experienced by medical students.

Such a pattern of reasoning employing the essential additional knowledge of diagnostic levels and syndromes is used in CLINAID. The inferential structure of its diagnostic unit also employs levels – as explained in Section 5.3 below. In the process of moving from ignorance to adequate knowledge CLINAID's inferential process passes dynamically through intermediate states involving various diagnostic levels. In these dynamic states, it has only partial information, hence the strategies of inference that guide repeated iterations through the levels will generate intermediate partial conclusions. The dynamics of inference is such that several partial conclusions can be kept under consideration until further diagnostic activity can distinguish between them. As more than one possibility is being considered at once, CLINAID implements a form of concurrent inference that depends on the context. This is made possible by employing relational inference mechanisms which have inherently parallel nature.

In terms of functional activity structures [4, 5], Inferential Structure (IHI) of CLINAID focuses its activity into a particular area of locality according to the context. Context is semantically controlled by syndromes. However, because the logical properties of a combination of premisses may be in conflict, the local contexts may clash. This, in general, leads to the phenomenon of paraconsistency [6], or in a more restricted situation at least to the requirement to deal with non-monotonic reasoning. The problem of inconsistency is avoided by employing *inference localised* within a specific context. Of course, the context in which the premisses are combined may change during the inferential process. Thus not only static logic components but also their dynamic interaction is *what matters.*

It has been observed that in the context of general medicine, the consequences of the simultaneous validity of 'Incompleteness' and of 'Locality of Inference' may in some contexts lead to 'dead ends' or 'blind alleys' of diagnostic inference. The inferential process *does not reach* the final conclusion because of the combinatorial explosion of the task, so that the chosen path has to be abandoned; or alternatively it reaches a *wrong conclusion* caused by the confusion of contexts. An interesting example is quoted [7]:

> "I have just taken the students over a patient with a very obvious carcinoma of the stomach who had vomited and bled. There is a certain syndrome that links his metabolic state, anaemia and everything together.

> They (the students) just see it as a list of sequences and they are searching through textbook images. They cannot group these things together and ask more pertinent questions. If you do, it makes a lot more sense, a lot more quickly."

The expert continues the explanation of how the diagnostic inference may end in a 'blind alley' by ignoring the proper context:

> "He (the patient) is starving to death, he is very seriously ill, he is an old man and you wouldn't expect to find bowel sounds. Well, they (the students) found no bowel sounds, but they go to a surgical list for absent bowel signs and they are quite lost. The answer is, he is not eating anything so you wouldn't expect his guts to be churning around."

The quote amicably shows how and why an accomplished expert uses certain higher order patterns of reasoning. We can see that in this context, the bowel signs were not diagnostically relevant. They were excluded dynamically, during the inference process, when it become apparent to the expert that they were *irrelevant in a specific context.* But outside this particular context, they still might be relevant. Excluding them inappropriately would cause what one might call *context-dependent incorrectness* of logical inference. Hence, when clinical judgement is concerned with matters that are outside of the narrow context located within a single medical specialty the context-dependence of medical reasoning cannot be ignored.

Ignoring this in the design of a knowledge-based system that is aimed at spanning a wider medical domain may result in a system that will exhibit unpredictable 'lapses of correctness of inference'. Namely, in the wrong context, the system would simply reach the wrong conclusion. This would not be detected unless the logic of inference can deal with a multiplicity of contexts. To deal with this problem adequately, it is necessary to design multi-context knowledge-based systems [2]. In CLINAID,we deal with this problem by partitioning the knowledge structures into multiple-body systems [8, 9] with concurrent inference over these.

Once the inferential process is focused into the body systems that are currently relevant, within the context that is controlled by introducing an appropriate questioning strategy [10, 11], syndromes begin to play an essential role. For example if dyspnea is the only symptom discovered then it could relate to either the cardiovascular system or the respiratory system or the endocrine or renal system. The possible syndromes which have dyspnea as one of their elements are next considered in each of the body systems and the most relevant questions will be asked. Then the questioning may shift to relevant physical signs if there are no further symptoms. The inferential process may reach a conclusion that one, or more than one body system could be involved. The knowledge-based system employing this multi-context process can then either suggest further investigations to resolve the diagnostic problem or the development of either further symptoms or new physical signs might be awaited if appropriate.

2.3. An Example of Multi-Context Inference Involving Several Body Systems

Let us look at a concrete example of clinical inference that involves several body systems. Symptom *Sore throat* may point to diseases in many body systems. The most likely of these will include:

1. an upper respiratory tract infection
2. rheumatic fever
3. collagen diseases (a large group)
4. leukemia
5. immune deficiency syndrome (a large group)

To decide which body system is affected we need to obtain a ranking order of likelihoods (plausibilities, possibilities and such like) of body system candidates. This is obtained by asking *questions* about the presence of other symptoms. It is a *constellation of symptoms* that makes one or other disease more likely.

Let us take *sore throat*, together with *running nose, eyes; headache, fever/chills*. If one or more of these are positive, this makes an *upper respiratory infection URI* most likely. Even if the answer is *no* to some questions this does not exclude the URI diagnosis.

We have, however to distinguish the context in which the answers appear: e g. if the patient is a child with *aching in the joints*, another diagnosis, namely, *rheumatic fever* becomes more likely.

In order to include context, it is not sufficient to present only symptoms; in many instances *risk factors* are also needed. These are obtained from the *patient history* and includes such items as past history, alcohol, drugs, diseases appearing in patient's family, relations, etc.

The likelihoods (plausibilities, possibilities) of this example are reinterpreted with respect to the context that is embedded within the structure containing *signs/symptoms, risk factors* and *body system* levels.

The expertise lies in utilizing this additional knowledge consisting of:

- knowing which question to ask next;
- the ability to interpret the answers in the right context;
- the competence in deciding which is the next body system to consider when the likelihood of the first candidate body system becomes less and less likely with the new questions presented.

2.4. Impact of Multiple Context Inference on Design of Medical Knowledge-Based Systems

Although it would superficially appear that the relation between signs, symptoms and illnesses is sufficient to adequately perform diagnostic inference, we have seen that this cannot be so in the broader medical context of multiple body systems. Sometimes it is also erroneously assumed that any medical diagnostic inference can be performed in a way similar to that used in the rule-based medical expert systems that proved successful in a very narrow medical knowledge domain, delimiting a tiny part of a single medical specialty. Investigation of the logical structure of broader categories of medical knowledge, however, shows that *this is not* an adequate way of dealing with the problem of diagnostic judgement in general. The example of general medical judgement presented in the previous section involving the need to identify the correct body system shows where the problem with multiple context comes from.

Indeed, the multiplicity of contexts leads to the same sign/symptom acquiring a *different meaning* in a different context, as will be shown by the detailed example in Section 7. This leads to a number of problems. By and large, these problems cannot be dealt with in a way that is logically correct and performance-wise adequate when classical rule-based systems or Prolog systems not supporting concurrent inference and using logic without types are employed.

As we mentioned above, in order to avoid the problems of inference caused by 'Incompleteness' and 'Locality', the expert often uses higher units of knowledge, namely 'syndromes' and other groupings, in moving towards a diagnosis. Introducing an appropriate strategy into the inference process helps to avoid the 'blind alleys' of inference and to eliminate the problems caused by excessive complexity. It is most essential to take the complexity aspect into account, as an inference process can rapidly grow and became unmanageable.

We are now in a better position to revisit the three problems effective clinical judgement has to deal with and to suggest a path to their solution:

- The Problem of INCOMPLETENESS:
  Not all signs and symptoms characterising the disease are always observable or present. Inference methods that can deal with incomplete information are essential.
- The Problem of LOCALITY OF INFERENCE:
  Not all signs and symptoms are relevant in a particular given diagnostic context. Means for handling relevance and irrelevance of premisses in multiplicity of contexts is required.
- The Problem OF COMPLEXITY OF INFERENCE:
  The complexity of exhaustive matching of all disease descriptors and indicators (e.g. signs, symptoms, tests, etc.) may be forbidingly high. Strategies for reduction of complexity of inference need to be employed.

Conceptually, levels of diagnostic inference employing additional constructs such as syndromes are used in inference, and the judgmental process is instantiated by suitable inferential strategies. That is the way an accomplished medical expert deals with the three problems of diagnostic inference. This process has been characterised by an instructive analogy [12]:

> "We can view the diagnostic process at different levels, as a small part of a chess game. Thus there may be an opening game, a middle game and the end game. Thus it may be possible to *see the different stages in a similar way* and so decrease complexity."

To deal with the different stages in a similar way, preserving the diversity of levels and at the same time dynamically imposing suitable inferential strategies over these within a knowledge-based system requires a unique range of methods that can be presented and manipulated in a unified computational framework. Many-valued logic based (fuzzy) relational computational methods and architectures provide the desired means.

In a nutshell, the relational approach employed by CLINAID can be characterised as follows. Inference methods that can deal with incomplete information and are capable of handling relevance and irrelevance of premisses in a multiplicity of contexts are provided by means of triangle and square products of relations. Fuzzy relational knowledge representation methods combined with fast fuzzy relational algorithms provide the means for eliciting, representing and verifying knowledge structures to be used in multi-context inference. Multi-context inference is performed by means of triangle and square products operating over the fuzzy relational structures. Strategies for reduction of complexity of inference that are to be employed while dealing with multiple contexts have to be parallel. Parallelism is, however, inherent in relational inference employing relational products.

3. An Overview of CLINAID Architecture

The majority of extant medical expert systems deal with a limited medical context, the largest domain of knowledge being just a single medical field, e.g. Internal medicine in CADUCEUS. The inherent limitation of such medical expert systems is in its essence conceptual and logical: their knowledge bases and inference engines cannot mix easily the knowledge from several fields without some adverse effects. CLINAID deals with this problem by introducing a multi-centre architecture in the Diagnostic Unit. The medical data and knowledge of each medical specialist field exhibit different logical properties. This in turn leads to the several kinds of many-valued logics on which the relational inference and data manipulation is based. Semantic and epistemological justification of the use of these logics for the ***interval-valued inference*** is provided by a theoretical device called the ***checklist paradigm*** [13].

4. Description of the Clinaid Architecture

The CLINAID architecture [9, 8, 14], consists of four main co-operating units (basic shell substratum):

1. Diagnostic Unit (comprized of several parallel co-operating centres)
2. Treatment Recommendation Unit
3. Patient Clinical Record Unit.
4. Co-ordination and Planning Unit.

The global configuration of this architecture, including the data and control flow interaction between its main parts is shown in Figure 1. Each unit of this configuration is a quite complex autonomous subsystem. The greatest degree of concurrency is achieved in the Diagnostic Unit which is comprized of a number of parallel co-operating centres. Each centre of the Diagnostic Unit deals with a different body system. It is processing its own input and may be co-ordinating several parallel threads of computation within its own structure in a multicontext fashion.

This parallel function is facilitated by relational representation of inference (cf. Section 6 below) which also supports interval-based reasoning [15] as explained in greater detail in Section 7.

As is apparent from Figure 1, also the other parts, namely the Treatment Recommendation Unit, Patient Clinical Record Unit and Co-ordination and Planning Unit have to interact concurrently. Each of these global units is at the same time a knowledge source and an information consumer. The operation of communicating knowledge sources is an important issue of its own standing (cf. [16]). As we are concerned in this paper mainly with

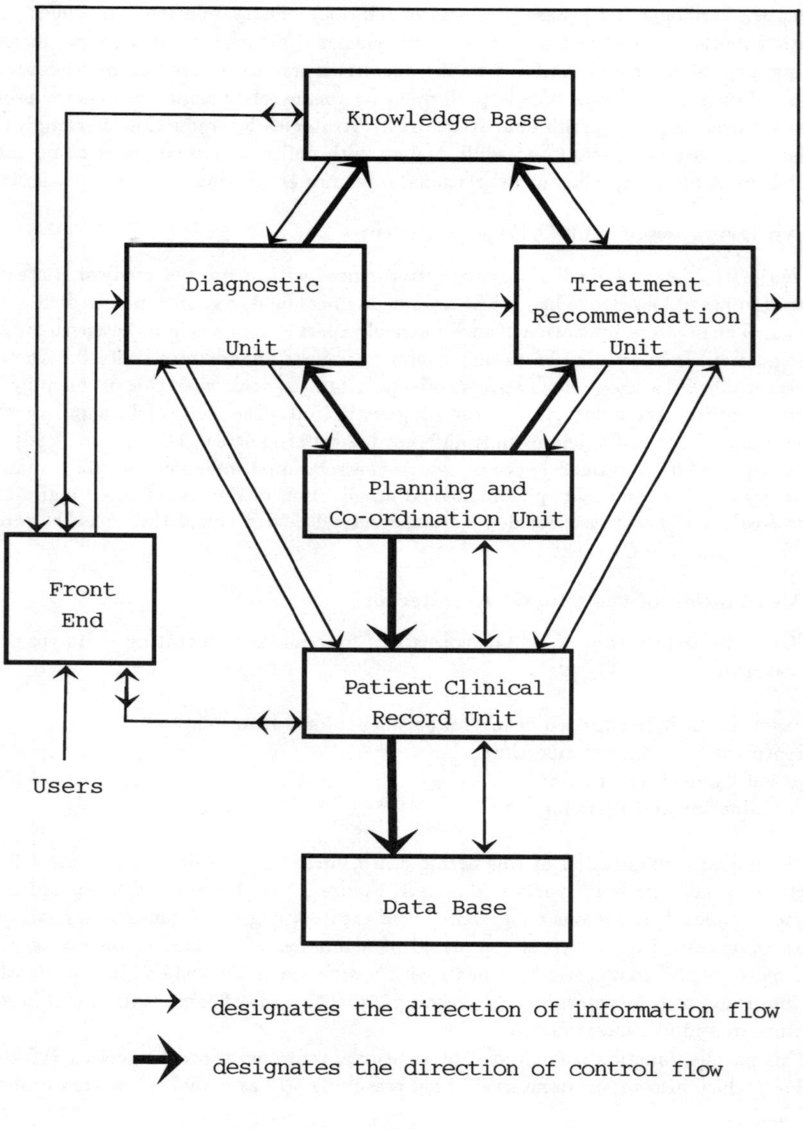

Figure 1: The basic configuration of Clinaid.

the interplay of issues of parallelism with context-dependent inference, we shall direct our presentation in subsequent sections towards a more detailed exposition of the multi-centre Diagnostic Unit that involve not only the cardiac but also other body systems. We shall proceed now with a brief outline of activities of the individual CLINAID units that helps to appreciate better the global functions of CLINAID and their dynamic interaction.

4.1. The Diagnostic Unit

The purpose of the unit is to assist in the diagnosis of diseases that are within its purview. During this activity it accepts the information required in a dynamic manner. It is not connected to the patient but relies on requests to the user (clinician) for further information as long as it lacks sufficient information to recommend a working diagnosis. As it acquires more and more information, it restricts the set of the most likely diseases to fewer and fewer. During this activity, the unit is in potential communication with the treatment recommendation unit. This is in order to deal with possible emergencies if necessary, before the working diagnosis is reached. Finally the unit either proffers a conclusion for the user's consideration or, if it still lacks sufficient evidence, an indication is given that the unit is unable to reach a final diagnostic conclusion. If a conclusion is reached then this conclusion is communicated to the Treatment Recommendation Unit.

During the inference process, the Diagnostic Unit requires the experts' knowledge and experience which is obtained from the Knowledge Base. Sometimes this unit also requires use of the patient's medical record when it works towards a diagnosis. All the signs, symptoms, the results laboratory tests and the conclusion are communicated to the Patient Clinical Record Unit. The occurrence of this communication depends on the context and circumstances. Patients records are updated dynamically as the clinical process proceeds, and in some situations this also requires concurrency [17, 18].

As CLINAID attempts to be a comprehensive medical consultation system, its knowledge base has to contain a large amount of medical expert knowledge. Taking the diagnostic unit as an example, CLINAID deals with a number of body systems, where each body system belongs to a different branch of medicine. The multiplicity of body systems in which the given signs and symptoms of a particular patient are interpreted, defines logically a multiplicity of contexts. It requires special precautions for the inferential system to deal with this multiplicity of contexts correctly, and this has to be reflected in the diagnostic unit architecture and the inferential procedures employed. Exactly how the relational products are used to deal with this challenge will be seen later in Section 5.

The average size of the knowledge structure of a body system of a comprehensive medical system indicates that the problems of efficiency and correctness of inference are not insignificant:

Signs/symptoms per body system	200-400 approximately
Diseases per body system	100-400 approximately
The total number of body systems......	11

Seven of the body systems listed in the CLINAID specification [8] are part of the following list:

1. Cardiovascular

2. Respiratory
3. Central Nervous System
4. Muscular and Peripheral Nervous System
5. Renal
6. Endocrine
7. Blood and Reticulo-endothelial
8. Reproductive
9. Skeletal
10. Gastrointestinal
11. Psychological

By comparison with INTERNIST and CADUCEUS, CLINAID faces a formidable problem. INTERNIST deals only with internal medicine and contains several hundred diseases. We are considering eleven body systems in the specification of our design. When the patient's signs and symptoms indicate candidate diseases from more than one system, the complexity of inference is formidable and parallelism is required for acceptable performance of the system. It will, however, be seen in the sequel that parallel inference can be performed also within one and each body system subunit of the diagnostic unit. Indeed, to have an acceptable speed of performance when a multiplicity of many-valued logic is used, some degree of real-time concurrency is inevitable.

4.2. The Treatment Recommendation Unit

The purpose of the second unit is to advise about treatment, taking into the account the working diagnosis and the possible adverse effects [19] of each member of the family of prima facie treatments appropriate for each individual patient. This unit accepts the conclusion of the Diagnostic Unit as its input data. It also sends a request for the pharmacological drug history to the patient record unit. In order to make a treatment recommendation, it needs the experts' knowledge from the Knowledge Base and the past history of the patient provided by the Patient Clinical Record Unit [20].

4.3. Co-ordination and Planning Unit

The fourth unit provides the overall control of the clinical management activities as well as all the necessary auxiliary matching functions such as generating and unifying the communication protocols. In addition it has to contain the log of the co-ordinating process to facilitate monitoring and auditing of the operation of the whole system.

We have seen that each of these four units fulfils a certain global task. The global tasks co-operate concurrently and for this purpose the units are connected to each other by appropriately matched data and control flow interfaces which are structured within an additional unit called "whiteboard." It should be noted that each unit of CLINAID may consist of a number of centres and thus itself form a multi-centre fuzzy knowledge-based system. The units themselves, each being already a multi-centre system, have also to co-operate in a concurrent manner. Hence, there is a two level hierarchy of concurrent activities – each unit can be viewed as an autonomous agent co-operating with other agents within a distributed structure of a *higher order*.

5. Knowledge Representation and Inference in Clinaid

5.1. Triangle and Square Types of Relational Products

Where R is a relation from X to Y, and S a relation from Y to Z, a ***product relation*** $R * S$ is a relation from X to Z, determined by R and S. There are several types of product used to produce product-relations [21, 22]. Each product type performs a **different logical action** on the intermediate sets, as ***each logical type*** of the product enforces a ***distinct specific meaning*** on the resulting product-relation $R * S$. When the relations are fuzzy, there is a further wide choice of realization for each of the four product kinds, because several many-valued logics provide ***implication operator*** and other connectives suitable for interval computation. In order to explain clearly the need for, and the significance of, different logical types of relational products, we begin with crisp relations, and then extend these to fuzzy.

Definition

Circle product:	$x(R \circ S)z \Leftrightarrow xR$ intersects Sz
Triangle Subproduct:	$x(R \lhd S)z \Leftrightarrow xR \subseteq Sz$
Triangle Superproduct	$x(R \rhd S)z \Leftrightarrow xR \supseteq Sz$
Square product:	$x(R \sqsubset S)z \Leftrightarrow xR = Sz$

Before the relational products can be of real service in interval computing, they must be fuzzified. For their fuzzification, the many-valued logic based (fuzzy) ***power set theories*** are essential [23, 24]. Once the concept of the fuzzy powerset is clearly understood, the way of fuzzifying formulas defining relational compositions becomes obvious. In order to switch over to the matrix notation that is more convenient computationally because of its explicit handling of logic values, we express the relational products in their pure logical form. In the logic formulas, R_{ij} will represent the fuzzy degree to which the statement $x_i R y_j$ is true.

$$(R \circ S)_{ik} = \bigvee_j (R_{ij} \bigwedge S_{jk})$$
$$(RS)_{ik} = \bigwedge_j (R_{ij} \rightarrow S_{jk})$$
$$(R \rhd S)_{ik} = \bigwedge_j (R_{ij} \leftarrow S_{jk})$$
$$(R \square S)_{ik} = \bigwedge_j (R_{ij} \equiv S_{jk})$$

The customary logical symbols for the logic connectives *AND, OR*, both ***implications*** and the ***equivalence*** in the above formulas represent the connectives of some many-valued logic, **chosen** according to the properties of the products required. The details of choice of the appropriate many-valued connectives are discussed in [25, 26, 27].

It is important to distinguish what we call ***harsh*** fuzzy products (defined above) from a different family, the family of ***mean*** products. Given the general formula $(R@S)_{ik} ::= \#(R_{ij} * S_{jk})$, a mean product is obtained by replacing the outer connective $\#$ by $\sum$ and normalizing the resulting product appropriately. The mean products provide an effective inference mechanism in CLINAID applications.

Representation of clinical knowledge structures requires not only quantitative but also qualitative notions. Product-relations formed by the relational products represent new entities composed from the original data. Their specific semantics defines the conceptual meaning which is partially dependent on the conceptual meaning of the original data-relations.

If R is the relation between *patients* and *individual symptoms*, and S a relation between *symptoms* and *diseases*, $R * S$ will be a relation between *patients and diseases*. The diagnostic clinical interpretation of each distinct logical type (e.g. the triangular square product types) of these product-relations has a **distinct clinical meaning** [26]:

$x(R \circ S)z$: x has at least one symptom of illness z.
$x(R \triangleleft S)z$: x's symptoms are among those which characterize z.
$x(R \triangleright S)z$: x's symptoms include all those which characterize z.
$x(R \square S)z$: x's symptoms are exactly those of illness z.

5.2. *The Checklist Paradigm in Interval Inference*

The triangle and square products may be based on a large variety of many-valued logic implication operators; a practical question then arises, as to which many-valued set or relational theory is the best for a particular application and/or knowledge domain, or inference task. Evaluation experiments performed in various applications [28, 29] conclusively show the importance of selecting a fuzzy knowledge representation structure or inference/decision making method that appropriately matches the data/knowledge structures dictated by the particular application. The most important point that emerges from empirical studies is that the technique that should be employed in a specific application will crucially depend on the nature of data and knowledge involved.

The interval inference in CLINAID is theoretically justified by the checklist paradigm. The checklist paradigm generates *pairs of* distinct connectives of the same logical type that determine the end points of intervals, thus providing formally and epistemologically justified systems of *interval-valued* approximate inference. The inequality restricting the possible values of measure m(F) expressing the logical values that fall within the interval, is written in its general form as: $contop \geq m(F) \geq conbot$. In this paper we employ $m(F) = m_1(F) = 1 - (\alpha_{10}/n)$. This choice yields the bounds [25]:

$$min(1, 1 - a + b) \geq m_1(PLY) \geq max(1 - a, b)$$

where the Lukasiewicz implication represents one bound while the other bound (plybot) is the Kleene-Dienes implication operator. Choosing for *con* the connective type **AND** we get for the same measure the bounds $min(a, b) \geq m_1(AND) \geq max(0, a+b-1)$. Further details and additional references may be obtained from a recent survey paper on the progress of the checklist paradigm methods [30].

5.3. *Dealing With the Inferential Context in CLINAID*

The diagnostic unit of CLINAID deals with a *multiplicity* of contexts provided by the several the body systems and other factors. Deep knowledge concerning *individual contexts* takes into account cross-contextual similarities and differences. We distinguish: a) the *context of different body systems*; b) the *context of different diagnostic levels* within the super-context of a specific body system.

There are hundreds of symptoms and physical signs which are related to different body systems. These symptoms and physical signs do not have the same importance in each body system, some play a more prominent role in one body system than in another. A few may distinctly identify a particular body system.

We have already explained that our method of dealing with complexity reduction is to subdivide the activities and so decrease the size of the problem to be resolved at any particular stage. This hierarchical manner of subdividing the activities reveals the structure of processes that can be executed in parallel and allows the inference to proceed rapidly. CLINAID uses classificatory knowledge in order to diagnose diseases. As more information is obtained from the patient and presented by the doctor to the system, groups of unrelated diseases can be eliminated from the diagnostic path. This process continues until the final diagnostic conclusion is reached.

The inferential process is performed in a hierarchical or heterarchical manner, involving the following levels:

1. Symptoms and Sign Level
2. Risk Factors Level
3. Body System Level
4. Syndrome Level
5. General Disease Level
6. Specific Disease Level
7. Aetiological Level

The strategy of clinical inference used over this diagnostic hierarchy is realized by means of fuzzy triangle products [21]. Within each specific body system of CLINAID, (e.g. cardiac or respiratory, etc.) the inferential levels have to be related appropriately. Each body system has specific conceptual semantics that assign the clinical meaning to the relational compositions.

At each level of the diagnostic process, different fuzzy relations are used to perform the inference because the *purpose* of each fuzzy relation is different. Hence internal information within each relation may also differ. For example, the use of symptoms and physical signs at level three (body system level) and four (syndrome level) are not identical. The symptoms and physical signs at level three represent symptoms and physical signs of the whole human body, thus forming a relation which can identify possible body systems. On the other hand, symptoms and physical signs of level four represent all the symptoms and physical signs a syndrome consists of, and are meant to identify the relevant syndrome(s). All this can be formalized and expressed as a stream of relational computations. The conceptual contents of the levels and their mutual interaction are expressed by means of mathematical relations. Such a relational description is presented in the next section.

6. The Relational Structures of a Diagnostic Centre Representing a Specific Body System

6.1. A General Outline

The relations are created, represented and computed according to the level-based classification given in the previous section. Only the items of information which are relevant for reaching the conclusion of a specific level are utilized when each level is activated. The relations employed within a diagnostic level are particular to that level. They are made redundant after the process has passed through that diagnostic level. In this way, a fraction of the entire knowledge is used at any one time, and therefore the complexity of such a structure and the processing time are sharply reduced.

The activation of levels within the specific body system represented in a centre of the diagnostic unit is ordered by the following sequence:

(body system) $\Rightarrow$ syndromes $\Rightarrow$ general diseases $\Rightarrow$ working diagnoses.

Signs and symptoms of a patient entered into the system are matched with the knowledge structures distributed within the individual levels of a specific centre. The stream of computations passes through the levels of the above sequence, in an iterative manner. This is depicted in Figure 2.

The knowledge represented at each level is captured in a relational structure and the inference is performed by the relational products composing the knowledge items of the levels with the information items entered into the level from its environment. Table 10.2 in [1] provides further details.

Complexity of clinical inference within the multiple context is reduced by the diagnostic hierarchy which uses *syndromes* as the main instrument. Syndromes are essential when dealing with a multiplicity of body systems of general medicine, as they help to focus the inference within a particular context, excluding those combinations of signs and symptoms that are irrelevant within the context the syndromes define.

A syndrome is defined as a cluster of signs and symptoms that appear together and characterise a specific group of diseases. This cluster consists of signs and symptoms that, when viewed in probabilistic/statistical terms, are mutually dependent.

The knowledge contained in syndromes and similar semantic constraints, additional to that contained in the relationship of signs and symptoms to diseases vastly reduces complexity of the inferential task as well as increasing its reliability. Without the application of such constructs the inferential process might have difficulty in reaching the final conclusion.

Semiotic Descriptors and Fuzzy Relational Knowledge Structures of Individual Diagnostic Levels

Let us list now, the medical meaning (semiotic descriptors) of all sets entering into the relations of individual levels.

B .... a set of body systems.
G .... a set of general diseases.
D .... a set of specific diseases.
I .... a set of investigations.
P .... a set of patients.
S .... a set of symptoms and physical signs.
Y .... a set of syndromes.

Definition of the relation 'symptoms and signs to body systems'

$SB \in \mathcal{F}(S \rightarrow B)$

The relation SB relates the set S of symptoms and physical signs to individual body systems B. The aim of this relation is to select the body systems relevant to presented patient information. Therefore, the symptoms and physical signs which form this relation are those which are suitable to identify relevant body systems efficiently. This relation is used in

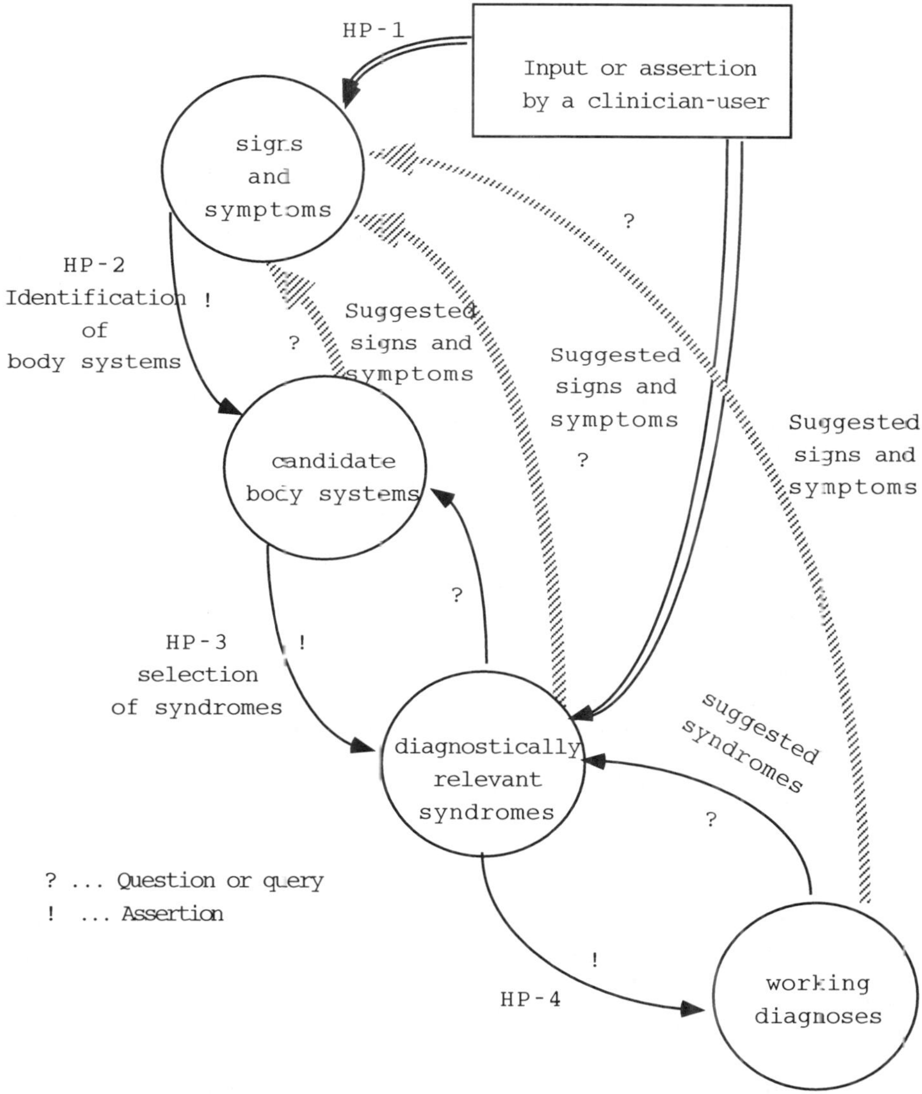

Figure 2: Activity graph of the dynamics of a body system.

those versions of CLINAID which use point based fuzzy reasoning. When the interval-based reasoning is involved, a more complex scheme using ternary relations is used. This will be described in sufficient detail in Section 7 where we present the clinical example diagnosing cardiac diseases.

Definition of the relation 'symptoms and signs to syndromes'

$SY_i \in \mathcal{F}(S \to Y)$

This is a family of fuzzy relations as there is a different relation SY_i for each of the body systems. The aim of this fuzzy relation is to identify possible syndromes. By identifying the appropriate syndromes, the complexity of search for diseases can be reduced, since a syndrome is a cluster of relevant symptoms and physical signs. The semantic type of each relation of this level is the same (from signs and symptoms to syndromes), regardless of which body system contains that fuzzy relation. But the domain and the range of each SY_i are different from the domains and ranges of other relations of this family since each belongs to a different body system. Also the degrees of symptoms, physical signs or general diseases differ, as these do not have the same certainty in each body system.

Definition of the relation 'syndromes to general diseases'

$YG_i \in \mathcal{F}(Y \to G)$

The fuzzy relation YG_i shows the degree of relevance of syndromes Y to different general diseases G. The aim of this fuzzy relation is to identify the general diseases of the patient. There is a separate relation for each body system.

Definition of the relation from 'general diseases G to investigations I'

$GI \in \mathcal{F}(G \to I)$

There are several possible types of investigation I, tests or examinations that can be performed to explore each general disease. In fact, the fuzzy relation GI shows for each general disease, the possible number of investigations with their degree of relevance. The aim of this fuzzy relation is to identify the possible investigations that can be performed for a particular general disease which ultimately can contribute to the identification of specific disease(s).

Definition of the relation from 'investigations results J to specific diseases D'.

JD $\in \mathcal{F}(J \to D)$

The results of the investigations, tests or examinations can lead to the identification of specific diseases. These investigation results can contribute by identifying specific diseases with a varying degree of certainty. The relation JD shows the results of investigations which yield specific diseases with different degrees of relevance(certainty). The aim of this relation, accepting the results of an investigation, is to be able to confirm, reject or change the priority of the specific diseases that might be in the current working diagnoses set.

If the etiological level is added, the current clinical state and the dynamics of the change of the patient have to be interpreted with respect to the causal relations displaying the causal factors which are statistically reflected in risk factors. These factors can be divided into the disease primary cause and the causes of the subsequent development. This kind of information cannot be dealt with by conventional rule-based technologies but requires a fundamentally different approach to causality as described in [31]. On a different level the interpretation can be linked to physiological models, and the causal factors interpreted with respect to the physiology related explanations, such as provided for cardiovascular diseases in [32]. In the neurological body system a link to the neurological substratum may sometime be helpful. In such cases a pair of substratum and functional structure is to be employed in the etiological level of the knowledge based system. Some guidelines as how to deal conceptually and formally with these is provided in [33, 34] and [5] chapters 3–5.

6.2. Inadequacy of Bayesian Inference

Although syndromes carry important medical information, they are usually neglected by the designers of medical ESs. There are several reasons for this. One of these is the fact that when Bayesian inference is used, the dependency of the syndrome's component substantially increases the complexity of Bayesian inference. This has the consequence that the resulting expert system cannot deal with the multiple contexts and works satisfactorily only within the narrow context of one body system. If, on the other hand, the designer opts for the inclusion of syndromes, it has the following serious consequences when Bayesian inference is used. Given m diseases and n signs & symptoms that are independent, one requires $P_{ind} = m.n + m + n$ probabilities. Without the assumption of independence, and given k dependent signs & symptoms simultaneously, one requires $P_{dep} = (m.n)^k + m + n^k$ probabilities. Taking for example one body system which contains for the purpose of this example 200 diseases and 200 signs & symptoms, $P_{ind} = 40,400$. Taking 10 dependent signs & symptoms that enter into 1 syndrome, $P_{dep} = 4.10^{40}$. This explains why excluding syndromes and/or using Bayesian inference is an inadequate, albeit common, approach. We believe that the unique design of CLINAID avoids this pitfall.

We have discussed the major limitation of conventional systems which are due to the mismatch of properties of the data with properties of the Bayesian statistics. The next issue is the multiplicity of contexts in which a given item of input data (patient's signs and symptoms) must be interpreted, in order to reach the conclusion–by deciding which of the competing hypotheses is the most plausible one.

If, however, one intends to employ Bayesian inference, a careful check and simulation has to be performed to establish that the domain in which it is to be used is adequate for it. Chard's method of simulation has to be used [35] to verify the degree of inaccuracy introduced.

7. Multi-context Inference in Clinaid Involving Interval-Valued Inference

In this section we present a clinical example clearly demonstrating the use of fuzzy interval logics in CLINAID. The main contribution of interval reasoning is to provide the limits by which the degrees of plausibility of logical conclusion must be bound. After outlining the necessary prerequisites in terms of the relational structures involved, we present the actual computations that clearly demonstrate the merit of our method. Our main concern in this paper is to show how the cardiac and other body systems are dynamically selected. This dynamic selection avoids the ambiguities of multiple contexts that may be created by apparent conflicts of incomplete input information.

7.1. Relationships Over the Basic Relational Structures of Clinaid

Global inferential activity of CLINAID consists of matching the relevant empirical findings with medical theories and normative facts ([2] Chapter 10 section 4, pp. 181-184). Empirical findings are obtained through communication with patients (syndromes), direct observations of patient by a clinician (signs) and by laboratory tests and investigations. Medical theories and normative facts are held in the knowledge bases of CLINAID and are represented mostly as many-valued logic based (fuzzy) relations. The match of the two described kinds of information is performed by relational compositions which are called circle and square products, and triangle sub- and super-products (cf. section 5.1 above). The types of products needed to deal with the example presented in this section are listed and explained below.

Let us list now, the medical meaning (semiotic descriptors) of all the sets entering into the relations of individual levels used in the sequel.

Name:	A set of:
B	body systems.
D	specific diseases.
V	variability index of observation events.
P	patients.
S	symptoms and physical signs.

Name:	Definition:	Relation
PVS	$\mathcal{R}(P \times V \times S)$	between *patients, variability index (time) of observation events* and *signs and symptoms*
VBS	$\mathcal{R}(V \times B \times S)$	between *variability index of observation events* and *signs and symptoms*
PS	$\mathcal{R}(P \to S)$	from *patients* to *symptoms and physical signs.*
PD	$\mathcal{R}(P \to D)$	from *patients* to *specific diseases.*
SB	$\mathcal{R}(S \to B)$	from *symptoms and physical signs* to *body systems.*
SD	$\mathcal{R}(S \to D)$	from *symptoms and physical signs* to *specific diseases.*

Now, we shall briefly explain the meaning and purpose of the relations employed in the inference. Given are two ternary relations, PVS and VBS, from which the composed relations PBS and PB are computed. The medical domain semantics (i.e. semiotic descriptors) is outlined below.

PVS is a ternary (3-place) relation relating the set of patients P with the set of all time instances V at which the observations of relevant signs and symptoms S are made. This relation belongs to the family of relations capturing the relevant empirical findings. VBS is a ternary relation relating the variability index of observational events V with the set of body systems B and the set of signs and symptoms S. This relation belongs to the family of relations capturing medical theories and normative facts. The VBS relation captures the relationship between signs and symptoms and body systems. In the example discussed here, the relationship of S and B does not depend on the variability index, as the relationship is stable in time.

The actual observations of patients captured by PVS relation have to be matched with the knowledge contained in the relation VBS over the set V. This yields the computation

$$PBS_{imk} = (PVS \triangleleft VBS)_{imk} = (1/cardV)\sum_{j=l}(PVS_{ijk} \to VBS_{lmk})$$

Table 1: Relation of Signs/symptoms to Body systems

Signs/symptoms	*Body systems*			
	RS	CVS	MS	HEM
SOB	.9	.9	.3	.6
PND	.1	.9	.1	.6
Cyanosis	.8	.8	.3	.3
Tachycardia	.5	.9	.2	.6
Fine basal creps	.2	.9	.2	.6
Ankle swelling	.3	.9	.2	.6
Hepatomegaly	.3	.7	.1	.6

$$PB_{im} = (PBS\square^{*}PBS)_{im} = (1/cardS)\sum_{k}(PBS_{imk} \wedge (PBS_{imk} \equiv PBS_{imk}))$$

where *card V, card S* are the cardinalities (sizes) of the sets of relevant elements, over which the relational composition (matching) is performed. The second product yielding the relation PB computes the degree of involvement of each body system relative to the composition over available symptoms and signs (and generally also over other observables) characterising individual patients. The connectives used by this method are divided into two classes: TOPCON and BOTCON, computing the top and bottom point of the interval of the possible values of the products. We have used the following connectives in the examples of the next section:

$$TOPCON: \quad a \rightarrow_5 = min(1, 1-a+b); \quad a \equiv b = min(1-a+b, 1-b+a).$$

$$BOTCON: \quad a \rightarrow_6 b = max(1-a, b); \quad a \equiv b = max(a+b-1, 1-(a+b)).$$

7.2. *The Use of Interval Relational Inference in CLINAID: An Example of Diagnosis of a Cardio-Vascular Problem*

In this section we present a sample result of working diagnoses computed from real clinical data. Table 1 presents a small fragment of the knowledge structure of CLINAID, capturing the relationship of signs/symptoms to several body systems. The first part of the example shows how the interval based inference helps in selecting the relevant body system in CLINAID, while the second part presents the actual working diagnoses within the Cardiac body system.

Let us assume that our clinical case is a patient that exhibits the following set S of signs and symptoms. The set S is a fuzzy set consisting of $s_1 = SOB/.8$ (Shortness of breath), $s_2 = AS/.6$ (Ankle swelling), $s_3 = HM/.7$ (Hepatomegaly), $s_4 = ANX/.6$ (Anxiety), $s_5 = JVPH/.8$ (Jugular venous pressure high), $s_6 = CMRM/.7$ (Cardiac murmurs), $s_7 = PLP/.7$ (Palpitations) and $s_8 = RVEP/.75$ (Right ventricular enlargement). From this set, and using the clinical knowledge structure of Table 1 one computes the relation PB that suggests the involvement of individual body systems. This relation is computed by the

Table 2: Interval-Based Diagnosis: Identification of Possible Body Systems of Patient p_1

Body Systems	$p_1 PB$		$1 - p_1 PB$	
RS	.5	.43	.57	.5
CVS	1.0	.67	.33	0
MS	.5	.33	.67	.5
HEM	.9	.2	.8	.1
value	max-positive	min-positive	max-negative	min-negative
Grounds for:	*Acceptance*		*Rejection*	

products $PVS \lhd VBS$ and $PBS\Box^* PBS$ listed above. The results of this computation are listed in Table 3.

It can be seen from Table 2 that there is ***high*** positive evidence for the involvement of cardiovascular system CVS, *low*, negligible positive and negative evidence (around .5) for respiratory system RS and ***substantial*** negative evidence for the involvement of the muscular system MS. There is, however, great uncertainty in indicating the possibility of the involvement of the hematological system HEM. From the clinical point of view, the wide interval [.2, .9] indicates that the given signs and symptoms are not as specific for HEM as they are for the cardiovascular system CVS. Hence, the CVS is the winning candidate body system.

The relevant syndromes in a specific body system are computed by the fuzzy triangle product $PY = PS \lhd SY$ from patients to syndromes given by the formula

$$PS_{ij} = (PS \lhd SY)_{ik} = (1/cardS)\sum_j (PS_{ij} \rightarrow SY_{jk})$$

The following syndromes are identified as the most plausible for patient p_1:
Acute cardiac failure (ACF), Left sided heart failure (LHF), Right sided heart failure (RHF), Murmurs (MRM) and *Dysrythmia (DSR)*. The intervals of the possibility of their occurrence are listed in the decreasing order as the fuzzy interval set of syndromes Y: $Y = \{ACF/[.72, .57],\ DSR/[.63, .43],\ MRM/[.56, .48],\ RHF/[.54, .47],\ LHF/[.38, .36]\}$.

Utilizing the same clinical information for the patient p_1, namely the fuzzy set S listed above, one can obtain the working diagnoses for this patient. Fixing l in order to select a specific candidate syndrome, one computes the working diagnoses, using the fuzzy triangle product $PDY = PS \lhd SDY$. This relational composition, the result of which ranges from patients to diseases is given by the formula

$$PDY_{ikl} = (PS \lhd SDY)_{ikl} = (1/cardS)\sum_j (PS_{ij} \rightarrow SDY_{jkl})$$

It can be seen from the results listed in Table 3 that the only significant candidate diseases are *Congestive Heart Failure (CHF)* within the fuzzy interval *[1.0, 0.76]* and *Heart Block* within *[0.89, 0.64]*. The winning candidate *CHF* is indeed the correct diagnosis. The intervals of the other diseases do not overlap with the interval *[1.0, 0.76]* at all, having their

Table 3: Working Diagnoses.

Syndrome: Disease	**Acute Cardiac Failure** (ACF/[0.72, 0.57]): Possibility of occurrence
Congestive Heart Failure	[1.0, 0.76]
Heart Block	[0.89, 0.64]
Myocardial Infarction	[0.73, 0.59]
Malignant Hypertension	[0.72, 0.59]
Cardiomyopathy	[0.73, 0.58]

Syndrome: Disease	**Murmurs in structural cardiac and blood vessel lesions** MRM/[.56, .48] Possibility of occurrence
Tricuspid Valve Disease	[0.73, 0.57]
Mitral Valve Disease	[0.71,0.54]
Pulmonary Valve Disease	[0.64, 0.54]
Occlusion of Superior Venae Calva	[0.64, 0.53]
Aneurysm of Aorta	[0.56, 0.48]
Aorta Valve Disease	[0.53, 0.46]

Syndrome: Disease	**Dysrythmia** DSR/[.63, .43] Possibility of occurrence
Atrial Fibrillation	[0.63, 0.44]
Tachycardia	[0.63, 0.43]
Bradycardia	[0.63, 0.43]

values significantly lower. For this reason these diseases can be disregarded from further consideration. It should be noted that this working diagnosis is based entirely on the small set of signs and symptoms listed above. Additional patient data confirming the working diagnosis should be obtained by further clinical investigations. The resulting laboratory-test patient data can be processed by CLINAID at the level of investigations.

8. Conclusion

The generic architecture of CLINAID is designed to operate in a multienvironmental situation and make decisions within a multiplicity of contexts. In this paper we have used several body systems to demonstrate interaction across body systems during the inferential process and context dependence of some signs and symptoms. We have shown on a concrete clinical example how interval based methods of inference help in dealing with diverse medical expert knowledge related to a number of body systems. In our example the *Cardiovascular, Respiratory, Hematological and Muscular* body systems were involved in the inferential process. We have shown how CLINAID selects the relevant body systems. We have also outlined how CLINAID generates further inferential refinements when the inference process homes into a specific subset of body systems. In this process the use of syndromes is essential. The final correct diagnosis of *Congestive Heart Failure* located in the Cardiovascular system was indicated by CLINAID as the final diagnosis winning by a substantial interval margin.

Acknowledgments

The figures in this article appear in *Knowledge-Based Systems for Multiple Environments*, L.J. Kohout, J. Anderson, and W. Bandler, editors, (Ashgate Publ. (Gower), Aldershot, U.K., 1992), and are reproduced with permission of the editors.

9. References

1. L.J. Kohout, J. Anderson, W. Bandler, S. Gao, and C. Trayner. CLINAID: A knowledge-based system for support of decisions in the conditions of risk and uncertainty. In L.J. Kohout, J. Anderson, and W. Bandler, editors, *Knowledge-Based Systems for Multiple Environments*, chapter 10. Ashgate Publ. (Gower), Aldershot, U.K., 1992.
2. L.J. Kohout, J. Anderson, and W. Bandler. *Knowledge-Based Systems for Multiple Environments.* Ashgate Publ. (Gower), Aldershot, U.K., 1992.
3. L.J. Kohout, A. Behrooz, J. Anderson, S. Gao, C. Trayner, and W. Bandler. Dynamics of localised inference and its embedding in activity structures based IKBS architectures. In *Proc. of Second IFSA Congress*, pages 740–743. International Fuzzy Systems Association, July 1987.
4. L.J. Kohout. Activity Structures: A methodology for design of multi-environment and multi-context knowledge-based systems. In L.J. Kohout, J. Anderson, and W. Bandler, editors, *Knowledge-Based Systems for Multiple Environments*, chapter 5. Ashgate Publ. (Gower), Aldershot, U.K., 1992.
5. L.J. Kohout. *A Perspective on Intelligent Systems: A Framework for Analysis and Design.* Chapman and Hall & Van Nostrand, London & New York, 1990.
6. L.J. Kohout. Paraconsistency in activity structures. In G.E. Lasker, editor, *Proc. of 3nd Internatinal Symposium on Systems Research, Informatics and Cybernetics*, Germany, August 12-18 1991.
7. L.J. Kohout, J. Anderson, W. Bandler, A. Behrooz, S. Gao, and C. Trayner. Activity structures based architectures for knowledge-based systems, part I: Dynamics of localised fuzzy inference and its interaction with planning. *Fuzzy Sets and Systems*, 44(4):405–420, 1991.

8. L.J. Kohout, W. Bandler, J. Anderson, and C. Trayner. Knowledge-based decision support system for use in medicine. In G. Mitra, editor, *Computer Models for Decision Making*, pages 133–146. North-Holland, Amsterdam, 1985.
9. J. Anderson, L.J. Kohout, W. Bandler, and C. Trayner. A knowledge-based clinical decision support system using new techniques. In A.H. Levy and B.T. Williams, editors, *Proc. of AAMSI Congress 1985*, pages 187–192, Washington, DC, May 1985. American Association for Medical Systems and Informatics.
10. S. Gao, L.J. Kohout, J. Anderson, and W. Bandler. Questioning strategy in fuzzy knowledge-based systems. In *Proc. Internat. Symposium on Fuzzy Systems and Knowledge Engineering, vol. 1*, pages 164–171, Guangzhou & Guiang, July 1987.
11. L.J. Kohout, S. Gao, and H. Kalantar. Design of questioning strategies for knowledge-based systems. In L.J. Kohout, J. Anderson, and W. Bandler, editors, *Knowledge-Based Systems for Multiple Environments*, chapter 11. Ashgate Publ. (Gower), Aldershot, U.K., 1992.
12. J. Anderson, W. Bandler, and L. Kohout. In *Reports on Clinaid.* Department of Medicine, King's College of Medicine and Dentistry, University of London, London, U.K., 1982.
13. L.J. Kohout and W. Bandler. Use of fuzzy relations in knowledge representation, acquisition and processing. In L.A. Zadeh and J. Kacprzyk, editors, *Fuzzy Logic for the Management of Uncertainty*, pages 415–435. John Wiley, New York, 1992.
14. J. Anderson, W. Bandler, L.J. Kohout, and C. Trayner. The design of a fuzzy medical expert system. In M.M. Gupta, A. Kandel, W. Bandler, and J.B. Kiszka, editors, *Approximate Reasoning in Expert Systems*, pages 689–703. North-Holland, Amsterdam, 1985.
15. L.J. Kohout and I. Stabile. Interval-valued information retrieval and inference in medical knowledge-based system Clinaid. In *Conf. on Numerical Analysis with Automatic Result Verification*, Lafayette, Lousianna, February 25 – March 1 1993.
16. L.J. Kohout and W. Bandler. The use of fuzzy information retrieval techniques in construction of multi-centre knowledge-based systems. In B. Bouchon and R.R. Yager, editors, *Uncertainty in Knowledge-Based Systems (Lecture Notes in Computer Science vol. 286)*, pages 257–264. Springer Verlag, Berlin, 1987.
17. L.J. Kohout, J. Anderson, W. Bandler, and A. Behrooz. Formalization of clinical management activities for a knowledge-based clinical system. In A.H. Levy and B.T. Williams, editors, *Proc. of AAMSI Congress*, Washington, DC, May 1986. American Association for Medical Systems and Informatics.
18. G. Marshal and L.J. Kohout. Concurrency in CLINAID. In L.J. Kohout, J. Anderson, and W. Bandler, editors, *Multi-Environmental Knowledge-Based Systems*, chapter 12 Ashgate Publ. (Gower), Aldershot, U.K., 1992.
19. L.J. Kohout, E. Keravnou, W. Bandler, C. Trayner, and J. Anderson. Construction of an expert therapy adviser as a special case of a general system protection design. In R. Trappl, editor, *Cybernetics and Systems Research 2*, pages 97–104. North-Holland, Amsterdam, 1984.
20. V. Kaliappan, L.J. Kohout, and J. Anderson. Design of a well-protected patient record unit for multi-centre knowledge-based system clinaid. In K.-P. Adlasnik, G. Grabner,

S. Bengtsson, and R. Hansen, editors, *MIE91 – 10th International Congress (Lecture Notes in Medical Informatics)*, pages 309–313, Berlin, August 19-22 1991. European Federation for Medical Informatics, Springer Verlag.

21. W. Bandler and L.J. Kohout. Relations, mathematical. In M.G. Singh, editor, *Systems and Control Encyclopedia*, pages 4000–4008. Pergamon Press, Oxford, 1987.
22. L.J. Kohout and W. Bandler. Fuzzy relational products in knowledge engineering. In V. et al. Novák, editor, *Fuzzy Approach to Reasoning and Decision Making*, pages 51–66. Academia and Kluwer, Prague and Dordrecht, 1992.
23. W. Bandler and L.J. Kohout. Fuzzy power sets and fuzzy implication operators. *Fuzzy Sets and Systems*, 4:13–30, 1980. Reprinted in: *Readings in Fuzzy Sets for Intelligent Systems*, D. Dubois, H. Prade and R. Yager (eds.), pages 88-96, Morgan Kaufmann Publishers, San Mateo, Calif., 1993.
24. W. Bandler and L.J. Kohout. Fuzzy relational products as a tool for analysis and synthesis of the behaviour of complex natural and artificial systems. In P.P. Wang and S.K. Chang, editors, *Fuzzy Sets: Theory and Applications to Policy Analysis and Information Systems*, pages 341–367. Plenum press, New York and London, 1980.
25. W. Bandler and L.J. Kohout. Semantics of implication operators and fuzzy relational products. *Internat. Journal of Man-Machine Studies*, 12:89–116, 1980. Reprinted in Mamdani, E.H. and Gaines, B.R. eds. *Fuzzy Reasoning and its Applications*. Academic Press, London, 1981, pages 219-246.
26. W. Bandler and L.J. Kohout. A survey of fuzzy relational products in their applicability to medicine and clinical psychology. In L.J. Kohout and W. Bandler, editors, *Knowledge Representation in Medicine and Clinical Behavioural Science*, pages 107–118. an Abacus Book, Gordon and Breach Publ., London and New York, 1986.
27. W. Bandler and L.J. Kohout. Fuzzy implication operators. In M.G. Singh, editor, *Systems and Control Encyclopedia*, pages 1806–1810. Pergamon Press, Oxford, 1987.
28. B. Ben-Ahmeida, L.J. Kohout, and W. Bandler. The use of fuzzy relational products in comparison and verification of correctness of knowledge structures. In L.J. Kohout, J. Anderson, and W. Bandler, editors, *Knowledge-Based Systems for Multiple Environments*, chapter 16. Ashgate Publ. (Gower), Aldershot, U.K., 1992.
29. L.J. Kohout and M. Kallala. Choice of fuzzy optimal logics for pattern classifiers by means of measure analysis. In *Proc. of 7th International Congress on Cybernetics and Systems*, Imperial College, London, September 1987.
30. L. J. Kohout and W. Bandler. Interval-valued systems for approximate reasoning based on checklist paradigm semantics. In P. Wang, editor, *Advances in Fuzzy Set Theory and Technology, vol. 1*, pages 167–193. Bookwrights Press, Durham, NC, 1993.
31. I. Stabile and L.J. Kohout. Causation in science, medicine and the law with particular reference to toxic tort litigation. In G.E. Lasker, editor, *Proc. of 6th Internatinal Conference on Systems Research, Informatics and Cybernetics*, Germany, 1992.
32. J.S. Flier. Diastolic dysfunction in congestive heart failure. *The New England Journal of Medicine*, 325(22):1557–1564, 1991.
33. L.J. Kohout. The functional hierarchies of the brain. In G.J. Klir, editor, *Applied General Systems Research: Recent Developments and Trends*, pages 531–544. Plenum

Press, New York, 1978.

34. L.J. Kohout. Representation of functional hierarchies of movement in the brain. *Internat. Journal of Man-Machine Studies*, 8:699–709, 1976.

35. T. Chard. The effects of dependence on the performance of Bayes' theorem: an evaluation using a computer simulation. *Computer Methods and Programs in Biomedicine*, 29:15–19, 1989.

DIAGNOSTIC ASPECTS OF DIASTOLIC DYSFUNCTION: REPRESENTATION IN D-LOG LANGUAGE

ANTONIO MUSCARI
Institute of Medical Pathology and Clinical Methodology, University of Bologna, S.Orsola Hospital, Via Massarenti 9, Bologna, 40138, Italy

1. Introduction

DIANA 2 / The Diagnostic Analyzer is an expert system for microcomputer designed to provide the physician with a diagnostic consultation tool in the field of internal medicine. Its knowledge base presently includes a dictionary of nearly 3500 terms and the description of 110 infectious and 50 cardiovascular diseases. A preliminary description of the system has been given elsewhere [1], [2]. Briefly, the programs are written in C language for the MS-DOS environment and the diagnostic algorithm essentially consists of "pattern matching" routines with a non-linear weight scoring system. Besides efficient algorithms, also an adequate scheme of representation of medical concepts and terminology is needed to obtain a reliable simulation of diagnostic reasoning. For this reason in DIANA 2 the description of medical terms, diseases and patient's complaints is based on rather complex coding mechanisms, which on the whole constitute the D-LOG language. The language also allows the system to provide detailed explainations on its behavior and to perform temporal evaluations. At present only the Italian version of DIANA 2 is available, and all the examples reported further have been translated from Italian. The second section of this paper illustrates the general features of the D-LOG language. To provide an example of how the language may be practically applied, in the third section the diagnostic aspects of the article by Grossman "Diastolic dysfunction in congestive heart failure" [3] are shown in D-LOG format. In the fourth section the history and complaints of an imaginary patient are proposed to illustrate how the system takes advantage of the D-LOG representation to provide a differential diagnosis, explainations and suggestions on further investigations. Finally, in the fifth section the distinctive features with respect to other methods of knowledge base representation are briefly discussed.

2. The D-LOG Language

2.1. Types of Information

The information that the D-LOG language is able to handle is classified into 9 Types, 5 of which are Data and 4 are Attributes. Data are items of information provided with essential pathologic significance or laboratory-instrumental investigation names. Attributes are items of information that are used to specify, localize or modify other items of information (Data or other Attributes). Data can be connected with multiple Attributes to describe even very complex expressions. Furthermore, since each element of the expression is analyzed separately, an exact correspondence between the whole expression reported in the knowledge base and the expression present in patient's history may not be necessary (*see Section 2.3, Necessity of the Attributes*). The names of Data and Attributes are respectively upper and lower case.

2.1.1. Data

Simple datum - Elemental datum whose instances can be represented by one of the following sets of statuses: present/absent or increased/decreased/normal or positive/negative. Its name must be chosen taking into account that the absent or normal or negative status always indicates the condition of normality. Examples: PAIN (pres/abs); BLOOD GLUCOSE (incr/decr/norm); STANDARD ECG (pos/neg).

Alternative datum - Elemental datum representing one of the possible instances of a set of mutually exclusive alternatives, which are considered by the diagnostic program as equivalent to statuses. Examples: NORMAL PUPIL SIZE / MONOLATERAL MYOSIS / MONOLATERAL MYDRIASIS / BILATERAL MYOSIS / BILATERAL MYDRIASIS; NORMAL BOWEL FUNCTION / CONSTIPATION / DIARRHEA.

Structure - Complex datum indicating an intermediate pathophysiologic condition that does not correspond to a final diagnosis. Its name is associated with a descriptive list consisting of elemental items of information or other lower-level structures. Examples: SHOCK:GENERAL FEATURES; CHRONIC CHOLESTASIS.

Disease - Complex datum indicating a possible final diagnosis. Its name is associated with a descriptive list consisting of elemental or complex items of information. Examples: INFECTIOUS MONONUCLEOSIS; GASTRIC CANCER.

Category of data - Complex datum indicating a set of data that share a common characteristic. Examples: ACUTE INFECTIONS; OCULAR ABNORMALITIES. Whenever the name of a Category of data is indicated in the descriptive list of a Structure or Disease, any datum in patient's history which is a member of the Category is considered concordant. In patient's history a Category of data can be used with the absent status: this is a convenient way to mean that all the Data that are members of the Category are absent or normal in the patient.

2.1.2. Attributes

Simple attribute - Elemental attribute allowing 1 of the 3 sets of statuses described for the Simple datum. For the attributes of localizing Kind the present status is implicitly assumed. If appropriate, a preposition can be associated with the attribute name. Examples: [in the] epigastrium; [for] pq interval (incr/decr/norm).

Alternative attribute - Elemental attribute representing 1 of the possible instances of a set of mutually exclusive alternatives. Examples: brown color / green color / red color ... ; [for] st segment elevation / st segment depression / normal st segment; generalized / circumscribed; single / multiple.

Category of attributes - Complex attribute indicating a set of attributes that share a common characteristic or localization. Examples: [in the] bones; [in the] abdominal regions; [in the] upper limb. A Category of attributes may be itself a member of a higher level Category. For example, "little finger" is a simple attribute of localizing Kind which is a member of the "fingers" Category which, in turn, is a member of the "hand" Category, which finally belongs to the "upper limb" Category. The links among attributes and categories of localizing Kind on the whole constitute a hierarchical representation of anatomy and body regions. Whenever the name of a Category of attributes is indicated in a Structure or Disease list, any attribute in patient's history which is a member of the Category is considered concordant (for instance, "PAIN in the little finger" would match with "PAIN in the upper limb").

Key-words of Special Procedures - Pre-defined attributes which direct the diagnostic processing to the correspondig Special Procedures. These are program routines designed to carry out complex tasks, including calculations, evaluation of rule sets and temporal reasoning.

2.2. *Global Parameters: Definition of Items of Information*

When a new item of information is defined, the following parameters are assigned to it. These parameters remain constant, independently of the contexts in which the item will be subsequently used.

Main name and synonyms - Any number of synonims may be associated with the main name.

Note - A free-text note may be associated with the item, to provide explainations on its significance and correct use.

Allowed statuses - Pres/abs or incr/decr/norm or pos/neg.

Normal alternative - In the case of alternative data or attributes it is necessary to state whether the item represents the condition of normality.

Intrinsic specificity - Integer ranging 1 to 4, which is inversely proportional to the number of diseases that may cause the presence of the item of information. The single values are so defined: 1= Unspecific information, which is sometimes present in normal subjects (e.g. HEADACHE, SKIN PALLOR); 2 = Information specific of the condition of disease, but too common to allow, *per se*, the formulation of a differential diagnosis (e.g. FEVER, VOMITING); 3 = Information specific of a reasonably small number of diseases, so that it allows, *per se*, the formulation of a differential diagnosis (e.g. NUCHAL RIGIDITY, JAUNDICE, SPLENOMEGALY); 4 = Information characteristic of a very small number of diseases (usually 1 only) (e.g. FTA ABS TEST positive). A score is associated with each specificity value, in this way: 1->1, 2->3, 3->20, 4->60. The scores of the items of information in patient's history which are compatible with the Structure or Disease under evaluation are summed up by the system to assess the overall score in favour of the diagnostic hypothesis.

Categories of which the item is a member - Each item may belong to more than 1 Category.

Cost - Integer ranging 1 to 8, which expresses the 'cost' of a Datum mainly in terms of discomfort or risk for the patient: 1 = Orally reported information or subjective complaint, 2 = Physical examination, ... , 8 = High-risk invasive investigation. Together with Intrinsic specificity and Necessity (*see further*), this parameter is used by the system to suggest further investigations.

Kind - This is an integer associated with each Attribute. Its 3 possible values are:1= Localizing; 2 = Investigation result; 3 = Specifying. It is used by the system mainly to ask the user further details concerning data already present in patient's history and to provide explainations.

2.3. Local Parameters: Using Items of Information within Descriptive Lists

After the definition is completed, the items of information can be used to compose lists (or frames) describing structures or diseases in the knowledge base. Attributes usually follow the data or the attributes to which they are referred. Nevertheless, a few attributes may be indicated just at the beginning of the list: in this case it is meant that they apply to every datum of the list. Alongside of the name of each item some parameters are usually indicated which affect only the local context.

Status - Only 1 of the allowed statuses can be indicated. When no status is indicated, the "pres" status is presumed. An "inverse status" may be added to mean that any status is allowed except the one indicated (Example: BLOOD GLUCOSE "not" incr = Blood glucose may be either normal or decreased). For diseases the "prec" status (= preceding) may be used in the place of the "pres" status to mean that the disease must have occurred before the current condition started. Differently from the "predisposing" Procedure (*see further*), the "prec" status does not imply that the disease must still be present while the current condition begins, nor it allows the addition of temporal specifications to change the default.

Necessity - This parameter expresses in a qualitative or semi-quantitative way the frequency of association of an item of information with its context.

Necessity of the Data - It indicates how often a datum is present in the presence of a given structure or disease. The allowed values are: 0 (= sometimes, approximatively 0-49 % of the cases), 50 (= often, 50-89 % of the cases) or 90 (= always, 90-100 % of the cases). The concept of "never" is represented by using the absent or normal or negative status associated with a Necessity of 90. For structures, the possible minimum number of items in the structure list that must be present in patient's history may be indicated by adding the specification "at least" (e.g.: MINOR DEPRESSION CRITERIA at least 3 90). When a datum in patient's history explicitly denies a datum with a Necessity of 90, also the structure in which it is included is considered denied. If also the other upper-level structures are necessary, this mechanism may cause a propagation of negative effects up to the disease under evaluation, which will therefore be considered an "improbable" diagnosis. The explicit negation of a datum with a Necessity of 50 causes less serious effects on the disease under evaluation, which will be penalized with respect to another disease only if the overall scores of the 2 diseases are equal. However, 3 or more denied data with a Necessity of 50 are considered equivalent to a denied datum with a Necessity of 90.

Necessity of the Attributes - It is regarded only if the datum to which the attributes refer matches with a datum in patient's history. This parameter indicates whether the attribute is necessary for the existance of the datum, and what should be the effects on the datum, and on the Necessity of the datum, in case of either explicit negation or omission of the attribute in patient's history. The following values are allowed.

0 = The attribute is not necessary.

90 = Necessary attribute. The datum is considered as explicitly denied if the attribute is explicitly denied.

91 = The attribute is strictly connected with the datum, of which it usually indicates a localization (but attributes of any Kind may be associated with this value). Often multiple attributes have the 91 value, indicating all the possible localizations. If none of such attributes is present in patient's history, the datum is discarded, but its necessity does not imply negative consequences for the list under examination. Example: in the ACUTE MYOCARDIAL INFARCTION disease the following expression is reported: "PAIN 50 in the sternal region 91 in the shoulder 91 in the upper limb 91 ... ". If patient's history includes "PAIN in the ankle to the left", PAIN is rejected but its necessity (50) does not cause a disadvantage for the hypothesis of MYOCARDIAL INFARCTION, since the possible presence of the expected PAIN has not actually been excluded.

92 = The attribute usually indicates one of the expected results of an investigation (which coincides with the datum) and in fact often multiple attributes have this necessity value. If none of such attributes is reported in patient's history, the datum is discarded and its necessity may cause a disadvantage for the list under examination. Example: In the PULMONARY VENOUS CONGESTION: SIGNS structure the following expression is reported: "CHEST X-RAY pos 90 for pulmonary venous congestion 92 for interstitial pulmonary edema 92 for alveolar pulmonary edema 92 ...". If patient's history just includes "CHEST X-RAY pos for lobar opacity", it is assumed that no other positive results were obtained by the investigation, and therefore CHEST X-RAY is rejected with subsequent rejection also of the hypothesis of PULMONARY VENOUS CONGESTION.

93 = If the single attribute with which this value is associated is not present in patient's history, the datum to which it is referred is discarded, and its necessity may cause a disadvantage for the list under examination.

Evidence - A necessary datum may be marked as Evident by an exclamation mark. This means that the datum is not of trivial importance and that it can be detected by simple inspection, so that it is assumed that the datum could not accidentally be omitted in patient's history by any physician. Therefore, if an Evident datum is not indicated in patient's history, it is regarded as denied, and its necessity implies a disadvantage for the list that includes it. An example of how evidence works is given further ("*Evaluation of a clinical case*").

Non-inheritability of attributes - Attributes have the property of *inheritability* : when they are indicated at the beginning of a descriptive list, without being preceded by a datum, they are transmitted to all the data of the list and even to all the data within the lower-level structures. The same applies to the attributes following the name of a structure. This propagation process may be interrupted by marking either the structure attribute that must not be transmitted to internal data, or the datum that must not inherit external attributes, with the '#' symbol .

2.4. *Special Procedures*

The Special Procedures are routines of the diagnostic program designed to perform complex processings, different from the normal procedures that perform comparisons between the elements of patient's history and the elements of Structures or Diseases. A Special Procedure becomes active when an appropriate key-word is found during processing of a descriptive list. Since most of the Special Procedures perform temporal assessments, it is opportune to briefly mention how time is represented in descriptive lists.

2.4.1. Time representation for Special Procedures

Many of the temporal Procedures check whether the temporal endpoints of the data present in patient's history are compatible with an allowed range of duration. The allowed range of duration is usually indicated alongside the Procedure key-word, and is expressed by 2 durations, minimum and maximum, separated by a right-pointing arrow (->). Durations are expressed by a number followed by the proper temporal unit: Y = years, M = months, D = days, h = hours and m = minutes. One of the 2 durations may be omitted.

Examples: 15D -> 2M = any duration between 15 days and 2 months is allowed; 30m -> = any duration greater than 30 minutes is allowed; -> 45m = any duration less than 45 minutes is allowed.

2.4.2. Temporal Procedures

1) Age of onset - This Procedure calculates how old the patient was when a given datum started, and verifies whether the resulting age is comprised within the expected

interval. The "age" key-word is usually inserted among the "initial" attributes of the disease, so that it applies to all the data describing the disease (except the "preceding" or "predisposing" ones). Alongside of the "age" key-word, at least 1 of 2 age ranges must be indicated: a range of "typical" age and/or a range of "necessary" age. Example: age 20Y -> 40Y (10Y ->) = the age of onset is typically comprised between 20 and 40 years, and in any case it must be greater than 10 years. An age comprised within the "typical" range involves the addition of 1 point to the datum weight. An age incompatible with the "necessary" range causes the rejection of the datum.

2) Datum duration and/or course - This procedure is designed to check the duration and the course of a single datum. The course may be continuous or intermittent (an indifferent course does not have to be specified). If the course is intermittent, the possible range of duration specified by this procedure is referred to the overall period during which episodes occur, and at least the range of duration of each episode or the range of duration of each interval must be specified in the following lines of the descriptive list. Example: duration 3D -> 1M intermittent course.

3) Episode duration - If the datum has been declared intermittent, by this procedure it is possible to check the mean duration of the episodes.

4) Interval duration - This procedure checks the mean duration of the intervals between the episodes of an intermittent datum.

If the course of patient's datum is compatible with the expected characteristics, 2 points are added to the datum weight.

5) Maximum duration - The "maximum duration" key-word may be indicated among the "initial" attributes of a structure or disease. In this way the corresponding Special Procedure will verify whether all patient's data compatible with the hypothesis of disease or structure under evaluation have a shorter duration than the expected one, and whether they are distributed within a temporal interval not exceeding the maximum duration expected. If the compatible data are dispersed in a too wide interval, the Procedure begins to reject the most remote data, until a temporal compatibility is reached. This procedure is especially useful in the description of acute conditions, in which it is important that symptoms or other data are sufficiently close in temporal terms. The Procedure has no effect on "preceding" or "predisposing" data.

6) Predisposition - The "predisposing" key-word is used to mark the data that favour the occurrence of a structure or disease, but that are not strictly part of it, from a logical point of view. By deafault, a patient's datum can be considered as predisposing to a structure or disease only if the oldest datum in patient's history which is compatible with the descriptive list started while the "predisposing" datum was present. The default may be modified by specifying a possible minimum period of persistence of the predisposing datum, necessary to allow the predisposition to occur, or a possible maximum period after the predisposing datum conclusion, beyond which the predisposing effect can no longer be present. Examples: TOTAL SERUM CHOLESTEROL incr 0 - predisposing 6M -> = to regard the increase in serum

cholesterol as a predisposing factor, it must have been present for at least 6 months before the beginning of the disease; USE OF DIURETICS 0 - predisposing -> 3D = to regard the diuretics as a predisposing factor, they must not have been discontinued more than 3 days before the beginning of the disease.

7) Causation - Any of the 4 allowed key-words ("may cause", "associated with", "may be associated with" or "contemporaneous with") may be used to mark a datum in a descriptive list. In this way the marked datum is considered the causal or fundamental element, and all the other data of the list (except those marked as "preceding" or "predisposing") are considered as effects or elements that cannot exist without the fundamental element. The diagnostic program rejects all the effects that, in the patient, had a period of presence not comprised within the period of presence of the causal datum, unless "Persistence" or "Delay" are specified.

8) Persistence - The "may persist" key-word is used to mark those effects that may persist after the cause is concluded. However, also these data must start while the cause is present.

9) Delay - The "retards" key-word may be associated with an effect to specify a minimum interval of time between the onset of the cause and the onset of the effect (necessary for the effect to be caused), and/or a maximum interval of time between the end of the cause and the onset of the effect (beyond which the effect can no longer be caused).

10) Complication - When a causal element is not indicated in a descriptive list, it is assumed that the temporal endpoints of a structure or disease are the time of onset of the most remote patient's datum and the ending time of the most recent patient's datum, which are compatible with data in the list that are not "preceding", "predisposing" or "complication", and which are comprised within the possible maximum duration. By default, the data marked with any of the 4 key-words "complication", "consequence", "possible effect" or "contemporary effect" must have their time of onset comprised between the 2 temporal endpoints of the condition under consideration. However, also in this situation the default may be modified by specifying possible necessary or allowed delays.

11) Sequence - When 2 or more data, within a structure or disease, often occur following a typical order of appearance, they may be marked as elements in sequence. In this case the minimum and maximum interval allowed between the onset of each element and the onset of the preceding element in the sequence must be indicated. If at least 2 data in patient's history comply with the sequence and intervals expected, each of them are given an additional 2 points.

12) Necessary phase - There are conditions in which a datum is necessary only during a limited temporal phase, while during the remaining period of presence of the condition the necessity of the datum is null. For example, an increase in SERUM CREATINE PHOSPHOKINASE is necessary for the diagnosis of ACUTE MYOCARDIAL INFARCTION but, if the measurement is too early or too late, this datum may be found normal; nevertheless, in this case the hypothesis of myocardial

infarction should not be penalized. The "necessary phase" key-word may be associated with a necessary datum, to specify during which phase the necessity of the datum is active, taking as reference the onset of the condition under consideration. Example: necessary phase 12h -> 2D = the datum is definitely necessary only during the period comprised between 12 hours and 2 days after the onset of the condition.

13) Daily rhythm - The typical recurrence of a datum during some phases of the day may be specified by the following key-words: "night", "day", "early in the morning", "morning", "afternoon" and "evening". If patient's datum is not associated with one of these key-words, the Procedure will verify whether the time of onset of the datum is compatible with the expected daily phase. In case of compatibility, 2 points are added to the datum weight.

14) Seasonal rhythm - The bahaviour of this Procedure is similar; in this case the allowed key-words are "spring", "summer", "fall", "winter" and "seasons of transition" (i.e. spring or fall).

2.4.3. Other Procedures

1) Sex - The "sex" key-word, followed by "male" or "female" and the value of necessity (0 or 90), is usually indicated among the "initial" attributes of a disease list. If patient's sex is the expected one, 3 points are added to the overall score of the disease under consideration. If patient's sex is not the expected one, and the necessity value is 90, the whole hypotesis of disease is rejected. The key-word "sex", with a necessity of 90, may also be associated with a single datum. If patient's sex is not the expected one, this datum will not be proposed by the system as a possible further investigation.

2) Amount - Although proper attributes may be specially defined to quantify any datum, for this purpose the use of the pre-defined key-words "small-medium amount" or "considerable amount" is generally sufficient (and recommended). Only 2 quantitative values are available, to facilitate the concordance of the estimates expressed in the list and in patient's history. By default, "small-medium amount" has a specificity of 1, and "considerable amount" has a specificity of 2. However, since the specificty of the datum may change according to its amount, this Procedure admits a "local specificity", which may be indicated following the value of necessity. Example: SGOT incr 90 - in considerable amount 90 s3 = SGOT has a rather low intrinsic specificity (2). However, since not many diseases may cause a considerable increase in SGOT, in this case the key-word has been assigned a high local specificity value (3).

3) Side - To specify a side of the body, 6 key-words are allowed ("right", "left", "middle", "bilateral", "homolateral" and "counterlateral"), followed by a necessity value (0 or 90). Only the first 4 key-words may be used in patient's history. The last 2 key-words are designed to mark, in a descriptive list, all the data expected to be located on the same side, and possibly those expected to be located on the opposite side, without explicitly specifying the affected side of the body (right or left). The Procedure

rejects the incompatible data in patient's history and keeps, among all the compatible combinations, the least unfavourable combination for the condition under consideration.

4) Result - The "result" key-word, followed by a status (pos or neg) and a necessity value (0 or 90), is used to specify which result is expected, with respect to a structure or disease, following the use of some type of treatment. Similarly to the Amount Procedure, a local specificity may be indicated. For example, this expression may be used in the descriptive list of the ANGINA PECTORIS Structure: USE OF NITROGLYCERIN - with result pos 90 s3 = a positive effect of nitroglycerin is necessary for the diagnosis of angina pectoris. Local specificity is high (3), since there are not many diseases that improve with nitroglycerin.

2.5. Patient's History

Patient's history is written in D-LOG format (i.e. as data variously specified by attributes), by using a word-processor-like interface which is able to check the correctness of the terminology used and possibly to suggest the appropriate corrections. The history may be organized into 2 sections, "Past history" and "Present problem", but only the latter is indispensable to obtain a diagnostic consultation, since the system will propose only diagnostic hypotheses that explain at least one of the data contained in the "Present problem" section. All the items of information in the history must be provided with their respective temporal references.

2.5.1. Time representation in patient's history

Within each section of the history, the items of information must be divided into homogeneous groups according to their temporal characteristics. This means that all the items of information that occurred during the same period of time constitute a temporal group. Each temporal group must be preceded by the definition of its temporal interval, i.e. by a starting and an ending time which must be written in 2 separate lines. The starting time is preceded by "Since ...", and must always be indicated. The ending time is preceded by "until ...", and may be omitted (in that case it is assumed that at the present time the elements of the group are still present). Time is expressed in the format "day/month/year hour:minute", but only the year, possibly in abbreviated form, is indispensable. It often happens that the time in which an event was detected is known, but the actual starting or ending time of the event is not known (typically in the case of physical findings or laboratory / instrumental investigations). In this case the time of detection should be followed by the '#' symbol, to inform the system about this type of uncertainty. In other situations it may happen that, even though the exact starting (or ending) time is not known, an interval is known which necessarily includes the starting (or ending) time. In this case the starting (or ending) time may be expressed in the form of a temporal interval. The temporal procedures, during their processings, take account of these elements of uncertainty.

Example:

```
Since 15/4/1993--20/6/1993
until 27/6/1993 #
CHEST X-RAY pos
 for lobar opacity
 on the right
```

= three radiograms were performed: on April 15 the lobar opacity was not present, while it was present on June 20 and 27. Therefore, the actual starting time must be comprised between April 15 and June 20, and the ending time cannot be earlier than June 27.

When the course of the events is of intermittent type, the characteristics of intermittence may be specified in the same line of the ending time, by indicating the mean duration of the episodes and the mean duration of the intervals between episodes. If these durations are not specified, it is assumed that the events had a continuous course. Example:

```
Since 1/1/1988
until 1/1/1989, episodes of 5m every 10D
PAIN
 substernal
 in considerable amount
 arising on effort
```

= during the specified period chest pain was intermittent, occurring on average every 10 days and lasting 5 minutes each time.

3. Diastolic Dysfunction in D-LOG Language

In this section the general concepts so far described will be put into practice to code in D-LOG language the diagnostic aspects of the article by Grossman (1991) "Diastolic dysfunction in congestive heart failure". Since the D-LOG language is associated with a diagnostic system, all the elements that cannot be assessed clinically or by laboratory/ instrumental investigations will not be represented. Table 1 in the quoted article lists the diseases that may cause diastolic dysfunction, and the mechanisms involved in each disease. All the diseases are complex items of information that may be represented in D-LOG language by the "Disease" Type. Diastolic dysfunction clearly belongs to the "Structure" Type, and it seems reasonable to represent it by 2 separate Structures (LEFT VENTR. DIASTOLIC DYSFUNCTION and RIGHT VENTR. DIASTOLIC DYSFUNCTION), since the manifestations of the 2 Structures are different and some diseases can cause only 1 of them. The chaining of pathogenetic mechanisms leading to diastolic dysfunction may be represented by nested intermediate Structures, so that a Disease description will include an intermediate Structure (= mechanism), and the intermediate Structure description will include other intermediate Structures or, as last level, the Structure concerning the appropriate (left and/or right) diastolic dysfunction. Inserting intermediate Structures involves some slowing in diagnostic processing, so that an intermediate Structure should be added to a description only if the mechanism to represent is sufficiently different from diastolic dysfunction. For instance, since in the article diastolic dysfunction is defined as "increased resistance to filling of one or both cardiac ventricles", mechanisms such as "increased resistance to ventricular inflow" or "increased resistance to atrial emptying" do not seem to deserve a separate description. Other mechanisms, such as "diastolic calcium overload" or "activation of renin-angiotensin system" concern biochemical tissue abnormalities that cannot be clinically detected, and therefore they will not be represented. In practice, there are only 2 mechanisms provided with sufficient autonomy, complexity and clinical significance: myocardial hypertrophy (of the left ventricle) and impaired myocardial relaxation. The latter corresponds to the physiologic type of abnormality (as opposed to the structural one) that may lead to diastolic dysfunction, and is typically a consequence of myocardial ischemia. In particular, the article emphasizes the difference between "demand ischemia", which may cause impaired relaxation and diastolic dysfunction, and "supply ischemia", which may mainly cause systolic contractile dysfunction. Demand ischemia is a condition that may occur in several situations, and therefore it seems to deserve a separate description (which should include diastolic dysfunction).

Table 1 - Structures and Diseases involving diastolic heart failure.

	L. V. H.	D. M. I.	R. V. D. D.	L.V. D. D.	L.V. S. D.
Structures :					
DEMAND MYOCARDIAL ISCHEMIA	-	-	-	Yes	-
LEFT VENTRICULAR HYPERTROPHY	-	Yes	-	Yes	-
Diseases :					
TRICUSPID STENOSIS	-	-	Yes	-	-
CONSTRICTIVE PERICARDITIS	-	-	Yes	Yes	-
RESTRICTIVE CARDIOMYOPATHY	-	-	Yes	Yes	-
MITRAL STENOSIS	-	-	-	Yes	-
CLASSIC ANGINA PECTORIS	-	Yes	-	-	-
HYPERTROPHIC CARDIOMYOPATHY	Yes	-	-	-	-
AORTIC STENOSIS	Yes	-	-	-	Yes
AORTIC INSUFFICIENCY	Yes	-	-	Yes	Yes
MITRAL INSUFFICIENCY	Yes	-	-	Yes	Yes
DILATED CARDIOMYOPATHY	-	-	-	Yes	Yes

L.V.H. = Left Ventricular Hypertrophy, D.M.I. = Demand Myocardial Ischemia, R.V.D.D. = Right Ventricular Diastolic Dysfunction, L.V.D.D. = Left Ventricular Diastolic Dysfunction, L.V.S.D. = Left Ventricular Systolic Dysfunction.

In conclusion, the main tools necessary to describe the diseases in Table 1 correspond to the following Structures: LEFT VENTRICULAR HYPERTROPHY, DEMAND MYOCARDIAL ISCHEMIA, LEFT VENTRICULAR DIASTOLIC DYSFUNCTION, RIGHT VENTRICULAR DIASTOLIC DYSFUNCTION and LEFT

VENTRICULAR SYSTOLIC DYSFUNCTION. Other lower level Structures will be described further. Table 1, which is derived from Table 1 in the quoted article, shows the Structures belonging to each disease. The LEFT VENTRICULAR HYPERTROPHY Structure contains DEMAND MYOCARDIAL ISCHEMIA and LEFT VENTRICULAR DIASTOLIC DYSFUNCTION. Therefore, all the diseases causing LEFT VENTRICULAR HYPERTROPHY may indirectly cause the other 2 conditions. In some diseases diastolic dysfunction may be caused by more than one mechanism.

3.1. Example of Disease Description: Aortic Stenosis

This example shows the description in D-LOG language of the AORTIC STENOSIS Disease and of some Structures, and sub-Structures, associated with it. Within each descriptive list, Structure names are marked with an asterisk (*).

```
 AORTIC STENOSIS

  age 25Y->
  sex male  0

 RHEUMATIC FEVER  prec  0

*SYNCOPE  0
  arising on effort  0
*LEFT VENTRICULAR HYPERTROPHY: SIGNS  90
 SYSTOLIC BLOOD PRESSURE  not  incr  50

 PULSE PALPATION  pos  50
  for pulsus tardus  91
  for pulsus parvus  91
 FIRST HEART SOUND  INTENSITY  not  incr  0
 SECOND HEART SOUND  INTENSITY  decr  0
 SPLITTING OF SECOND HEART SOUND  0
  with paradoxic splitting  0
  decreases during inspiration  0
  in the aortic area  0
*THIRD HEART SOUND  0
*FOURTH HEART SOUND  0
*AORTIC EJECTION SOUND  0
 HEART MURMUR  90
  in systole  90
      mid  0
  crescendo-decrescendo  0
  low-pitched  0
  with rough character  0
  in considerable amount  0  s3
  in the right upper sternal border  91
  in the aortic area  91
```

```
  in the mitral area  0
  in the apex area  0
  with radiation into the neck  0
 CARDIAC THRILL  0
  in systole  90
  in the right upper sternal border  91
  in the aortic area  91

 STANDARD ECG  pos  0
  for right axis deviation  93
 CHEST X-RAY  pos  0
  for aortic valve calcifications  92
  for ascending aorta calcifications  92
  for aortic arch calcifications  92
  for cardiac silhouette: right upper convexity  92
  for ascending aorta dilatation  92
 CAROTID PULSE WAVE RECORDING  pos  50
  for slow rising wave  93
  for notched upstroke wave  0
 MONODIMENSIONAL ECHOCARDIOGRAPHY  pos  90
  for aortic valve stenosis  92
  for aortic box  decr  92
  for bicuspid aortic valve  92
  for aortic valve calcifications  0
  for aortic knob dilatation  0
 DOPPLER ECHOCARDIOGRAPHY  pos  90
  for aortic valve stenosis  92
  for systolic transaortic gradient  92
 LEFT HEART CATHETERIZATION  pos  90
  for aortic valve stenosis  92
  for systolic transaortic gradient  92

*LEFT VENTRICULAR SYSTOLIC DYSFUNCTION  0
  complication  5Y->
 INFECTIVE ENDOCARDITIS 0
  complication
```

Besides LEFT VENTRICULAR HYPERTROPHY (which may cause LEFT VENTRICULAR DIASTOLIC DYSFUNCTION), the list includes LEFT VENTRICULAR SYSTOLIC DYSFUNCTION, which may also occur in the late phases of the disease.

```
 LEFT VENTRICULAR HYPERTROPHY: SIGNS

 CARDIAC APEX BEAT AMPLITUDE  incr  0
 CARDIAC APEX BEAT LATERAL DISPLACEMENT  0
 CARDIAC APEX BEAT DOWNWARD DISPLACEMENT  0
 CARDIAC DULLNESS AREA  incr  0
*FOURTH HEART SOUND  0
```

```
*LEFT VENTRICULAR DIASTOLIC DYSFUNCTION  0

 STANDARD ECG  pos  50
  for left ventricular hypertrophy  92
  for left axis deviation  92
  for left anterior hemiblock  92
  for left bundle branch block  92
  for left ventricular strain  92
  for st segment depression  92
      with downsloping st segment  0
 STANDARD ECG  pos  0
  for r wave amplitude incr  92
  in the anterior-lateral leads  91
  in the upper lateral leads  91
*LEFT BUNDLE BRANCH BLOCK: SIGNS 0
*VENTRICULAR PREMATURE BEATS: SIGNS  0
 CHEST X-RAY  pos  50
  for left ventricular hypertrophy  92
  for left ventricular volume incr  92
  for cardiac silhouette: left lower convexity  92
  for cardiomegaly  92
 MONODIMENSIONAL ECHOCARDIOGRAPHY  pos  90
  for left ventricular hypertrophy  93
 TWO-DIMENSIONAL ECHOCARDIOGRAPHY  pos  90
  for left ventricular hypertrophy  93
```

<u>LEFT VENTRICULAR DIASTOLIC DYSFUNCTION</u>

```
*PULMONARY VENOUS CONGESTION: SIGNS  90
*LEFT ATRIAL ENLARGEMENT: SIGNS  50
```

Pulmonary venous congestion is the main clinical manifestation of left ventricular diastolic dysfunction. The left atrium is also often enlarged.

<u>PULMONARY VENOUS CONGESTION: SIGNS</u>

```
*ATRIAL FIBRILLATION AND COMPLICATIONS  0  #
 predisposing

 DYSPNEA  50
  arising on effort  0
  subsiding with rest  0
  with orthopnea  0
  at night
 COUGH  0
*HEMOPTYSIS  0
*CARDIAC ASTHMA  0
*ACUTE PULMONARY EDEMA  0
```

```
 CYANOSIS  0

 PULMONARY CRACKLES  50
  crepitant rales  90
  at the pulmonary base  90
  bilateral  0
*TRANSUDATIVE PLEURAL EFFUSION  0
  on the right  0

*RESPIRATORY ALKALOSIS  0
*RESPIRATORY ACIDOSIS  0
 ARTERIAL GAS ANALYSIS  pos  0
  for po2 decr  93

 CHEST X-RAY  pos  90
  for pulmonary venous congestion  92
  for interstitial pulmonary edema  92
  for alveolar pulmonary edema  92
 RIGHT HEART CATHETERIZATION  pos  90
  for pulmonary capillary wedge pressure  incr  93
```

The most necessary elements for the diagnosis of this condition are the radiologic aspects and the increase in pulmonary capillary pressure. If both are missing in patient's history, the system will suggest to perform a CHEST X-RAY, which has a lower Cost with respect to RIGHT HEART CATHETERIZATION. Since crepitant rales may be confused with pleural friction rubs, the user is offered the opportunity to adopt the more general term PULMONARY CRACKLES, which may possibly be further specified with the attribute "crepitant rales" or "pleural friction rub". The "right" key-word, referred to the TRANSUDATIVE PLEURAL EFFUSION Structure, indicates the most frequent, althogh not obligatory, localization of the effusion. It is transmitted to the internal elements of the Structure, through all its hierarchical levels. In his article Grossman underscores how atrial fibrillation, causing the loss of "atrial kick", may often lead to acute congestive heart failure. Therefore, the ATRIAL FIBRILLATION AND COMPLICATIONS Structure has been added to the descriptive list of PULMONARY VENOUS CONGESTION as an independent predisposing element.

```
ACUTE PULMONARY EDEMA

  with sudden onset  0
  maximum duration  2D

 SYSTOLIC BLOOD PRESSURE  incr  0  #
  in considerable amount  0  s3
  predisposing
```

```
 DYSPNEA  90  !
  in considerable amount  90
  with orthopnea  90
 COUGH  50
  productive  0
 EXPECTORATION  0
  with light color sputum  91
      pink color  0
  with blood-tinged sputum  91
 RESTLESSNESS  0
 ANXIETY  50
 PALPITATIONS  0
 SKIN PALLOR  0
 CYANOSIS  0
 DIFFUSELY COLD SKIN  0
 SWEATING  incr  0

 HEART RATE  incr  50
 PULMONARY RALES  90
  bilateral  90
  at the pulmonary base  0
  in considerable amount  0
 CHEST RESONANCE  decr  0
  bilateral  90
*THIRD HEART SOUND  0
*FOURTH HEART SOUND  0
*RESPIRATORY ACIDOSIS  0

 CHEST X-RAY  pos  90
  for alveolar pulmonary edema  93
  for interstitial pulmonary edema  90
  for pulmonary venous congestion  90

*TRANSUDATIVE PLEURAL EFFUSION  0  #
  on the right  0
  duration  ->1M
  complication
```

A maximum duration of 2 days has been arbitrarily assigned to acute pulmonary edema: in fact a maximum duration must necessarily be assigned, otherwise the system might refer to an acute pulmonary edema even symptoms very distant in time. An elevated blood pressure may independently favour the onset of acute pulmonary edema, so SYSTOLIC BLOOD PRESSURE incr has been inserted in the list as a predisposing element. The '#' symbol, which is automatically added to predisposing data, prevents this datum from inheriting attributes so that, for example, it will not undergo the check of the maximum duration allowed for acute pulmonary edema. DYSPNEA has been considered necessary and evident (exclamation mark): it is therefore assumed that in the presence of acute pulmonary edema dyspnea must be absolutely present and that it cannot pass unnoticed. As a consequence, if in patient's history DYSPNEA is omitted, the hypothesis of acute pulmonary edema is automatically rejected. The possible TRANSUDATIVE PLEURAL EFFUSION may persist even after the conclusion of acute pulmonary edema, so that pleural effusion is marked as a "complication". However, it cannot last more than 1 month.

```
LEFT ATRIAL ENLARGEMENT: SIGNS

*ATRIAL FIBRILLATION AND COMPLICATIONS  0
 DYSPHAGIA  0

 STANDARD ECG  pos  50
  for p wave duration  incr  92
  for abnormal p wave morphology  92
      for notched p waves  91
      for biphasic (+--) p waves  91
  for left atrial volume  incr  92
 CHEST X-RAY  pos  50
  for left atrial volume  incr  92
  for sharply indented esophagus  92
 MONODIMENSIONAL ECHOCARDIOGRAPHY  pos  90
  for left atrial volume  incr  93
 TWO-DIMENSIONAL ECHOCARDIOGRAPHY  pos  90
  for left atrial volume  incr  93
  for left atrial thrombosis  0
```

4. Evaluation of a Clinical Case

The history of an imaginary patient is here proposed, to illustrate the most significant features of the diagnostic program. The patient (male sex, 49 years old) reported that, during the month of January 1980, he presented episodes of precordial sharp pain lasting on average 6 hours, associated with a mild increase in systolic blood pressure. On that occasion a chest X-ray and a standard ECG were performed and both were normal. Afterwards he did not complain any chest pain and blood pressure was always normal. The patient showed other ECG recordings, performed in the following years. In 1985 the ECG was still normal, but since 1987 left axial deviation and an increase in R wave amplitude in the anterior-lateral leads were present, likely due to left ventricular hypertrophy. On December 14, 1992 the ECG was substantially unchanged, but on February 7, 1993 notched P waves were also present in the inferior leads. Furthermore, the patient reported that since February 3, and for only 2 days, he had been affected by symptoms probably due to acute bronchitis: cough with yellowish expectoration and slight fever. On March 19, 1993 the patient was admitted to hospital for severe dyspnea occurring at rest, with orthopnea and palpitations. The physical examination showed the presence of pulmonary rales diffused to both sides, dullness associated with bronchial breathing at the right pulmonary base, a moderately low blood pressure, considerable tachycardia with arrhythmic heart sounds and a gallop rhythm. Moreover, a loud "rough" systolic murmur was present, which was especially intense at the right upper sternal border and which radiated to the neck. The ECG now showed, besides the signs of left ventricular hypertrophy, also an atrial fibrillation with elevated ventricular rate.

This history was written in D-LOG language by using the appropriate data and attributes, and submitted to the diagnostic section of DIANA 2. This suggested that AORTIC STENOSIS was the most probable diagnostic hypothesis, with an overall score of 174 points and no necessary data discordant, followed by HYPERTROPHIC CARDIOMYOPATHY and AORTIC INSUFFICIENCY (both with 140 points and some necessary data discordant).

The system is able to provide detailed explainations on its behavior, in relation to any diagnostic hypothesis. There are 2 levels of explaination. In the first level patient's history is shown, and a short message is displayed alongside each element of the history. Considering the hypothesis of AORTIC STENOSIS, the first level explainations would be the following:

```
HYPOTHESIS OF AORTIC STENOSIS                           174 points

20/3/1993  7:00
IMAGINARY PATIENT
male sex                                 OK
date of birth 16/2/1944 (49 years old)

Past  History

Since 1/1/1980
until 1/2/1980, episodes of 6h every 2D
PAIN                                 (1) Episode incompatible
 in precordial area                      Ok, but datum discarded
 sharp                                   Status incompatible

Since 1/1/1980
until 1/2/1980
SYSTOLIC BLOOD PRESSURE incr         (2) Cannot be predisposing
 in small-medium amount                  Status incompatible
CHEST X-RAY  neg                         Status incompatible
STANDARD ECG  neg                        Status incompatible

Since 15/3/1985--8/7/1987
STANDARD ECG pos                         OK
 for left axis deviation                 OK
 for r wave amplitude  incr              OK
 in the anterior-lateral leads           OK

Since 14/12/1992--7/2/1993
until 7/2/1993 #
```

STANDARD ECG pos		OK
for abnormal p wave morphology		OK
for notched p waves		OK
in the inferior leads		Not found

Since 3/2/1993
until 5/2/1993

COUGH	(3)	OK
EXPECTORATION	(4)	Maximum duration
incompatible		
with light color sputum		Ok, but datum discarded
yellow color		Status incompatible
FEVER		Not found
in small-medium amount		Not found

Present Problem

Since 19/3/1993 21:00

DYSPNEA		OK
in considerable amount		OK
arising at rest		Status incompatible
with orthopnea		OK
PALPITATIONS		OK

Since 20/3/1993 2:30 #

PULMONARY RALES		OK
bilateral		OK
CHEST RESONANCE decr		OK
at the pulmonary base		OK
on the right		OK
BRONCHIAL BREATHING	(5)	OK
at the pulmonary base		OK
on the right		OK
SYSTOLIC BLOOD PRESSURE decr		OK
HEART RATE incr		OK
in considerable amount		OK
ARRHYTHMIC HEART SOUNDS		OK
ADDITIONAL HEART SOUND		OK
HEART MURMUR		OK
in systole		OK
in considerable amount		OK
with rough character		OK
in the right upper sternal border		OK
with radiation into the neck		OK
STANDARD ECG pos		OK
for atrial fibrillation		OK

Discordant Necessary Data (NP = Not Penalizing)

CHEST X-RAY pos	(6)	Status incompatible (NP)

Conditions Definitely Incompatible With Patient's History

COMA (7)
SYNCOPE
HEMOPTYSIS
LEFT BUNDLE BRANCH BLOCK: SIGNS
PREMATURE VENTRICULAR BEATS: SIGNS

Some of the explanatory messages are easily understandable; others might require further explainations, i.e. a second level of explaination. This may be obtained by pointing the cursor on the message to be explained and then by pressing the return key. In the example some messages are marked with the numbers from (1) to (7). The corresponding second level explainations would be the following.

(1) "*PAIN was DISCARDED since in AORTIC STENOSIS it should have an intermittent course with episodes lasting less than 45 minutes, while in patient's history episodes had a longer duration: 6 hours. PAIN might be caused by AORTIC STENOSIS according to the following chaining of events: AORTIC STENOSIS -> LEFT VENTRICULAR HYPERTROPHY: SIGNS -> DEMAND MYOCARDIAL ISCHEMIA -> ANGINA PECTORIS -> PAIN*".

(2) "*SYSTOLIC BLOOD PRESSURE incr was DISCARDED since it stopped on 1/2/1980, while to predispose to ACUTE PULMONARY EDEMA it should persist until the onset of ACUTE PULMONARY EDEMA (which might coincide with the onset of DYSPNEA, which occurred on 19/3/1993 at 21:00). SYSTOLIC BLOOD PRESSURE incr independently contributes to the occurrence of ACUTE PULMONARY EDEMA, which in turn might be caused by AORTIC STENOSIS according to the following chaining of events: AORTIC STENOSIS -> LEFT VENTRICULAR HYPERTROPHY: SIGNS -> LEFT VENTRICULAR DIASTOLIC DYSFUNCTION -> PULMONARY VENOUS CONGESTION: SIGNS -> ACUTE PULMONARY EDEMA*".

(3) "*COUGH was ACCEPTED since it might be caused by AORTIC STENOSIS according to the following chaining of events: AORTIC STENOSIS -> LEFT VENTRICULAR HYPERTROPHY: SIGNS -> LEFT VENTRICULAR DIASTOLIC DYSFUNCTION -> PULMONARY VENOUS CONGESTION: SIGNS -> COUGH. Its overall weight is 4 points, including 3 for specificity (2) and 1 for age of onset*".

This example illustrates a typical situation of error in temporal reasoning. In this case cough is likely due to an intervened episode of acute bronchitis, but the system has interpreted this symptom as a consequence of the pulmonary venous congestion caused by left ventricular hypertrophy, which had already been present for some years.

Solving this type of problem without causing worse inconvenients than the problem itself is not easy.

(4) "*EXPECTORATION was DISCARDED since ACUTE PULMONARY EDEMA has a maximum duration of 2 days, while between the onset of EXPECTORATION and the end of PULMONARY RALES a longer interval elapsed: 1 month and 14 days. EXPECTORATION, within ACUTE PULMONARY EDEMA, might be caused by AORTIC STENOSIS according to the following chaining of events: AORTIC STENOSIS -> LEFT VENTRICULAR HYPERTROPHY: SIGNS -> LEFT VENTRICULAR DIASTOLIC DYSFUNCTION -> PULMONARY VENOUS CONGESTION: SIGNS -> ACUTE PULMONARY EDEMA -> EXPECTORATION*".

(5) "*BRONCHIAL BREATHING was ACCEPTED since it might be caused by AORTIC STENOSIS according to the following chaining of events: AORTIC STENOSIS -> LEFT VENTRICULAR HYPERTROPHY: SIGNS -> LEFT VENTRICULAR DIASTOLIC DYSFUNCTION -> PULMONARY VENOUS CONGESTION: SIGNS -> TRANSUDATIVE PLEURAL EFFUSION -> PLEURAL EFFUSION -> BRONCHIAL BREATHING. Its overall weight is 25 points, including 20 for specificity (3) and 1 for age of onset. The rest of the weight derives from attributes*".

The items marked with OK are those compatible (directly or indirectly) with the hypothesis of AORTIC STENOSIS, and contribute to the overall score of 174 points. By pointing the cursor on the compatible data their weights are shown, so that it is possible to understand how the overall score was reached. The same procedure may be applied to attributes, to verify their contribution to the overall score.

(6) "*CHEST X-RAY pos occurs often (necessity of 50), but not always, in the presence of LEFT VENTRICULAR HYPERTROPHY which, in turn, occurs in the presence of AORTIC STENOSIS. Therefore the incompatibility of CHEST X-RAY with patient's history would imply only a partial disadvantage for the hypothesis of AORTIC STENOSIS. On the other hand, CHEST X-RAY pos is necessary only during the period of presence of LEFT VENTRICULAR HYPERTROPHY: SIGNS, which might be comprised between the onset of STANDARD ECG pos and the end of THIRD HEART SOUND (since 15/3/1985--8/7/1987 until now). Since the period of presence of CHEST X-RAY neg is earlier in patient's history (since 1/1/1980 until 1/2/1980) the existence of a possible compatibility during the necessary period cannot be ruled out, and therefore no penalty is applied. As far as the reason of incompatibility is concerned, CHEST X-RAY pos is not concordant with patient's history since this includes CHEST X-RAY neg, which has a different STATUS. CHEST X-RAY pos might be caused by AORTIC STENOSIS according to the following chaining of events: AORTIC STENOSIS -> LEFT VENTRICULAR HYPERTROPHY: SIGNS -> CHEST X-RAY pos*".

In the presence of left ventricular hypertrophy chest radiograms often show some changes in cardiac profile, and this would be in contrast with the CHEST X-RAY neg datum. By identifying the likely temporal endpoints of left ventricular hypertrophy in the patient, the diagnostic program can correctly decide that the available CHEST X-RAY must be ignored, because it was performed too many years ago.

(7) "*UNCONSCIOUSNESS occurs always (necessity of 90) in the presence of COMA. Therefore the incompatibility of UNCONSCIOUSNESS with patient's history implies an absolute disadvantage for the hypothesis of COMA. As far as the reason of incompatibility is concerned, UNCONSCIOUSNESS is a relevant and immediately evident datum in the presence of COMA. Therefore its omission in patient's history cannot be fortuitous, and it has been considered absent. COMA might be caused by AORTIC STENOSIS according to the following chaining of events: AORTIC STENOSIS -> LEFT VENTRICULAR HYPERTROPHY: SIGNS -> LEFT VENTRICULAR DIASTOLIC DYSFUNCTION -> PULMONARY VENOUS CONGESTION: SIGNS -> RESPIRATORY ACIDOSIS -> COMA*".

In the last section of the first level explainations, the user is informed about which Structures, potentially caused by AORTIC STENOSIS, were considered definitely absent in the patient by the diagnostic program. In the case of COMA (which might be caused by a severe respiratory acidosis), rejection occurred automatically, since the UNCONSCIOUSNESS datum was not included in patient's history, while in the knowledge base it was marked as necessary and evident for the hypothesis of coma.

On request, the program may suggest further investigations to test any diagnostic hypothesis or to discriminate among the diseases in differential diagnosis. The choice is offered between a complete list of investigations (all the data provided with high specificity and/or necessity), or only a few investigations optimized according to cost/benefit criteria, taking also into account the level of diagnostic precision presently reached (invasive investigations are not proposed if several diagnoses are still possible or if the overall scores reached are low). In the present case only 3 "optimized" investigations are proposed by the program: DOPPLER ECHOCARDIOGRAPHY, CHEST X-RAY and PLEURAL FLUID EXAMINATION. For each investigation proposed, detailed explainations concerning the reason of the request may be obtained, similarly to what was previously described. The results of the investigations that the user decides to perform may be added to patient's history, and a new differential diagnosis may then be obtained.

5. Discussion

The D-LOG language has some similarities with the methods of knowledge base representation of other diagnostic consultation systems, such as INTERNIST/QMR [4],

[5], DXplain [6] and HELP/ILIAD [7], [8]. Structures, for example, resemble the 'clusters' of ILIAD. A scoring scheme with non-linear weights is also used by INTERNIST/QMR and DXplain. The "Alternative" types of information are equivalent, to some extent, to some "Properties" of INTERNIST/QMR [9]. A hierarchical representation of anatomy is also implemented in DXplain [6]. On the other hand, a few features of D-LOG can be considered as distinctive, and the most significant differences will be briefly discussed here.

Data and attributes - In the D-LOG language the resolution of the information into atomic elements reaches a considerable level of detail. There is no pre-defined hierarchy of attributes reserved for specific data: the same attribute may be linked with different data, if this may contribute to describe meaningful concepts. In the presence of a given disease, if a datum may present with multiple localizations and needs a quantification or other specifications, all these elements may be added in a natural way to the datum, without the need of foreseeing all the possible, or just the most characteristic, combinations. The user, in turn, is not forced to choose among some pre-defined combinations, but can describe patient's situation in a natural and accurate way.

Intrinsic specificity - Differently from ILIAD's Specificity and the Evoking Strength of QMR and DXplain, which are local, disease-dependent, parameters, intrinsic specificity is a global parameter associated with the item of information independently of the context. From this point of view, intrinsic specificity resembles the Import Value of INTERNIST/QMR [4], although the Import Value is used for the opposite purpose (penalizing the diagnostic hypotheses that do not explain an "important" element in patient's history, rather than increasing the score attributed to the diagnostic hypotheses that explain a "specific" element). If 2 diseases may cause the same symptom, ILIAD, QMR and DXplain will consider as most probable the disease in which the symptom has the highest Specificity or Evoking Strength, while DIANA 2 will show the 2 diseases with an equal score. The first behavior is more similar to that of the physician, who tends to disregard the less typical situations in favour of the more typical ones. On the other hand, the second bahavior is perhaps more effective in forcing the user to take into account even the situations that he or she does not know or tends to forget. The expert compiling the descriptive lists of diseases and structures is relieved from the task of attributing a local parameter, which can hardly be found in the literature, to each item in the list. Finally, also an automatic attribution of intrinsic specificity to each item of information could be easily obtained *a posteriori*, after the knowledge base has become sufficiently large, just by counting the number of diseases in which the item is present.

Necessity - The necessity of the data in DIANA 2 has a significance similar to the Frequency in QMR and DXplain, but only 3 values are allowed and they are not algebrically summed, as a negative score, to the overall score of the disease which is being processed. In this way the explainations are facilitated, since the user is allowed to separately consider the elements in favour of (score associated with the Intrinsic specificity of the compatible data) and the elements against (necessity of the incompatible data) the diagnostic hypothesis. The necessity of the attributes is a new parameter, which is used to state the kind of link existing between the attribute and its datum. Finally, D-LOG features related to the concept of necessity are Evidence, which allows the necessity of some data not explicitly indicated in patient's history to be activated, so that the program can automatically disregard the most unlikely situations, and Necessary phase, a temporal procedure that defines the period of a disease within which a datum is necessary.

Temporal aspects - In patient's history the representation of time is separated from the data, and this allows the DIANA 2 system to perform the main temporal assessments needed to reach diagnostic conclusions. This characteristic is not commonly present in other diagnostic consultation systems. Among the studies concerning the automatic solution of temporal problems, those by Kahn and coworkers are especially noteworthy [10], [11], [12]. In particular these Authors have recently developed an extension of the Time Oriented Databank (TOD) model, called the Extended Temporal Network (ETNET) which, besides allowing efficient storage and retrieval of patient-specific temporal information, may embody rules useful to solve temporal problems within a medical expert system [12]. Differently from ETNET, the D-LOG language does not allow the knowledge engeneer to write rules, it does not include key-words to express sophisticate relative timings, it does not imply the ability to automatically recognize intermittence (mean episodes and intervals must be declared *a priori* by the user), nor was it designed as a query-language to allow the user to retrieve information from a data-base, but it is mainly used to describe diseases and lower-level conditions in a knowledge base. On the other hand, ETNET was developed in conjunction with ONCOCIN [9], an expert system that provides therapy advice to physicians caring for patients who are receiving experimental cancer treatments. Therefore, the temporal problems faced by ETNET are to some extent different from those related to diagnosis. For example, differently from D-LOG, ETNET does not admit uncertainty in the definition of the temporal endpoints of the events, and this may not cope with some descriptive needs, especially those concerning patient's past history. Similarly, ETNET does not recognize as effects those events that start after the causal event is concluded, or those persisting beyond the causal event conclusion. On the whole, even though the D-LOG language is far from being able to manage all the temporal aspects of medicine, it has proven to be a sufficiently valid tool in the description of several temporal concepts of diagnostic relevance. In this respect, the use of key-words such as "predisposing", "may cause", "maximum duration", "retards" and so on, which induce the system to perform the corresponding temporal evaluations, is a unique feature of the D-LOG language: some similar terms are also present in the description of diseases in INTERNIST/QMR [4], but they are not associated with a true capacity of temporal reasoning.

The DIANA 2 system and its cardiological knowledge base have recently become available in Italy as the informatic appendix of a cardiology textbook for students [13].

6. References

1. A. Muscari, Consulenza diagnostica analitica mediante personal computer: DIANA 2, un sistema estensibile nel campo della medicina interna. *Medicina e Informatica* **7** (1990) 180-189.
2. A. Muscari, DIANA 2 / The Diagnostic Analyzer: diagnostic consultation in internal medicine by personal computer, in *Lecture Notes in Medical Informatics - MIE 91*, eds. K. -P. Adlassnig, G. Grabner, S. Bengtsson and R. Hansen (Springer-Verlag, Berlin, 1991) pp. 241-245.
3. W. Grossman, Diastolic dysfunction in congestive heart failure. *N Engl J Med* **325** (1991) 1557-1564.
4. R.A. Miller, H.E. Pople and J.D. Myers, INTERNIST-1, an experimental computer-based diagnostic consultant for general internal medicine. *N Engl J Med* **307** (1982) 468-476.
5. R.A Miller, F.E. Masarie and J.D. Myers, Quick Medical Reference (QMR) for diagnostic assistance. *MD Computing* **3** (1986) 34-48.
6. G.O. Barnett, J.J. Cimino, J.A. Hupp and E.P. Hoffer, DXplain: an evolving diagnostic decision-support system. *JAMA* **258** (1987) 67-74.
7. T.A. Pryor, R.M. Gardner, P.D. Clayton and H.R. Warner, The HELP system. *J Med Syst* **7** (1983) 87-102.
8. H.R. Warner, P. Haug, O. Bouhaddou, et al., ILIAD as an expert consultant to teach differential diagnosis, in *Proceedings Symposium on Computer Applications in Medical Care*, ed. R. Greens (IEEE Computer Society Press, Washington D.C., 1988) pp. 371-376.
9. F.E. Masarie, R.A. Miller and J.D. Myers, INTERNIST-1 Properties: representing common sense and good medical practice in a computerized medical knowledge base. *Comput Biomed Res* **18** (1983) 458-479.
10. M.G. Kahn, J.C. Ferguson, E.H. Shortliffe and L.M. Fagan, Representation and use of temporal information in ONCOCIN, in *Proceedings Symposium on Computer Applications in Medical Care*, ed. M.J. Ackerman (IEEE Computer Society Press, New York N.Y., 1985) pp. 172-176.
11. M.G. Kahn, S. Tu and L.M. Fagan, TQuery: a context-sensitive temporal query language. *Comput Biomed Res* **24** (1991) 401-419.
12. M.G. Kahn, L.M. Fagan and S. Tu, Extensions to the time-oriented database model to support temporal reasoning in medical expert systems. *Methods Inf Med* **30** (1991) 4-14.
13. A. Muscari, *Cardiologia al computer - Un sistema esperto per l'apprendimento e la diagnosi* (ETAS Libri / RCS Medicina, Milano, 1994).

IMPROVED NONINVASIVE DIAGNOSIS OF CORONARY ARTERY DISEASE USING NEURAL NETWORKS

METIN AKAY
YASEMINE M. AKAY
WALTER WELKOWITZ

Biomedical Engineering Department
Rutgers University
Piscataway, New Jersey 08855

1. Introduction

One-third of all deaths in the world are due to coronary artery disease (CAD) [2-5, 44, 45, 46, 51]. For this reason, early detection of coronary artery disease is one of the most important medical research areas. The most reliable way to diagnose CAD is with an invasive procedure, cardiac catherization (cath). With this method, a catheter is inserted into an artery (usually brachial or femoral) and advanced to the heart. Once in the heart, dye can be released to observe the cardiac structures, including coronary arteries [17, 19, 47, 48]. Although direct assessment of coronary occlusions is conclusive only through coronary angiography, this method is expensive, and has an element of risk (mortality rates range from 0.2%-7%) [17, 19, 47, 48]. For these reasons, **a reliable noninvasive method** is required for early detection of coronary artery disease.

Previous studies showed that coronary stenoses produce sounds due to turbulent blood flow in partially occluded arteries [1-5, 44, 45, 46, 51]. During diastole, coronary artery blood flow is maximum and the sounds associated with turbulent blood flow through partially occluded coronary arteries are loudest [1-5, 44, 45, 46, 51]. If these signals could be reliably detected , they would provide a simple, noninvasive approach to the detection of coronary artery disease.

Studies involving turbulent blood flow have been carried out in many components of the cardiovascular system and it has been widely reported that turbulence produced by stenoses produces sounds due to the vibration of the surrounding structures[11,13,14,18,24,25,27,31,34]. These sounds have been detected and analyzed, and the results generally show that the high frequency energy increased when the degree of stenosis was increased [24,25,27,31]. However, for severe obstructions, (above 95% occlusion), sounds may not produced due to the very low blood flow. Considering small blockages, occlusions as small as 25% narrowing have been detected and used as a noninvasive measure to assess arterial narrowing in vessels of the neck, thorax, and abdomen[24,25,27,31]. The auditory component associated with coronary stenosis is similar to that found in partially occluded carotid arteries, but is much attenuated by the intervening tissue[15,24,25,27,31]. It is also masked by the comparatively loud valve sounds. These loud valve sounds can be eliminated by isolating diastolic portions of the acoustic signal using a time window synchronized with the cardiac cycle[45].

The principle objective of the previous angioplasty and normal/abnormal studies done by our group was to evaluate the diagnostic capability of the acoustic approach in detecting coronary artery disease. In the previous study, heart sounds of 23 angioplasty patients were recorded before and after angioplastic surgery. In addition, two normal patients were used to add complexity to the study[3,4,5]. The most apparent spectral features associated with corrective surgery were a consistent decrease in the high frequency power above 300 Hz[3,4]. The relatively low frequency (100-200 Hz) peak did not change with the surgery. The amplitude of this peak was almost the same before and after angioplastic surgery. Though the exact cause of it is unknown, this peak may be due to low frequency produced by aortic pumping or ventricle filling. Angioplasty generally produced a consistent shift away from the unit circle in the second and third pole pairs obtained with the autoregressive (AR) method. A parallel normal/abnormal study showed that the percentage of spectral energy above 300 Hz differed between normal and diseased patients with the energy over 300 Hz being greater in diseased patients[3,4]. Again, in almost all subjects, it was found that the second and usually the third poles of the normal patients were farther from the unit circle than those of coronary artery disease patient[3,4].

The principal objective of this study is to use the combination of the additional signal components found in heart sounds of patients with coronary artery disease and the physical examination variables to improve the diagnostic accuracy of nonivasive detection of coronary artery disease.

Details of the other evaluations using recordings taken in **a soundproof and patient's bedside (noisy room)** room have been described elsewhere[3,4]. Results from these studies showed that the percentage of spectral power above 300 Hz is associated with coronary artery disease. Again, in almost all subjects, it was found that the second and usually the third poles of normal patients and many post- angioplasty patients were farther from the unit circle than those of CAD patients [3,4,45,51].

In this study, the neural network was applied to noninvasive detection of coronary artery disease using the model parameters of the AR method applied to isolated diastolic heart sounds associated with coronary artery disease as well as the physical examination variables of the patients in order to fully capture all relevant informations related to the disease state of the patients, relying on their nonlinear and multilayered architecture[5].

2. Methods

2.1 Adaptive Line Enhancer (ALE) Method

The Adaptive Line Enhancer (ALE)[6,10,15,20,30,39] method has been widely used in many fields including biomedical signal processing[3,4,6,10,15]. A particular advantage of this method is that it does not require a reference (noise) signal. The input signal, x(n), provides its own reference signal which is a delayed replica of this signal. The only difference between the primary and reference signals is the delay **d**. If the delay is properly chosen, the noise in the reference signal, r(n), is uncorrelated with the primary noise signal v(n). The output of the adaptive line enhancer estimates the desired signal y(n)[39]. The computational algorithm of the ALE can be summarized as follows[6,39]:

$$x(n) = y(n) + v(n) \tag{1}$$

$$r(n) = x(n-d) = y(n-d) + v(n-d) \tag{2}$$

$$\widehat{y(n)} = \sum_{p=0}^{m} h_p(n) r(n-p) \tag{3}$$

$$\widehat{y(n)} = \sum_{p=0}^{m} h_m x(n-p-d) \tag{4}$$

$$e(n) = x(n) - \widehat{y(n)} \tag{5}$$

$$h_p(n+1) = h_p(n) + 2\mu e(n) x(n-p-d) \tag{6}$$

for $p = 0, 1, 2, ..., m$

where x(n) represents the primary signal
y(n) represents the desired signal
r(n) represents the reference signal
v(n) represents the primary noise signal
$h_p(n)$ represents the adaptive filter weights
m represents the adaptive filter order
d represents the delay

In this study, we utilized the least mean square (LMS) implementation of the line enhancement method. We selected the delay $d = 5$ for ALE (see Fig. 3 in (3)) since this value is large enough so that the v(n) in the primary signal will be uncorrelated with $v(n-d)$ in the reference signal. The ALE filter order was taken as $m = 10$ based on our previous findings (see Fig.1(a) in [3]).

2.2 *Autoregressive (AR) Method*

The AR method is the most widely used modelling method to estimate parameters associated with biomedical signals. In the AR model, called the all-pole method, each sample of the biomedical signal can be expressed as a linear combination of previous samples and an error signal v(n)[1,3,6,12,16,23,28,36,38,39,45,51].

$$x(n) = -\sum_{p=1}^{m} a_p x(n-p) + v(n) \tag{7}$$

where $x(n)$ is the input signal
a_p is the AR coefficients
$v(n)$ is the estimated error signal
m is the AR model order

The power spectral density (PSD) function of the AR method, $S_{AR}(w)$, can be calculated as follows:

$$S_{AR}(w) = \frac{\sigma_e^2}{[1 + \sum_p^m a_p e^{-jwp\Delta t}]^2} \tag{8}$$

where σ_e^2 is the noise power
w is the frequency
Δt is the sampling interval

The details of the Modified Yule-Walker AR method has been described elsewhere[6].

The transfer function of the AR method, $H(z)$, can be calculated as follows[14]:

$$H(z) = \frac{1}{A(z)} \tag{9}$$

where $A(z)$ represents filter function.

The coefficients of the AR model, $\underline{a}(m)$, can be calculated accurately and efficiently using the modified Yule-Walker(MYW) method [6,16]. The overdetermined type MYW ARMA method shows better performance than the other block processing AR methods when the poles of A(z) are sufficiently close to the unit circle The first step in the procedure is to calculate the estimated autocorrelation functions. The MYW method calculates the AR coefficients using a set of linear equations of the autocorrelation function (ACF), $R_{yy}(k)$, recursively[15].

The AR coefficients, $a_(m)$, can be calculated using the following equation[6,16,39]:

$$R_{yy}(k) = \sum_{p=1}^{m} a(p) R_{yy}(k-p) \tag{10}$$

where $p = 1, \cdots, m$
k represents the highest order of the ACF.
m represents the highest order of the AR process.

To get the most accurate results, it has been proven that the higher order samples of the ACF (Autocorrelation function) should be utilized. Another key point to note is the requirement that the AR filter, A(z), has all of its zeros within the unit circle in order to guarantee the stability of H(z). For the initial estimation, one chooses $a(0) = 1$.

Instead of $k = m$ ACF (k is the highest order of the samples of the ACF), $k \geq m$ can be used to get an accurate estimate of the AR coefficients. By using this inequality, more equations will be available than unknowns. The extraction of AR parameters, $\underline{a}(m)$, can be carried out in general by solving the equation[8,9,39]:

$$\begin{vmatrix} R_{yy}(0) & R_{yy}(1) & \cdots & R_{yy}(m-1) \\ \cdots & & & \\ \cdots & \cdots & \cdots & \\ \cdots & \cdots & \cdots & \\ R_{yy}(k-1) & & & R_{yy}(k-m) \end{vmatrix} \begin{vmatrix} a(1) \\ \\ \\ \\ a(m) \end{vmatrix} = \begin{vmatrix} R_{yy}(1) \\ \\ \\ \\ R_{yy}(k) \end{vmatrix} \qquad (11)$$

This equation can be solved by using either the Levinson recursion technique, or the least squares algorithm[3,16,39]. A study using the AR method has shown that for filter order, m, greater than 10 the minimal mean-square error as a function of filter order was relatively stable. Based on the data in Fig.1a, 1b in [3] and our initial empirical findings, filter orders between 10 or 15 were judged sufficient to represent the signal records. Further, our results were insensitive to the filter orders within this range. For these reasons, a filter order of $m = 10$ and an autocorrelation order of $k = 15$ were chosen as adequate to represent the original signal.

2.3 Patient Analysis

The object of this study was to evaluate an improved method for the acoustical detection of diastolic heart sounds associated with the diagnosis of coronary artery disease. Diastolic heart sound recordings were made in **both soundproof and noisy rooms**. Patients were selected from those undergoing catherization and/or angioplasty at the Cardiodynamics Laboratory of Robert Wood Johnson University Hospital. Diastolic heart sounds were recorded from the 4th intercostal space on the chest of patients using a specially designed high sensitivity accelerometer[40] in conjunction with a portable digital pulse code modulation (PCM) data recorder (TEAC, RD-11OT). The output of a finger plethysmograph was also recorded as a timing reference to aid in locating the diastolic period. Next, the data are loaded from the digital tape to computer (HP 9000) using standard data acquisition system (3852A, HP). These sounds were recorded while the patients held their breath and were supine[1,5,44,45,46,51]. All of these patients were cath-proven as normal or abnormal.

For each patient 10 cardiac cycles were digitized (sampling frequency =4kHz). As detailed elsewhere[1,5,44], the diastolic heart sounds were passed through an anti-aliasing analog filter set for a cutoff frequency of 1200 Hz and a highpass digital filter set for a cutoff frequency of 180 Hz.

2.4 Neural Networks

Recent developments in the field of artificial neural networks have made them a powerful tool to analyze signals. The application of artificial neural networks(ANNs) has opened a new area for solving problems not resolvable by other signal processing techniques. A number of ANN algorithms and their applications have been widely reported[21,22,26,33,35,41,50]. Among the many neural network models, **Multi-Layer Perceptrons** which are considered the most useful learning models[41] have been used in the biomedical field[29,33,37,52].

A multi-layer perceptron can be trained by adjusting the connection weights and changing the unit threshold values. These networks can be trained by using a recently developed **fast backpropagation** algorithm which has proven to be extremely useful in training these networks[26,50]. The backpropagation is actually a generalization of the least mean square (LMS) algorithm which uses a gradient search technique to minimize a cost function equal to the mean square difference between the desired and the actual network outputs[41]. In these methods, the output error which can be expressed as the difference between the desired output and the actual network output from a training trial is propagated backwards through the network to update the connection weights. The output of each layer tends to be in binary form despite the analog signal at the input of the networks[41].

$$\Delta W_{ij}(t) = \eta \delta_j x_j \tag{12}$$

$$W_{ij}(t+1) = W_{ij}(t) + \eta \delta x_j \tag{13}$$

where $W_{ij}(t)$ corresponds to the weight from node i of
first layer or from an input to node j of second layer
at the time t
x_j corresponds the output of the output of the jth unit
of the secondary layer
η corresponds to learning rate control constant.
δ corresponds to the error

The error term δ_j can be estimated as follows(41):

$$\delta_j = (r_j - x_j)\frac{\partial x_j}{\partial net_j} \tag{14}$$

The error equation for the hidden layer can be written as follows(41):

$$\delta_j = \frac{\partial x_j}{\partial net_j}\sum_k \delta_k W_{kj} \tag{15}$$

where r_j corresponds to the desired response of the jth node

As a summary, the error terms for the any output layer and the hidden layer can be written, respectively, as follow[41]:

$$\delta_j = (r_j - x_j)x_j(I - x_j) \tag{16}$$

$$\delta_j = x_j(I - x_j)\sum_k \delta_k W_{kj} \tag{17}$$

The error term for hidden units includes all weights and error terms related to the second layer. The updating process starts with the output layer. Then, each previous layer is updated by propagating backwards through all the layers, by processing one layer at each time t. In order to increase the speed of convergence, a momentum term can be added to the updating equation. The momentum term also smoothes the updating process. The overall updating can be summarized as follows[41]:

$$W_{ij}(t+1) = W_{ij}(t) + \eta\delta_j x_j + \alpha(W_{ij}(t) - W_{ij}(t-1)) \tag{18}$$

where $0 < \alpha < 1$.

In this study, the neural network was trained by using backpropagation algorithm. The learning coefficient, η, and the momentum factor, α, of the neural network were set at 0.5 and 0.1, respectively. Initial weights of the neural network were random. Details of ANNs have been described elsewhere[26,41,43,50].

3. Results

3.1 Feature Extraction

For each patient, the feature pattern consists of 15 parameters. Of these parameters, 6 were obtained from the analysis of the diastolic heart sounds associated with CAD. The parameters obtained from the diastolic heart sounds were the model parameters (the power spectral density function peaks and the poles) of the AR method applied to the diastolic heart sounds of patients in the data base.

For each patient, individual spectra were obtained from each diastolic cycle using the AR method. Since there was some slight change in parameter values from period to period, the average PSD function and the poles of the MYW AR method was calculated by averaging the autocorrelation lags over 10 cardiac cycles. Before the analysis, the DC component from each record was eliminated (period by period). The ALE method was used to eliminate the background noise. The most apparent spectral feature associated with corrective surgery was a consistent decrease in the amplitude of the second and the third (or in some patients, the first) power spectral peaks[1,3]. The other definitive parameters were the amplitudes of the pole pairs. Surgery produced a consistent shift away from the unit circle in the second and the third pole pair, the pole pair associated with the second (between 300 and 500 Hz) and third (around 600 Hz) spectral peaks. They were numbered according to the phase of the pole pairs. For example, the pole pair with smallest radian frequency was called the first pole pair. The pole associated with frequencies between 300 and 500 Hz was called the second pole. These complex conjugate pole pair fell closer to the unit circle for the patients with coronary artery disease. For the normal patients, the amplitudes of the second and third poles were considerably smaller than their counterparts in the diseased patients.

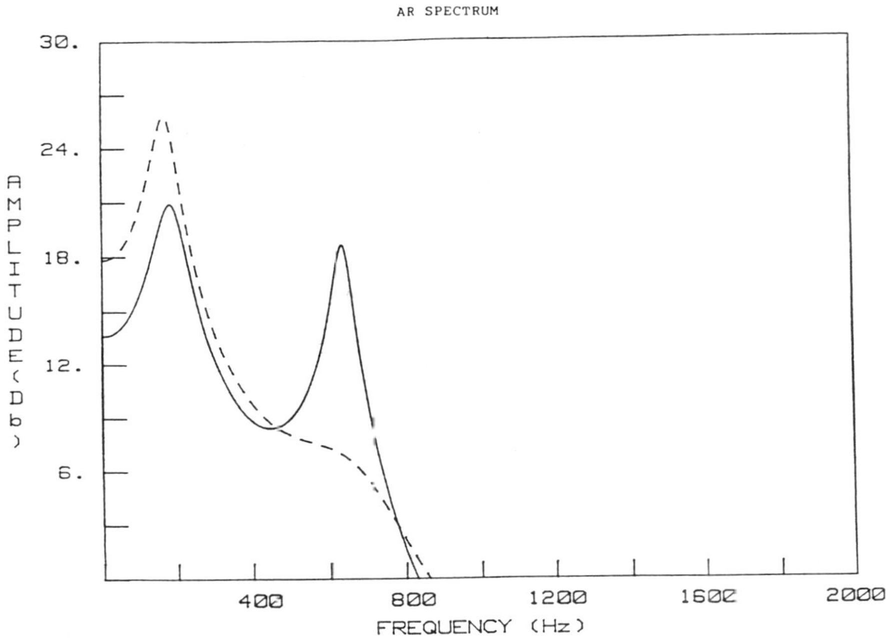

Figure 1: PSD functions obtained from the AR model applied to the isolated diastolic heart sounds of abnormal patient and normal patient after adaptive line enhancement. Solid line: Abnormal. Dashed line: Normal.

The amplitudes of the three power peaks (p1, p2, and p3 at respective frequencies of approximately 200 Hz, 400 Hz, 600 Hz) and the amplitudes of the poles of the AR (z1, z2, and z3) for all patients were the diastolic heart sound parameters of the feature vectors. The amplitudes of the peaks were coded as analog values between 0 and 1 since the amplitudes of the poles lie between 0 and 1 on the basis of stability. Figures 1 and 2 show the poles and the PSD functions obtained using the AR model applied to the isolated heart sounds (over 10 periods) of typical diseased and normal patients, respectively after adaptive line enhancement.

The remaining 9 parameters were taken from physical examination records.

The physical examination parameters of the feature pattern were sex (s), age (a), systolic blood pressure (sbp), diastolic blood pressure (dbp), smoking

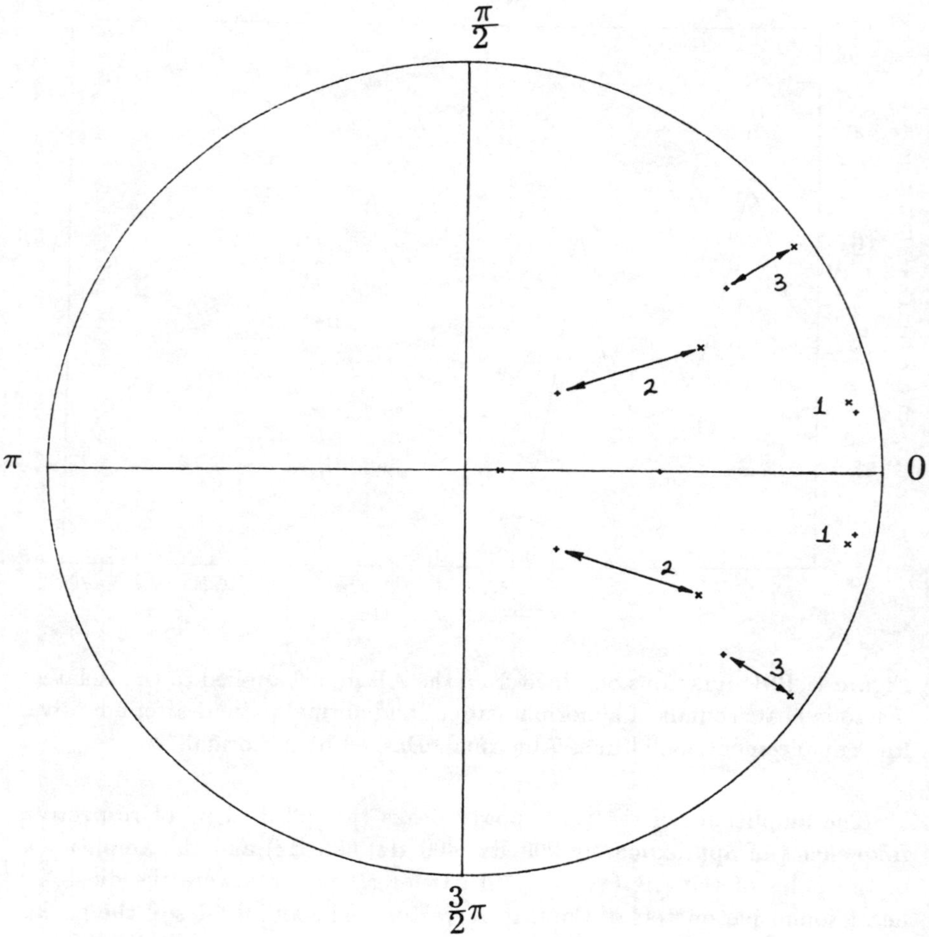

Figure 2: Poles obtained from the AR model applied to the same patients in Fig.1. X: Abnormal. +: Normal.

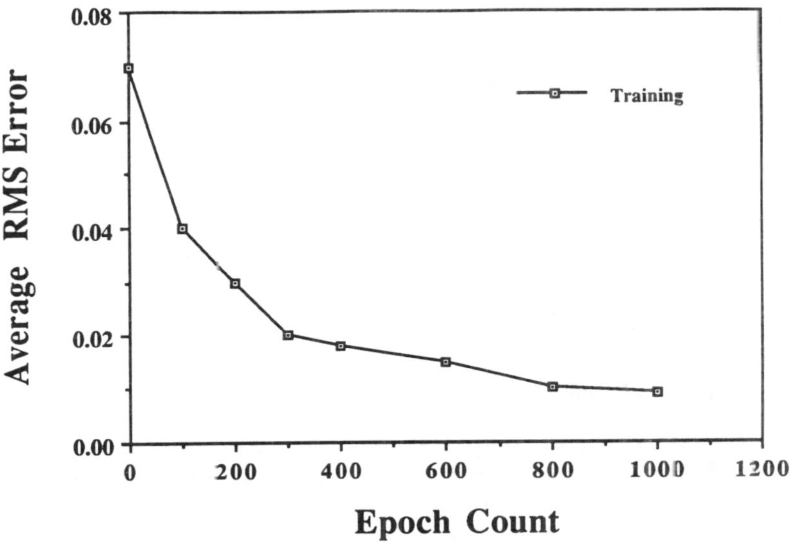

Figure 3: Average RMS error versus epoch count for training set

habit (sh), body weight (bw). These parameters are significant to the diagnosis of coronary artery disease [7,17,19,47]. Four preprocessed parameters such as normalized systolic blood pressure (nsbp), normalized diastolic blood pressure (ndbp), and the body mass index (bmi) [19,47] were also added to the physical examination parameters since they are also useful to the diagnosis of coronary artery disease. The normalized systolic and diastolic pressures were calculated since blood pressures are strongly dependent on age. The empirical formulas was used as follows[7,47]:

$$nsbp = sbp - 3.7 - 0.08(age)^2 + 0.331(age) \tag{19}$$

$$ndbp = dbp + 9 + 0.005(age)^2 - 0.53(age) \tag{20}$$

Finally, the body mass index which takes into account the body weight and height was calculated as follows[35]:

$$bmi = \frac{weight}{(height)^2} \tag{21}$$

The parameters a, dbp, sbp, nsbp, ndbp, bmi were coded as analog values between 0 and 1. The remaining physical examination parameter s, smoking habit was coded in binary manner where 1 represents a male as well as smoker since the risk factor for a man and a smoker is much higher than that of a woman and a non-smoker.

The feature pattern, all parameters inclusive, was utilized as the input to the neural network. Twelve patients were randomly selected for use as training cases for the neural network. Of these 6 were normal, and 6 were abnormal patients. A three layer **backpropagation** network was used. The network was run on a Sun system. Several configurations were tested. A network with 15 input nodes, 12 hidden layer nodes, and 2 output nodes showed the best performance. Using more than 12 hidden layer nodes did not improve the network performance. This network was trained until the averaged root-mean square (RMS) error per pattern at the output was less than 0.01.

3.2 Network Output Representation

The target values for the output was coded as 0 for the subsequently confirmed absence of coronary artery disease and 1 for the confirmed presence of coronary artery disease. The testing of the network was achieved by using the weights derived in the training test and applying the new patterns to the network to which it has not been exposed. Performance was scored as correct if the activation of the output unit was equal to or greater than 0.75 when the target was 1 or if the activation of the output was equal to or less than 0.25 when the target was 0. The network was tested on 100 patients. All of these patients, except for 5 pseudo-normals (who were not cath-proven) were either cath-proven normal or abnormal patients. All training was done in a supervised fashion, which means that the inputs and desired outputs were known during the training process.

The winner-take-all decision rule used in this study meant that the input pattern vector was set to the class belonging to the output node whose value is the biggest. Detection rate (sensitivity) was defined as the number of the correctly diagnosed abnormal patients divided by the total number of the abnormal patients in the test set. Specificity was defined as the number of the correctly diagnosed normal patients divided by the total number of the normal patients in the test set.

The learning coefficient, η, and the momentum factor, α, of the neural network were set at 0.5 and 0.1, respectively. Initial weights of the neural network were random. Figure 3 shows the average RMS error per pattern for training set used in this study. As shown in Figure 3, the trajectory of the test set qualitative errors decreases very rapidly first, then does not decrease after 800 epochs.

Results showed that 10 of 63 abnormal (a sensitivity of 84%), and 4 of 37 normal cases (a specificity of 89%) were correctly diagnosed.

4. Discussion and Conclusion

In this study, Neural Networks were proposed to improve the sensitivity and the specificity of the acoustical approach proposed by our group to an acceptable level. The Neural Networks were applied to the combination of the physical examination variables and the model parameters of the AR method applied to the diastolic heart sounds associated with coronary artery disease. The network had a detection rate of 84% and a false alarm rate $(1 - specificity)$ of 11%, whereas the previous study only using the PSD characteristics of the AR method showed a detection rate of 76% and a false alarm of 16% (3). The network correctly identified four patients with 100% occlusions as well as three other mis-diagnosed patients who were incorrectly diagnosed by using the spectral estimation methods (3).

These results compare quite favorably with other noninvasive methods for detecting CAD. For example, the sensitivity of the Cardiointegram (CIG) technique developed by TEICHHOLTZ et al.[49], was found to be 73% with a specificity of 78%. This approach was considered to be a moderately useful noninvasive method to detect CAD.

This new approach described above is based on the diastolic heart sound measurements associated with turbulence due to stenoses and the physical examination variables such as age, sex, diastolic and systolic blood pressures, and weight.

Results showed that neural networks were potentially capable of differentiating normal patients from abnormal patients. In addition, the diagnostic capability of this approach is much better than any available noninvasive approach.

Acknowledgment

The authors wish to thank Drs. JL Semmlow, J. Kostis for providing data, and J. Redling, D. Shen, A. Smith, and V.Padmanabhan for collecting and preprocessing the data used in this study.Address correspondence should be made to Dr. Metin Akay.

References

1. AKAY, M., SEMMLOW, J.L., WELKOWITZ, W., BAUER, M., KOSTIS, J.(1990) *Detection of Coronary Occlusions using AR modelling of Diastolic heart sounds*,IEEE Trans. on Biomed. Eng. BME.37:366-373.

2. AKAY, M., SEMMLOW, J.L., WELKOWITZ, W., BAUER, M., KOSTIS, J. (1990) *Noninvasive detection of coronary occlusions using Eigenvector methods before and after angioplasty*, IEEE Trans. on Biomed. Eng. BME.37:1095–1105.

3. AKAY, M. (1990) *Noninvasive Detection of Coronary Artery Disease using Advanced Signal Processing Methods*, Ph.D. Dissertation, Rutgers University, Piscataway, NJ.

4. AKAY, M., WELKOWITZ, W., SEMMLOW, J.L., KOSTIS, J.(1990) *Application of the ARMA method to Acoustic Detection of Coronary Artery Disease*, Med. Biol. Eng. Comput.29:365-372.

5. AKAY, M and WELKOWITZ (1993) *Acoustical Detection of Coronary Occlusions using Neural Networks.* J of Biomedical Engineering, vol.15, pp.469-473, November 1993.

6. AKAY, M(1994) *Biomedical Signal Processing.* Academic Press, NY.

7. BLINOWSKA, A., CHATELLIER, G., BERNIER, J., LARVIL, M (1991) *Bayesian Statistics as Applied to Hypertension Diagnosis*, IEEE Trans on BME.38:699-706.

8. BRUZZONE, S.P., KAVEH, M. (1984) *Information Tradeoffs in using the sample autocorrelation function in ARMA parameter estimation,* IEEE Trans. Acoustics, Speech, Signal Processing.32:701-715.

9. BOX, G. and PIERCE, D.(1970) *Distribution of Residual Autocorrelation in Autoregressive-Integrated Moving Average Time Series Models.* J.Am. Statist.Assoc.64:122-145.

10. CHEN, J., VANDEWALLE, J., SANSEN, W., VANTRAPPEN, G.,and JANSSENS. J.(1989) *Adaptive method for cancellation of respiratory artifact in electrogastic measurements.*Med. Biol. Eng. Comp.27:57-63.

11. CHENG, T.O. (1970) *Diagnostic Murmur Caused by Coronary Artery Stenosis.* Ann. Intern. Med.72:543-546.

12. DAVID, J-Y., S. A. JONES, D.P. GIDDENS (1991),*Modern Spectral Analysis Techniques for Blood Flow Velocity and Spectral Measurements with Pulsed Doppler Ultrasound.* IEEE Trans. BME,38:589-596.

13. DOCK, W., ZONERAICH, S.(1967) *A Diastolic Murmur Arising in A Stenosed Coronary Artery.* Am. Journal of Medicine.42:617.

14. DUNCAN, G.W., GRUBER, T.O., DEWEY, C.F., MYERS, G.S.

and LEES, R.S. (1975) *Evaluation of Carotid Stenosis by Phonoangiography.* New England J. of Med.27:1124-1128.

15. FERRARA, E.R.and B. WIDROW,(1981) *Adaptive filtering for signal enhancement*, IEEE Trans. ASSP,29.

16. FRIEDLANDER, B. and PORAT, B (1984) *Modified Yule-Walker of ARMA Spectral Estimator,*IEEE Trans.Aerospace, Electron., Syst.20: 158-172.

17. GANONG, WF (1981), *Review of Medical Physiology*, Los Altos, CA, Lange Medical Publication.485-488.

18. GIDDENS, D.P. et al. (1976) *Measurements of Disordered Flows Distal to Subtotal Vascular Stenoses in the Thoracic Aortas of Dogs.* Circulation Research. 39(1):112-119.

19. GUYTON, AC (1987), *Textbook of Medical Physiology.* W.B. Saunders Company, PA.

20. HAYKIN, S.,(1986) *Adaptive Filter Theory*, Englewood Cliffs, Prentice Hall, NJ.

21. HUANG W, LIPPMANN R, (1987), *Comparison between neural network and conventional classifiers.* In proceedings of the 1987 IEEE International Conference on Neural networks.485-494.

22. IWATA, A, NAGASAKA Y, SUZUMURA N, (1990), *Data Compression of the ECG Using Neural Network for Digital Holter Monitor*, IEEE EMBS Magazine.53.

23. IYER, V.K., P.A. RAMAMOORTHY, Y. PLOYSONGSANG, (1989) *Autogressive Modeling of Lung Sounds: Characterization of Source and Transmission.* IEEE Trans. BME.36:1133–1136.

24. LEES, R.S. et al. (1970) *Phonoangiography: A new Noninvasive Diagnostic Method for Studying Arterial Disease*, Proc. Natl. Acad. Sci.67:935-942.

25. LEES,R.S., MYERS, G.S. (1982) *Noninvasive diagnosis of arterial disease.* Adv. Intern.23:475-509.

26. LIPPMANN R, (1987), *An introduction to computing with neural networks*, IEEE ASSP Magazine, 4-22.

27. KARTCHNER, M.M., MCRAE, L.P., MORRISON, F.D. (1973) *Noninvasive detection and evaluation of carotid occlusive disease,* Arch. Surg., 106:528-535.

28. KAY, S.M. and MARPLE, S.L. (1981) *Spectral Analysis: A Modern Perspective.* Proc. IEEE, 69:1380-1419.

29. KELLY MF, PARKER PA, SCOTT RN, (1990), *The Application of Neural Networks to Myoelectric Analysis: A preliminary Study*, IEEE Trans. on Biomedical Eng.37:221-230.

30. KENTIE, M.A., VAN DER SCHEE, E.T., GRASHIUS, J.L., and SMOUT, A.J.P.M.,(1981) *Adaptive filtering of canine electrogastrographic signals-Part1; System Design.* Med. Biol. Eng. Comput.19:759-764.

31. KHALIFA, A.M.A. and GIDDENS, D.P. (1981) *Characterization of poststenotic flow disturbances.* J. Biomechanics.14:275-296.

32. KRUPP, MA (1982), *Current Medical Diagnosis and Treatment*, Los Altos, CA, Lange Medical Publications.193-210.

33. KUROGI, S. (1991) *Speech Recognition by an Artificial Neural Network using findings on the Afferent Auditory System*, Biological Cybernetics.64:243–250.

34. KURTZ, K.J. (1984) *Dynamic Vascular Auscultation*, Am. J. Med. 76:1066–1074.

35. LARVIL, M., CHATELLER , G., DEGOULET, P., SAUQUET, D., JEUNEMAITRE, X., MENARD, J., ROVANI, C. (1988)*ARTEL: An expert system in hypertension for the general practitioner, in Lecture Notes in Medical Informatics.* Berlin: Springer-Verlag.314-321.

36. MAKHOUL, J.,(1981) *Spectral Linear Properties and Applications*, Trans. ASSP.29:282-296.

37. MARMAROU RM, WHITE MW, MARMAROU A, (1990), *Classification of Somatosensory of Evoked Potentials Recorded from Patients with Severe Head Injuries.* IEEE BME Magazine.43-49.

38. MARPLE, S.L.(1976)*Conventional Fourier, Autoregressive, and Special ARMA Methods of Spectrum Analysis*, Engineer's Dissertation, Stanford University.

39. ORFANIDIS,S.J.,(1985) *Optimum Signal Processing*, Mac Millan, New York.

40. PADMANABHAN, V., FISHER, R., SEMMLOW, J.L., WELKOWITZ, W., and KOSTIS, J.(1989) *High Sensitivity PCG Transducer for Extended Frequency Applications*, Proc. IEEE Frontiers in Medicine, Seattle.57-59.

41. RUMELHART D, HUNTON GE, WILLIAMS RJ, (1986), *Learning Internal Representations by Error Propagation, ch.8, pp. 318-362, volume I of Parallel Distributed Processing; Explorations in the microstructure of cognition*, MIT press, Cambridge, Mass.

42. SANGSTER, J.F. et al. (1973) *Diastolic Murmur of Coronary Artery Stenosis*, Br. Heart J.35:840-844.

43. SEJNOWSKI T, ROSENBERG CR (1986) *NET talk: A parallel Network that learns to read aloud,* Johns Hopkins Univ. Technical Reports, JHU/EECS-86/01.

44. SEMMLOW, J.L., WELKOWITZ, W., KOSTIS, J., MACKENZIE, J.W. (1983) *Coronary Artery Disease-correlates Between Diastolic Auditory characteristic and Coronary Artery Stenoses,* IEEE Trans. Biomed. Eng.30:136-139.

45. SEMMLOW, J.L., AKAY, M., WELKOWITZ, W. (1990) *Noninvasive detection of CAD using parametric analysis methods,* IEEE, EMBS Magazine.9:33-37.

46. SHEN, D., J. SEMMLOW, W. WELKOWITZ(1990), *Automated Identification of Artifact-free Diastolic Heart Sounds*, Proc. IEEE Frontiers in Medicine, PA, 569-570.

47. SOX, H.C., BLATT, M.A., HIGGINS, M.C., MARTON, K.I. (1988), *Medical Decision Making*, London, Butterworth.

48. STOLZENBERG, J (1980), *Stress-Thalium-201 Scanning in CAD*, Med. Clin. North Amer., 64(2): 149-162.

49. TEICHHOLTZ , L.E.(1984)*Cardiointegram Detection CAD using in Normal Resting Electrocardiograms,* J. Am. Coll. Cardio. 3.598.

50. VOGL, T.P., MANGIS, J.K., RIGLER, J.K., ZINK, W.T., ALKEN, T.L.,(1988) *Accelerating the convergence of the back propagation method*, Biological Cybernetics.59:257-263.

51. WELKOWITZ, W., AKAY, M., WANG, J-Z., SEMMLOW, J., KOSTIS, J.,(1990) *A Model for Disturbed Coronary Artery Flow with Phonocardiographic Verification*, Activation, Circulation and Transport In the Cardiac Muscle, S. Sideman and R. Beyer, Eds. Kluwer Academic Publishers, Massachusetts.

52. XUE Q, HU Y, TOMPKINS WJ, (1990), *A Neural Network Weight Pattern Study with ECG Pattern Recognition*, IEEE Engineering in Medicine and Biology 11 th Annual Int. Conf.2023.

FUZZY NEURAL NETWORK-BASED ADAPTIVE REASONING WITH EXPERIENTIAL KNOWLEDGE

HONG DING* AND MADAN M. GUPTA
Intelligent Systems Research Laboratory, College of Engineering,
University of Saskatchewan, Saskatoon, Saskatchewan, Canada S7N OWO

1. Introduction

The goal of medical diagnostic problem solving is to find a parsimonious set of disorders in a given realm as a diagnostic solution to explain why a set of observed symptoms are present, absent or unknown by using an expert's knowledge. This problem can be formalized as a four-touple: DP = $< D, M, K, M^* >$ with a solution $D^* \in D$, where D is a finite non-empty set of disorders, M is a finite non-empty set of manifestations (or symptoms), K is the diagnostic knowledge about the relationship between D and M, and $M^* \in M$ is a subset of observed manifestations. A number of diagnostic methodologies have been proposed to reach this goal, such as fault tree analysis [1], knowledge-based systems [2], and neural networks [3].

Knowledge-based systems (KBSs) provide 'knowledge' processing techniques to find the diagnostic solution, and such systems have shown a number of advantages compared to conventional diagnostic methods. According to the different levels of knowledge sources which are used in a KBS, knowledge-based diagnostic methods can be classified [4] as: structure-based diagnosis, behavior-based diagnosis, function-based diagnosis and experience-based diagnosis. The former three levels are usually called model-based diagnosis[1].

On the other hand, according to the constructive features of knowledge sources, two types of knowledge sources are commonly used, which are differently interpreted in diagnostic problem-solving. The first is experiential knowledge which maps from effects to causes and is employed in experience-based diagnosis. The second is causal knowledge which maps from causes to effects and may be employed in various levels of diagnoses. For example, structurally causal knowledge (i.e., causal structural connections), functionally causal knowledge (i.e., causal functional relations), and

---

* Dr. Ding is on leave from the Huazhong University of Science and Technology, P.R. China

1 However, the concept of models in model-based approaches, in the authors' opinion, is quite extensive, including physical models, state models and computational (cognitive or mathematical) models of the system to be diagnosed.

empirically causal knowledge, could all be investigated for the diagnosis of digital circuits or general composite systems [4], [5]. In medical diagnosis, however, difficulties are experienced in the extraction of the former three levels of knowledge sources because biological knowledge about human organization is not yet available. It is for this reason that the experience-based diagnostic approach has received more attention than the others.

If only the experience-based diagnosis is taken into account, the domains of *effects* and *symptoms* are the same and are denoted by M in the following discussion, and the domains of *causes* and *disorders* are denoted by D. In this case, the diagnostic knowledge K can be stated as a mapping from M to D (experiential associations), or from D to M (causal associations)[2]. Furthermore, in order to deal with the uncertainty of diagnostic knowledge and to emulate the diagnostic processes employed by human experts, fuzzy set theory has been widely used in this area for handling linguistic vagueness and data imprecision. However, it has been recognized that fuzzy logic-based KBSs, generally called **fuzzy expert systems**, for diagnostic problem solving have three intrinsic problems: knowledge acquisition bottlenecks, slow responses and weak adaptations to external changes.

On the other hand, with the emergence of a new generation of neural networks technology, much attention has been paid to the combination of neural networks with fuzzy logic systems, called **fuzzy neural networks** (FNNs), and this innovative technology of FNNs has successfully been applied to some diagnostic problems [6]. In this combination, the learning and adaptive capabilities of neural networks and the competitive aspects of fuzzy logic play important roles. In this article, the emphasis will be on knowledge acquisition and adaptation of knowledge processing using a FNN-based approach.

This paper is arranged as follows: In Section 2, we briefly characterize the knowledge processing approaches available for medical diagnosis, including fuzzy expert systems and fuzzy neural networks. We devote Section 3 to the development of an adaptive process for the acquisition of membership functions of fuzzy sets, which could be integrated into a fuzzy neural system or even a fuzzy expert system. A fuzzy neuronal model with composite fuzzy MAX-MIN neurons for combining the diagnostic process of fuzzy reasoning with the experiential knowledge is described in Section 4. An example of medical diagnosis is given in Section 5, and Section 6 summarizes the studies presented in this article.

2. Knowledge Processing Approaches to Medical Diagnosis

During the past decade, knowledge processing technology (KPT) for problem solving has been widely studied and applied in many fields. Generally speaking, KPT includes several issues such as knowledge acquisition, knowledge organization, knowledge utilization and knowledge integration, in which the knowledge acquisition has always been recognized as the *bottleneck* of problem solving. It is a bottleneck not only in the transfer of expertise, but also in dealing with quantitative sensor-based data using

---

[2] Because of the high complexity of relationships between D and M in complex systems to be diagnosed (such as human bodies and industrial equipment) and the complex mechanism of occurence and propagation of disorders, these sets of knowledge sources are naturally organized into various hierarchies or levels of abstraction [5, 7]. Because the focus of this articles is on the adaptation of fuzzy diagnostic reasoning process, for the sake of simplicity, only the mapping situation within a hierarchy is considered in the discussion to follow.

qualitative methods. Conventional knowledge-based techniques suffer deeply from the problems of inflexibility and slow response to external input information. In this section, a brief discussion is given of fuzzy expert systems and fuzzy neural computational models for handling diagnostic tasks with imprecise data and linguistic vagueness.

2.1 Fuzzy Expert Systems

2.1.1 Fuzzy uncertainties and knowledge representation

Fuzzy expert systems have been recognized as one of the most promising AI-based methods for handling linguistic vagueness and data imprecision. The general structure of a contemporary fuzzy expert system is shown in Fig. 1. The dotted-line box, the **knowledge acquisition** and **information perception** (KAIP) module, receives external inputs and transfers them into internal representation in the expert system [6]. The inputs to this system may come from both sensor-based data and linguistic statements through a multilevel man-machine interface. At the same time, the working conditions of the sensors are established and monitored using an operating environmental unit associated with the interface. In practical applications these working conditions of the sensors are also sent to the KAIP module as input information.

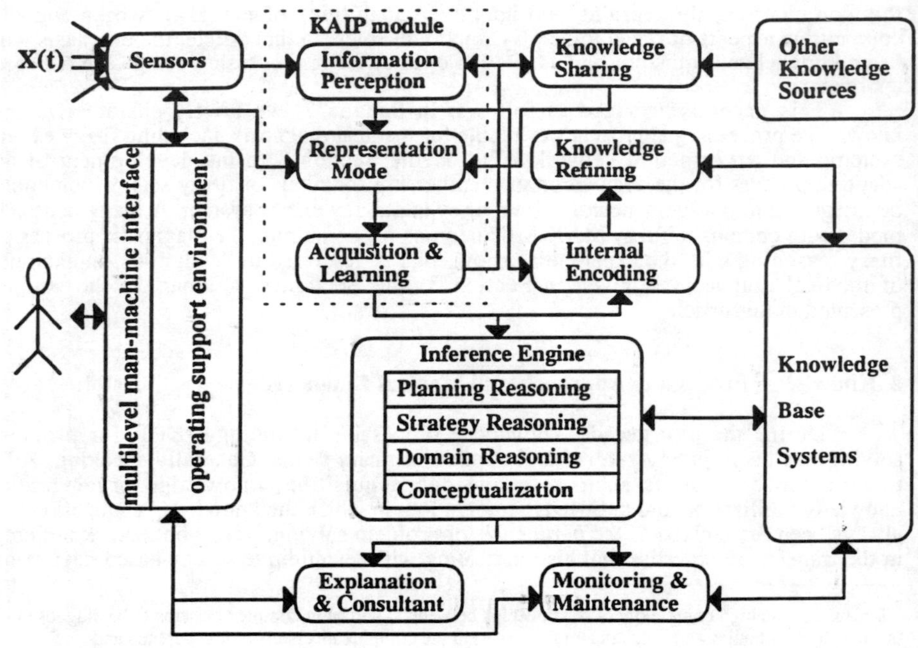

Fig. 1 A general architecture of fuzzy expert system

The only reason why fuzzy set theory should be combined with such expert systems is that knowledge sources in the *knowledge base system* and external inputs to the expert system are inherently shrouded with linguistic vagueness and numerical imprecision. In order to deal with such uncertainties fuzzy representation and fuzzy reasoning methods are introduced.

The fuzzy representation includes two steps. One is the definition of the membership functions of a fuzzy set for each variable in the input or output realms. The other is the formation of mapping from one universe to another, i.e., the acquisition of fuzzy associations. In the medical diagnosis, the definition of membership functions is supposed to be *given* and remains unchanged during the process of problem solving After that, two types of fuzzy associations are commonly used. One is *symptom-to-disorder* assertion, called experimential knowledge, mapping from symptoms to disorders, and denoted by $\{< m_j, d_i > | j = 1, 2, \ldots, N_m; i = 1, 2, \ldots, N_d\}$, where N_m is the number of symptoms; and N_d is the number of disorders. A mapping pair $<m_j, d_i>$ recalls the degree to which the disorder d_i occurs under the presence of a given truth value of the symptom m_j. In this type of association, both symptoms and disorders are represented by fuzzy sets, and the recalling mapping is crisp, i.e., $< m_j, d_i > \in (0, 1)$. Both the input and output fuzzy sets are supposed to be known, and this knowledge can be represented by fuzzy-if-then-rules [8]. If the mapping is uncertain but known, i.e., $< m_j, d_i > \in [0,1]$, and only the input fuzzy sets are known, the knowledge can be represented by a fuzzy relational matrix [9], where the element $< m_j, d_i >$ in the matrix is the possibilistic strength to which the occurrence of disorder d_i is recalled from the given truth value of the presence of the symptom m_j.

The order type of association is the *disorder-to-symptom* relations, called causal knowledge, which maps disorders to symptoms. This mapping depicts the intrinsic causal relations and is usually represented by mapping networks. In this case, because the diseases and symptoms are fuzzy sets, the causal mapping is generally evaluated by the possibilistic strength of the presence of a symptom which could be caused by the occurrence of a disease. In practice, however, we are only given an observation (fuzzy sets) of symptoms M^* and a mapping network of $\{< d_i, m_j > | i = 1, 2, \ldots, N_d; j = 1, 2, \ldots, N_m\}$, where M^* is usually only a subset of M (the realm of input symptoms). The causal relation $< d_i, m_j >$ indicates the possibility to which the disorder d_i could cause the manifestation m_j. Obviously, the $< m_j, d_i >$ in the matrix and the $< d_i, m_j >$ in the causal network have the same meaning in most cases.

2.1.2 Fuzzy reasoning

By employing the if-then fuzzy association we can use fuzzy modus ponens such as MAX-MIN and MAX-product methods to conduct the fuzzy reasoning [18]. For the fuzzy relational matrix, the extension principle is widely being used. However, in the diagnosis of multiple diseases, the conventional extension principle is not appropriate. We need to determine the degree to which any subset of diseases in the given realm accounts for or explains the presence of a given subset of symptoms M^* with the help of causal associations. Yager gave an explanatory model approach to this problem by using fuzzy logic [10].

In this paper, only the issues pertaining to adaptive fuzzy reasoning with the experiential knowledge represented by if-then rules are of concern. Studies on competitive and cooperative fuzzy reasoning with the causal knowledge represented by mapping networks will be addressed in [11].

We will now explain the diagnostic problem using the fuzzy expert system and the fuzzy-neural approaches using a simple example. In the medical diagnosis, the following logic assertions describe a typical if-then fuzzy rule on the ECG measurements (Fig. 2 gives a typical ECG measurements).

IF The 'Q' duration' is ***HIGH AND***
The 'Q/R amplitude ratio' is ***HIGH***
THEN The 'Lateral Myocardial Infarction' is ***SERIOUS*** (1)

The general form of such rules can be modeled as

$$R_p: \ \textit{IF} \quad x_1 \text{ is } T_1\,(x_1) \text{ AND} \ldots x_N \text{ is } T_M\,(x_N)$$
$$\textit{THEN} \quad y_1 \text{ is } S_1\,(y_1) \text{ AND} \ldots y_K \text{ is } S_L\,(y_K) \tag{2}$$

where $x_i \in X$ ($i = 1, 2, \ldots, N$) are input variables (e.g., the 'Q duration'), $y_k \in Y(k = 1, 2, \ldots, K)$ is an output variable (e.g., a disorder), and $T_j(x_i)$ indicates the jth fuzzy set (i.e., the jth linguistic term such as **HIGH**) that x_i belongs to. There are many kinds of fuzzy reasoning with these rules [8]. In a standard situation the inference engine in Fig. 1 must match the premises of each rule in the fuzzy if-then rule base with the input linguistic terms (fuzzy sets) and then perform implication. For example, using the pth fuzzy rule R_p, we obtain its implication for each output variable y_k as

$$\mu_{x \times R_p}(y^P) = \sup_X \left(\mu_{T_1(x_1)}(x_1)\, \Theta \ldots \Theta\, \mu_{T_p(x_N)}(x_N)\, \Theta\, \mu_{S_L(w)}(w)\right) \tag{3}$$

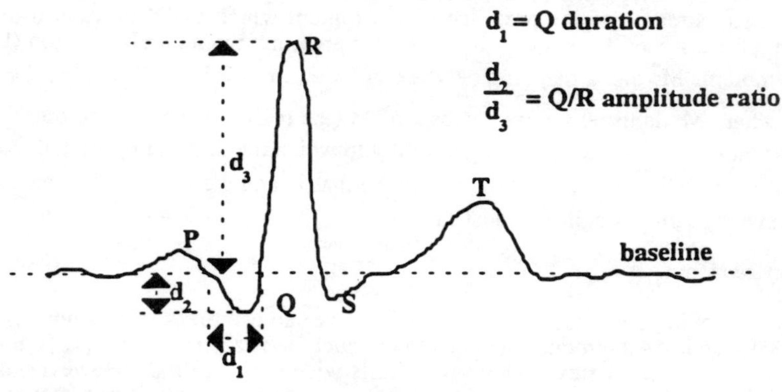

Fig. 2 Typical ECG waves

where "Θ" is a fuzzy operator which commonly employs the fuzzy intersection (i.e., Fuzzy MIN) or algebraic product, and w is the variable that represents the supporting values of the output fuzzy set $S_L(w)$. If there are several fired rules with the same output variable, the results implied by each of the rules should be combined as

$$\mu_{T_k(y)}(y) = (+)\,(\mu_{x \times R_p}(y^p) \mid p = 1, 2, \ldots, L) \tag{4}$$

where "(+)" is the fuzzy aggregation operator[3], and L is the number of rules with the same output variable, where $\mu_{x \times R_p}(y)$ in (4) is also a membership function curve. If a real-valued degree to which y is in $T_k(y)$ (e.g., the degree of occurrence of a disease) is required to be a final result, a defuzzification process is needed after the implication of each rule. Among the commonly used defuzzification strategies, the center of gravity method gives a fairly good result

$$\bar{y} = \frac{\Sigma\, \mu_{T_k(y)}(y) \cdot y}{\Sigma\, \mu_{T_k(y)}(y)} \tag{5}$$

The above describes the general inference process of if-then fuzzy rules in a fuzzy expert system. It is easy to see that the performance of a fuzzy expert system is heavily dependent upon the adaptation of an inference strategy and the learning ability of the system for new rules when the non-routine diagnosis is required.

2.1.3 Some Problem with Conventional Fuzzy Expert Systems

Now let us examine some problems in conventional fuzzy expert systems for medical diagnosis. First the membership functions of fuzzy sets in the fuzzy representation are always supposed to be *given* or assumed to be some specific shapes in almost all of the current diagnostic applications. There is no optimization and adaptation at all. Second, if the knowledge base is very large, the fuzzy reasoning with either if-then rules or causal mapping would be time consuming. In addition, since this kind of reasoning process is based on matching search techniques [18], a rapid response to changes in the operating environment is impossible. Third, for a fuzzy expert system, if the inputs are noisy or corrupted with the wrong information, the system can do nothing about this unreliable or mistaken information which will directly affect the performance. It is almost certain that the wrong results will be given by the system under such a situation. That is to say, this system is rarely fault-tolerant. Finally, the fuzzy reasoning model is almost static and is not able to adapt itself to improve its performance. One typical example is that this system may produce a solution to a given problem but always makes the same mistakes under the same situation. These problems faced by the conventional fuzzy expert system approach motivates us to develop a fuzzy-neural computational approach with learning and adaptive capabilities, which will be presented in the remainder of this paper.

---

[3] Fuzzy aggregation is a collective operation representing a fuzzy phenomenon, and can be modeled using fuzzy MAX, bounded sumation or some other form of t-conorms.

2.2 Fuzzy Neural Computational Models

As we have discussed above, the representation of fuzzy sets and the acquisition of fuzzy associations are heavily dependent upon an expert's prior knowledge about the diagnostic problem. If the number of fuzzy associations is very large (the fact is that sufficient fuzzy associations are often required to approximate the fuzzy uncertainty and cover complicated situations in the medical diagnosis to meet the required accuracy), the response of the fuzzy expert system is sometimes too slow to be applicable. When the situations vary, the developers or users of the expert system usually need to go back and modify the knowledge base and even the reasoning model, or to replenish the new fuzzy associations by themselves, which is often a difficult and time-consuming task. On the other hand, the neural networks-based approach performs well with respect to the perception of the environment. It also has effective learning abilities regarding past knowledge, as well as good adaptation with respect to current changes in the operating environment. Consequently, the integration of fuzzy expert systems and neural networks has been considered to be a promising approach.

Generally, current studies in this area can be classified into two categories: the **Fuzzy-Neuro approach** employing non-fuzzy neuronal models, and the **Neuro-Fuzzy approach** employing fuzzy neuronal models. In the fuzzy-neuro approach, fuzzy systems are approximated by using conventional neural models, while the non-fuzzy approach employs fuzzy logic to design fuzzy neuronal models. Obviously, the former approach mainly enhances the abilities of fuzzy systems, while latter mainly benefit the neural network technology [13].

2.2.1 Non-Fuzzy Neuronal Models

The fuzzy-neuro approach employs non-fuzzy neuronal models. A standard non-fuzzy neuronal model is usually a feedforward layered neural network except that in most cases the input x(t) to the network is fuzzy information, usually represented by an n-dimensional vector of real-valued membership grades, i.e., $\mathbf{x}(t) \in [0, 1]^n$. If it is assumed that the output $\mathbf{y}(t)$ of the network is an m-dimensional vector, $\mathbf{y}(t) \in [0, 1]^m$, the network actually performs a nonlinear fuzzy mapping from an n-dimensional hypercube $I^n = [0, 1]^n$ to an m-dimensional one $I^m = [0, 1]^m$:

$$x(t) \in [0, 1]n \xrightarrow{\text{FNNs}} y(t) \in [0, 1]^m \tag{6}$$

The weights in this network are real numbers, i.e., $w(t) \in [-\infty, \infty]$. The learning algorithm for this kind of networks can be any appropriate learning algorithm usually employed for standard neural networks [12].

In practical applications, an element $x_i(t)$ ($i = 1, 2, \ldots, n$) in x(t) usually represents the degree to which an input fuzzy variable $\bar{x}_i(t)$ belongs to a fuzzy set, while $y_j(t)$ ($j = 1, 2, \ldots, m$) in y(t) represents the degree of a fuzzy output variable $\bar{y}_j(t)$ in a fuzzy set. This approach will be used in the following section to approximate adaptively and functionally membership functions of fuzzy sets in the medical diagnosis.

2.2.2 Fuzzy Neuronal Models

The neuro-fuzzy approach employs neuronal models. The computational procedure of a fuzzy neuron includes two kinds of basic operations: i) synaptic fuzzy operations and ii) somatic fuzzy operations from the viewpoint of biological organization, as shown in Fig. 3(a).

1) Synaptic Fuzzy Operation The synapse in a fuzzy neuron is a storage element of the past experience (knowledge) which learns from the neuronal environment and continuously adapts its strength. The knowledge appears in a form of synaptic fuzzy weights. A synaptic fuzzy weight may be a real-valued fuzzy membership grade over the unit interval [0, 1] or it may be a fuzzy set represented by a continuous fuzzy membership curve, which depends upon the notion of fuzzy neuronal inputs. The synaptic fuzzy operation provides a *fuzzy similiarization* between the past experience (stored or memorized) in the synapse represented by a fuzzy weight vector w(t) and a fuzzy input vector x(t) at the time t as

$$u_i(t) = w_i(t) \Theta x_i(t), i = 1, 2, \dots, n \tag{7}$$

where "Θ" is the fuzzy synaptic operation. If the x(t) is an n-dimensional fuzzy vector bounded by a membership grade over the unit interval [0, 1], w(t) is also an n-dimensional fuzzy weighting vector represented by a graded membership over the unit interval [0, 1]. If x(t) is a vector of fuzzy-sets, w(t) will also be a weighting vector of fuzzy sets.

2) Somatic Fuzzy Operation The synapse transmits signals to the soma after the synaptic fuzzy operation. The somatic fuzzy operations are then performed on them through a two-step process as described below.

i) Fuzzy Aggregation The fuzzy aggregation operation is actually a fuzzy mapping from u(t) =

$$v(t) =(\oint (u_i(t) \mid i = 1, 2, \dots, n), v(t) \in R \tag{8}$$

where "$\oint$" means fuzzy aggregation (e.g., fuzzy addition) or, in terms of the fuzzy inner product, we directly have [13]

$$v(t) = w(t) (\cdot) x(t) \tag{9}$$

ii) Nonlinear Fuzzy Activation with Thresholding This is nonlinear activation with thresholding in the soma of a biological neuron that makes the neuronal process have some intriguing properties. For a fuzzy signal obtained from the fuzzy aggregation, we define the thresholding and nonlinear mapping as follows:

Thresholding process: $\quad z(t)\ v(t) (-) \theta(t), \quad z(t) \in R \quad (10)$

Nonlinear activation: $\quad y(t) = f_f[(z(t)], \quad y(t) \in R \quad (11)$

where "(-)" is a fuzzy thresholder (e.g., fuzzy subtraction) and $f_f[\cdot\,]$is a nonlinear function for fuzzy activation. If z(t) is real-valued membership degree over the interval [0, 1], the well-known sigmoidal function or Gaussian function may not be suitable activation functions. Mostly, $f_f[\cdot\ ]$ should be defined within a unit square, such as a sinusoidal function as shown in Fig. 4. If the z(t) is a fuzzy set represented by a fuzzy number, the sigmoidal function may still be appropriate.

From the viewpoint of information processing, the procedure of fuzzy neuronal computation addressed above can also be depicted by two operations: *fuzzy confluence*

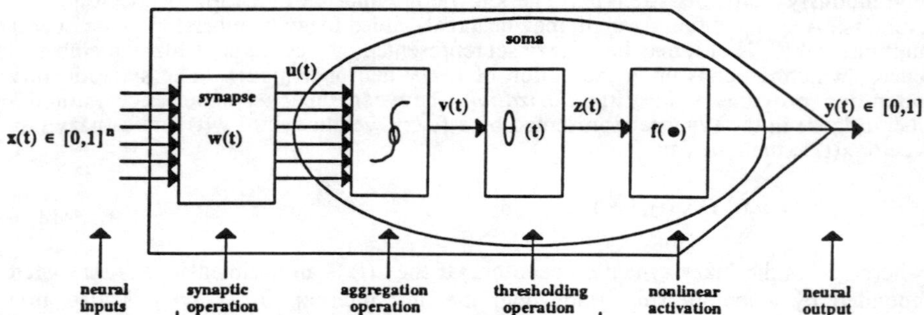

(a) Details of synaptic and somatic operations

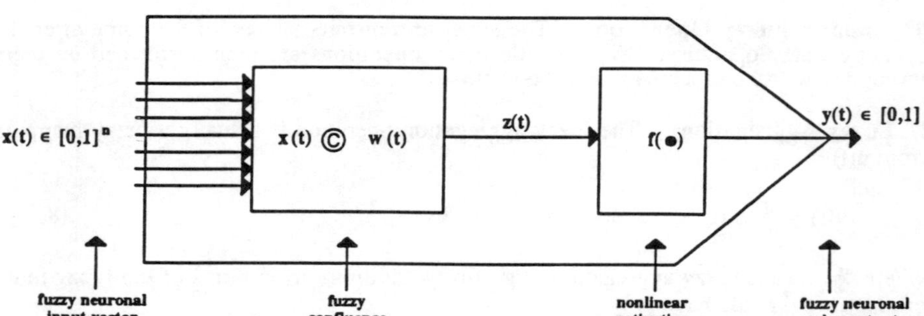

(b) Equivalent confluence and nonlinear activation operations

Fig. 3 A generalized morphology of fuzzy neuronal model, where $x(t) \in [0,1]^n$: fuzzy neuronal inputs $w(t) \in [0,1]^n$: fuzzy synaptic weights, ©: confluence operator.

operation and *nonlinear activation.* The confluence operation includes the synaptic operation for similiarization, the aggregation operation for summation and the thresholding operation for bias normalization as shown in Fig. 3(b). The main objective of the fuzzy confluence operation is to detect and measure the commonality or similarity between the neuronal input vector x(t), and the strength of the synaptic weighting vector w(t) which represents the accumulated past experience. The nonlinear activation that follows is to evaluate the measurement and then to output the graded degree of the commonality. More importantly, it is the nonlinear activation that makes the confluence measurement more robust and flexible. The adaptive ability of a fuzzy neuron is ensured, on the other hand, by the process of self-adjusting the synaptic weights w(t) by using an appropriate learning algorithm.

From the viewpoint of fuzzy neural computations, different neuronal morphology may be developed to implement the basic fuzzy neuronal operations and thus the scheme to detect and measure the commonality between the neuronal input x(t) and the prior knowledge in w(t) [13].

In this morphology, when the input x(t) is a vector of real-valued degrees of membership degrees, fuzzy neural networks with these neurons are called fuzzy-valued neural networks which are used to deal with the quantized fuzzy information. On the contrary, when x(t) is a vector of fuzzy sets, the corresponding network is called a fuzzy-sets neural network and is used to handle the continuous fuzzy information.

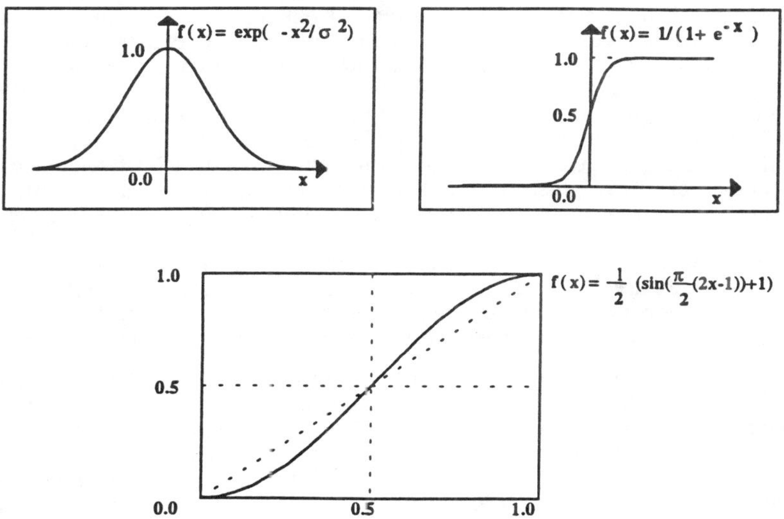

Fig. 4 Three kinds of nonlinear activation functions in fuzzy neurons

In most current applications of the fuzzy-neural approach to diagnostic problems, the non-fuzzy neuronal model is employed. The grades of presence of observed symptoms are taken as inputs to such a model, and its outputs directly represent the occurring degrees of potential diseases. This approach may enhance the fault-tolerant capability of fuzzy reasoning with the experiential knowledge, but does little for the adaptive learning of structural diagnostic knowledge represented by fuzzy if-then rules.

3. ADAPTATION OF FUZZY MEMBERSHIP FUNCTION

In the practical application of fuzzy logic systems, the membership function of variables in fuzzy sets are generally supposed to be *given*, or are often assumed to be such regular shapes as triangular, trapezoid or Gaussian functions. This assumption may not be reasonable. In practice, some empirical studies of pointwise measurements ($\{x_i$, $\mu(x_i)\} \mid i = 1, 2, \ldots, N$) are not too difficult to carry out. An intuitive problem is how to adaptively model the membership function $\mu(x_i)$ using the given measuring points. In order to solve this problem a two-step adaptive process, **Adaptive Fuzzy Set Ranking** and **Fuzzy Approximation,** is developed in the following section.

3.1 Adaptive Fuzzy Set Definition (Ranking)

The objective of this step is to partition the given domain into a number of fuzzy sets represented by linguistic terms according to a given set of measurements of this domain. An intuitive approach to this partitioning is to use fuzzy cluster techniques. Many types of fuzzy clustering methods could be used for this purpose [9], but to obtain an adaptive clustering, a modified Kohonen self-organization feature mapping network [9] is employed. The different with a standard Kohonen's network in which the neighborhood connection between two nodes in the Kohonen layer is determined by the index of topologic locations, the proposed clustering algorithm localizes the connection using the squared averaging distance between the individual weight of nodes and the input. The following gives an adaptive clustering algorithm for ranking fuzzy sets. At first, several parameters including individual weights, are initialized. The starting values of the learning ratio of about 0.1 and the neighboring ratio of 0.2, which are related to the possible number of fuzzy clusters and their overlapping degrees, are commonly recommended. A basic diagram of the proposed algorithm for applications is given in Fig. 5.

In this proposed algorithm the distances (differences) between the input and individual weights are used to control both the adaptation of the weights and the size of the neighborhood. Only those nodes centered around the winner in the neighborhood size of D_n will be updated for a given input. During an adaptive process, the neighboring ratio λ is kept a constant while the learning ratio η is linearly reduced. After the learning in the modified Kohonen network is completed, linguistic terms need to be given to describe the final clusters determined by the individual winners and their neighborhoods. The relative distances of the nodes in the neighborhood to the winner node are considered as being discrete sampling values of the membership function of the fuzzy cluster (set) related to this winner. Suppose that K fuzzy sets are clustered, named as S_i with the minimal distance nodes being d^i_{min} (i = 1, 2, ... K), the real-valued membership of each input x_m in each fuzzy set S_i can be derived by

$$u_{S_i}(xm) = \frac{d^i_{min}}{D_m}, \quad m = 1, 2, \ldots, M; \quad i = 1, 2, \ldots, K \tag{12}$$

The next step is to approximate the continuous membership functions using these discrete points. Sometimes, in order to approximate the trapezoid-like membership function of a fuzzy set, a prior parameter δ is defined to control the area around the winner to have the same membership degrees with that of the winner.

3.2 Functional Approximation

The functional approximation plays an important role in many areas, such as control, decision making, diagnosis, signal processing and image processing. Abstractly speaking, this can be considered as a mapping from one domain to another. The well-known polynomial scheme and neural network-based scheme are pointwise approximators, while a fuzzy expert system is a set-wise approximator to the mapping. All of them have been proved to be universal approximators to any continuous functions to any degree of accuracy [15, 16].

1. Initialize the architecture of a modified Kohonen map network with an input node in the input layer and N output nodes in the Kohonen layer; and initialize the weights w_{mj} of connection between the jth node (j = *1, 2, ..., N*) and the input (measurement) x_m in the mth training sample to small random values; choose the neighborhood ratio λ ($\equiv 0.2$) and the learning ratio η ($\equiv 0.1$).
2. Compute the second-order distance to the jth output node
$$d_{jm} = (x_m - w_{jm})^2$$
and compute the averaging squared distance
$$D_m = \frac{1}{N}\sum_{j=0}^{N-1} d_{jm}$$
where the subscript m indicates the mth input pattern (measurement).
3. Select the minimal distance node, i.e.,
$$d_{min} = MIN\{d_{jm} \mid j = 0, 1, ..., N-1\}$$
as the winner.
4. Compute the neighborhood size
$$D_n = \lambda(D_m - d_{min}) + d_{min}$$
5. Learn for the winner and all nodes in the neighborhood area (i.e., $d_{jm} \le d_n$)
$$w_{mj}(t+1) = w_{mj}(t) + \eta(x_m - w_{mj}(t))$$
6. Repeat steps 2-5 until no significant changes in the weights.
7. Assign linguistic terms to each clusters determined by each winner and its neighborhood.

Fig. 5 The proposed algorithm for adaptive fuzzy set ranking

In the case of this presentation, a set of samples $\{x_m, \mu_{s_i}(x_m)\}$, m = 1, 2, ..., M; i = 1, 2, ..., K, from the fuzzy set clustering in the previous subsection, is given so that the non-fuzzy neuronal network approach to the approximation is recommended. For each fuzzy set S_i, what we need to do is to learn a non-fuzzy neuronal network based on the desired training samples of mapping $\{x_m, \mu_{s_i}(x_m)\}$ using the gradient descent learning mechanism. Here, the single input to the network is the universes of discourse of fuzzy sets, while each output node represents the approximation of membership function of each fuzzy set, as shown in Fig. 6. Actually, this process corresponds to a nonlinear regression. The nonlinear functions in such a network can be sigmoidal functions or Gaussian functions. The hidden nodes and output nodes are fuzzy connected. In the case of neural networks using Gaussian functions, normalized Gaussian functions are usually used, and the hidden layer has the same number of nodes with that of the output layer, which equals the number of fuzzy sets to be approximated.

The Gaussian neurons in each layer can be described by the following operations:

Layer 1: $x_{1,m} = x_m, \quad y_{1,m} = x_{1,m}$ (13)

Layer 2: $x_{2,j,m} = (y_{1,m} - w_{2j}), \quad y_{2,j,m} = \exp\left(-\dfrac{x_{2,j,m}}{2 \cdot \sigma_{2,j}^2}\right)$ (14)

Layer 3: $x_{3,i,j,m} = y_{2,j,m}, \quad y_{3,j,m} = \dfrac{x_{3,i,j,m}}{\sum_{j=1}^{k} x_{3,i,j,m}}$ (15)

where x is an input to a neuron while y is the output of that neuron. The numbers of the subscript of x and y represent the ordering of network layers, m denotes the mth training sample; and j and i the number of the neurons in the hidden layer and the output layer respectively. The parameters to be learnt are $w_{2,j}$ and $\sigma_{2,j}$. Fig. 7 shows an example of

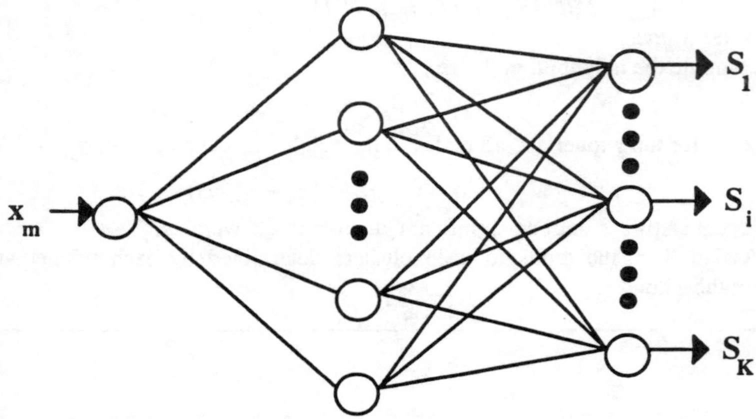

Fig. 6 Fuzzy membership function approximation using a *FNN* with a single input node and *K* output nodes, where x_m is the *m*th input to the *FNN*, S_i denotes the *i*th fuzzy set and *K* is the number of potential fuzzy sets

membership functions of the fuzzy sets **LOW, MEDIUM** and **HIGH** of the 'Q duration' in ECG measurements with Gaussian functions. By integrating these two steps an automatic and adaptive module can be obtained for the acquisition of membership functions of possible fuzzy sets from the given sampling data, as shown in Fig. 8, which could be integrated into any fuzzy neural systems or even fuzzy expert systems.

4. ADAPTATION OF EXPERIENTIAL KNOWLEDGE

An important application of fuzzy neuronal models in fuzzy expert system is to approximate structurally the fuzzy reasoning with if-then fuzzy rules. By this approximation the experiential knowledge can be adaptively acquired through the neural learning mechanism. In order to provide this kind of adaptive learning capability in a fuzzy expert system, a fuzzy neuronal model with composite fuzzy MAX-MIN neurons is proposed as shown in Fig. 9. In the following, we first describe how the three-layered fuzzy neuronal network works and then a learning scheme for the network is given. The basic structure of nodes in this network can be defined by the generalized morphology of fuzzy neuronal operations given in Section 2.

For the convenience of discussion let us denote $x_{l,j,i}$ as the input to the lth neuron in the ith layer from the jth neuron in the (i - 1)th layer, while $y_{l,i}$ is the output of the lth neuron. The inputs x(t) to the network is a vector of real-valued (quantized) membership degrees to which each input variable $x_i(t)$ belongs to each fuzzy set $T_j(x_i(t))$:

$$x(t) = [\mu_{T_1(x_1(t))}(x_1(t)), \ldots, \mu_{T_1(x_2(t))}(x_2(t)), \ldots, \mu_{T_M(x_N(t))}(x_N(t)]^T$$

where M is the number of fuzzy sets, and N is the number of input variables. Now let us describe the fuzzy neuronal information processing in each layer in terms of neuronal operations in Fig. 3.

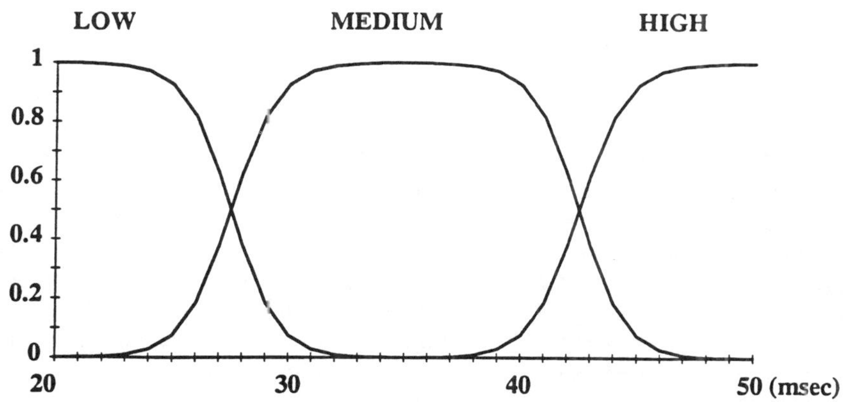

Fig. 7 Membership functions of fuzzy sets of 'Q duration'

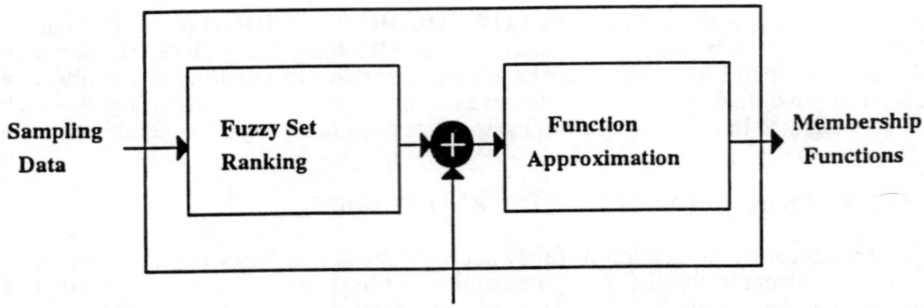

Fig. 8 Automatic and adaptive acquisition module of membership functions

Layer 1: The neurons in this layer perform linear transmissions of input values to the next layer, i.e.,

$$y_{1,j}(t) = x_{1,j,j}(t), \quad i = 1, 2, \ldots, N_1 \tag{16}$$

where N_1 is the number of input nodes ($N_1 \geq N$, the maximum of N_1 is $M \times N$).

Layer 2: The neurons in this layer are used to conduct premise matchings of $y_{1,i}(t)$ with precondition of if-then fuzzy rules stored in this network. Here, each node serves as a fuzzy if-then rule. The weight in this layer is unity. The fuzzy neuronal operations are described using equations (7-11).

$$x_{2,j,i}(t) = y_{1,j}(t), \quad u_{2,j,i}(t) = x_{2,j,i}(t) \tag{17a}$$

$$v_{2,i,l}(t) = \Theta\{(u_{2,j,i}(t), \ T_l w)) = \mid j = 1, 2., \ldots, N_1;$$

$$l = 1, 2, \ldots, L; \ i = 1, 2, \ldots, N_2\} \tag{17b}$$

$$y_{2,i,l}(t) = v_{2,i,l}(t) \tag{17c}$$

where w is the variable that represents the support values of membership function of the consequence for the lth output fuzzy set in the rule R_p "Θ" is the intersection by a fuzzy MIN operator, N_2 is the number of fired nodes (i.e., fired rules) in the hidden layer, and L is the number of output nodes. The membership function of each consequence $T_l(w)$ is transmitted through a feedback link from the output layer to the hidden layer with a unit linking weight. Therefore, $v_{2,i,l}(t)$, $y_{2,i,l}(t)$ are whole membership functions of fuzzy sets, not real-valued degrees of membership. This neuron has a different outputs $y_{2,i,l}(t)$ ($l = 1, 2, \ldots, L$) of implied membership functions to different nodes in layer three. This reflects that each output node will have different implied membership functions.

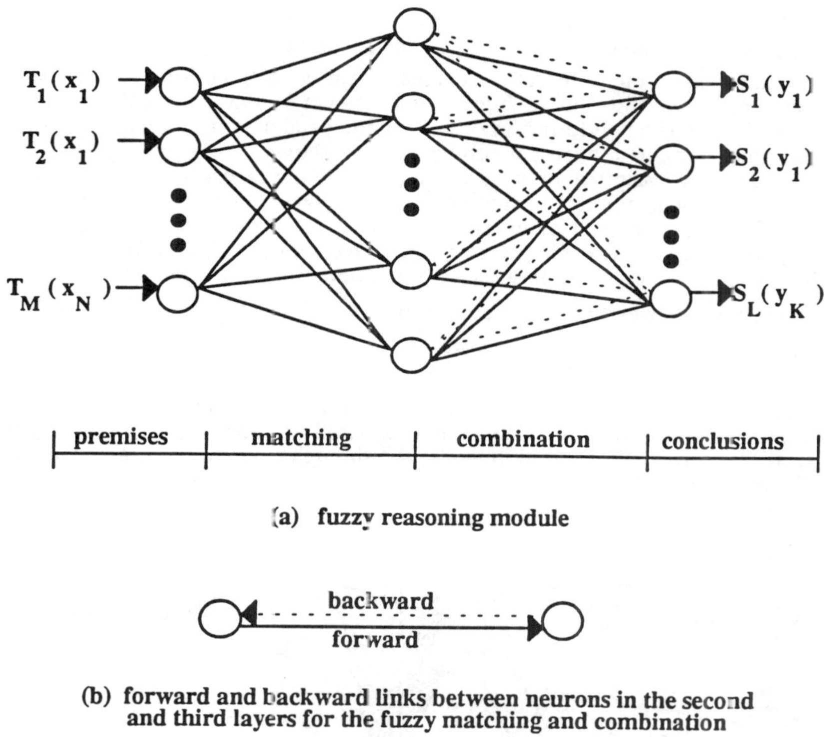

Fig. 9 Approximating fuzzy reasoning by using fuzzy neuronal models

Layer 3: The nodes in this layer use the fuzzy combination operation to integrate the individual membership functions implied by the fired rules which have the same variable of consequence. The weight in this layer is still unity

$$x_{3,i,l}(t) = y_{2,i,l}(t), \quad u_{3,i,l}(t) = x_{3,i,l}(t) \tag{18a}$$

$$v_{3,l}(t) = (+)\ \{u_{3,i,l}(t) \mid i = 1, 2., \ldots, N_2\}$$

$$l = 1, 2, \ldots, L;\ i = 1, 2, \ldots, N_2\} \tag{18b}$$

$$y_{3,l}(t) = v_{3,l}(t) \tag{18c}$$

where "(+)" is the union by the fuzzy MAX operator, and $v_{3,l}(t)$, $y_{3,l}(t)$ are whole membership functions.

Using this architecture of fuzzy neuronal models, the fuzzy reasoning is simply the forward mapping from the inputs $\{x_{1,j,j}(t)\}$ to the outputs $\{y_{3,l}(t)\}$.

Consider now the integration of the adaptive acquisition module of the membership functions into this architecture, as shown in Fig. 10. In this combined architecture, the first layer performs fuzzy set clustering and the definition of membership functions ,which itself is a neuronal sub-network as shown in Fig. 6. Layers 2 and 3 structurally emulate fuzzy mapping by if-then rules while layers 4 and 5 provide the defuzzification which includes a number of sub-networks for each output variable described below. Connections within layers 1, 2 and 5 are unipolar in a forward manner while the connecting links within layers 3 and 4 are bipolar, i.e., in a forward manner when the network operates and in a backward manner when the network learns. The forward and backward weights are represented by w_{il}^{3}, w_{ij}^{4} and w_{il}^{-3}, w_{ij}^{-4}, respectively.

In the operation mode the network receives the inputs $\mathbf{x}(t) = (x_1(t), x_2(t), \ldots, x^N(t))^T$, automatically ranks the input into different fuzzy sets and then acquires their membership functions using the first layer based on the discussion given in Section 3. After that, the network performs fuzzy reasoning based on equations (16)-(18). Finally, the defuzzification is conducted within the layer 5 through a number of sub-networks for each variable, as demonstrated in Fig. 11.

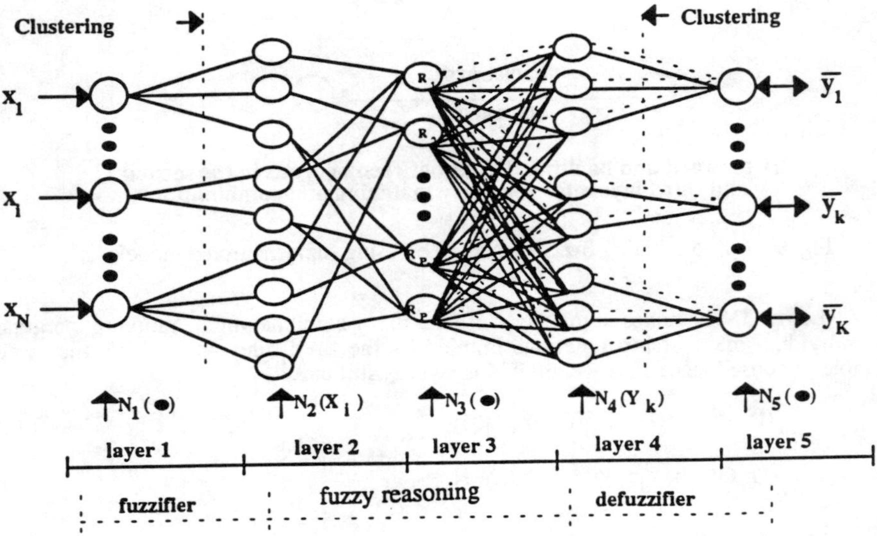

Fig. 10 Approximating fuzzy expert systems by using neuronal models

A defuzzification sub-network for the jth variable y_j has three layers with M nodes ($M = N_4(y_j)$) in the input layer, two nodes in the hidden layer, and one output node for crisp value, which is described as follows:

Layer 1: $y_{i,1,j} = x_{i,1,j}$, $i = 1, 2, \ldots, M;\ j = 1, 2, \ldots, K$ (19)

Actually, $x_{i,1,j}$ is the $y_{3,l}$ in (18) when $(i + \sum_{k=1}^{j-1} N_4(y_k))$ equals to l, and is also the membership function of the ith linguistic term related to the jth output variable y_j, which is discretized by a real-valued fuzzy vector using the fuzzy-set-as-vector [13].

Layer 2: $x^i_{1,2,j} = y_{i,1,j} \cdot w^{(1)}_{i,2,j}, \quad y_{1,2,j} = \sum_{i=1}^{M} x^i_{1,2,j}$ (20a)

$$x^i_{2,2,j} = y_{i,1,j} \cdot w^{(2)}_{i,2,j}, \quad y_{2,2,j} = \sum_{i=1}^{M} x^i_{2,2,j} \qquad (20b)$$

where $w^{(2)}_{i,1,j}$ is the vector of support values of membership function $y_{i,1,j}$, and $w^{(2)}_{i,2,j}$ is a unit row vector with the same dimension as y^3_j.

Layer 3: $x^1_{3,j} = y_{1,2,j}, \quad x^2_{3,j} = y_{2,2,j}$ (21a)

$$\bar{y}_j = y_{3,j} := x^1_{3,j} / x^2_{3,j} \qquad (21b)$$

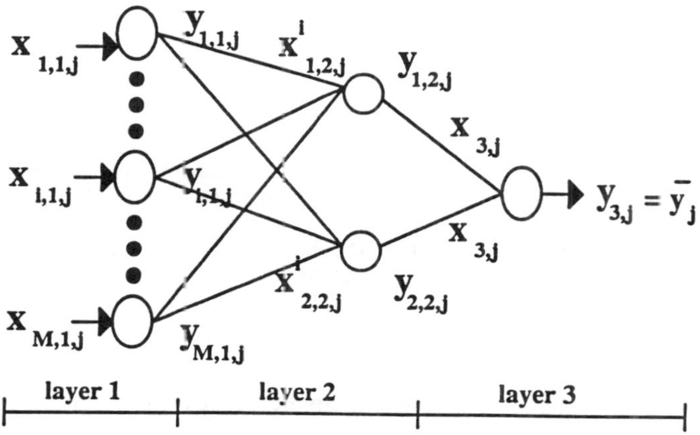

Fig. 11 A fuzzy neuronal sub-network for defuzzification

Obviously, the weight in this layer is also unity.

Now let us derive a two-phase learning scheme for the proposed fuzzy neuronal network in the learning mode. In the first phase the automatic adaptation and acquisition module is used to acquire the membership functions of fuzzy sets in both the input domain and the output domain, i.e., $T_j(x_j)$, j = 1, 2, ..., N_2 (x_i), i = 1, 2, ..., N; $S_l(y_k)$, l = 1, 2, ..., N_4 (y_k), k = 1, 2, ..., K where $N_2(x_i)$ and N_4 (y_k) are the number of linguistic terms related to variables x_i and y_k. After that, using the membership function as desired samples, the sub-network (layers 2, 3, and 4) in Fig. 10 is trained in the second phase, where the input and output of the sub-network of the samples are real-valued fuzzy vectors of discretized membership functions. Recalling that in Fig. 10 and Fig. 11, there is no synaptic weights to be adapted in the network of fuzzy reasoning. The learning task in this phase is the optimization of the architecture (i.e., connections) within layers 2 and 3 because layer 5, as shown in Fig. 10, is structurally fixed. The objective of the optimization is to compact maximally the information into if-then rules encoded by each hidden nodes in the layer 3 while still preserving the required mapping performance.

Initially, the network is considered as a most redundant situation; that is, there are $\prod_{i=1}^{N} (N_2(x_i))$ rule nodes in the layer 3. The inputs of each rule node come from one possible combination of linguistic terms (fuzzy sets) input variables under the constraint that only one fuzzy set related to each input variable can be an input of the rule node. The links between the nodes in layer 3 and the nodes in layer 4 are fully connected. All the initial links among layers 3, 4 and 5 are supposed to be unity (i.e., each *symptom-to-disorder* assertion is initially supposed to be truth). During the optimization process, it is assumed that each link varies in a binary fashion, i.e., 0 (representing no connection) or 1 (representing a valid connection). Some nodes and links of the initial structure are expected to be deleted or combined. In order to optimize the connections a genetic algorithm [17] is employed. Each link is encoded by one bit. The optimization function is defined by averaging the squared error over the whole sampling space.

$$E(w) = \frac{1}{N} \sum_{i=1}^{N} \sum_{j=1}^{K} (\bar{y}_{i,j}(t) - y^{d}_{i,j}(t))^2$$

where N is the number of training samples, W serves as the connection links, and $y^d_{i,j}$ is the desired output of the jth variable in the ith training sample. When the learning is complete, a recombination principle for connections between nodes is employed, i.e., a zero link means that this connection is not necessary and will be ignored. If all input links of a rule node are zero connections then the rule node will be deleted. If the input links of rule node A are included in the input links of rule node B then the rule node A will be combined into B.

5. AN EXAMPLE OF MEDICAL DIAGNOSIS

Let us consider now a simple example of medical diagnosis based on ECG measurements by using the proposed architecture of FNNs. We take the 'Q duration' and the 'Q/R amplitude ratio' as input variables, and the disease 'Lateral Myocardial Infarction' as the only output variable of the network.

First, we utilize 20 training samples for ranking the fuzzy domains of these variables with the help of the automatic and adaptive acquisition module given in Fig. 8. As a result, three types of fuzzy sets are defined for each variable as shown in Fig. 12. After that, we can reduntantly determine the number of nodes in each layer of the network. For example, for the model of FNN in Fig. 10, there are two nodes in the first layer, six nodes in the second layer, nine nodes in the third layer, three nodes in the fourth layer and one node in the output layer.

Another 20 training samples about the relationship among these variables are employed then to optimize the architecture of FNNs by using a genetic algorithm with a population size of 50, a crossover ratio of 0.8 and a mutation ratio of 0.6. After more than 150 generations, the reproduction process converges to a fittest population (i.e., having a optimized architecture) as shown in Fig. 13. After the recombination of the potential connections, this optimized architecture includes three hidden nodes which represent three fuzzy if-then rules, as shown in Table 1.

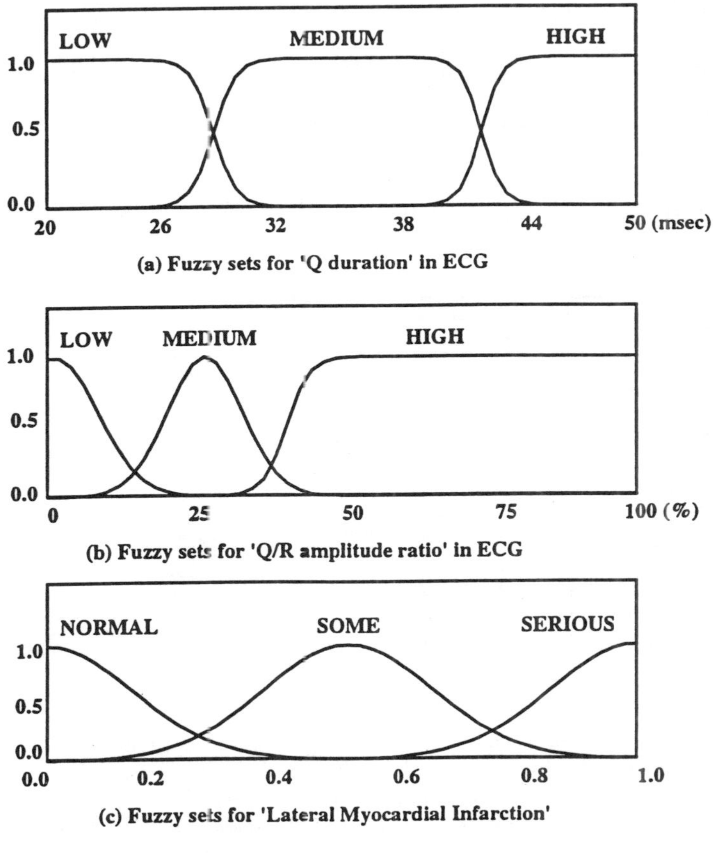

Fig. 12 Membership functions of fuzzy variables for medical diagnosis

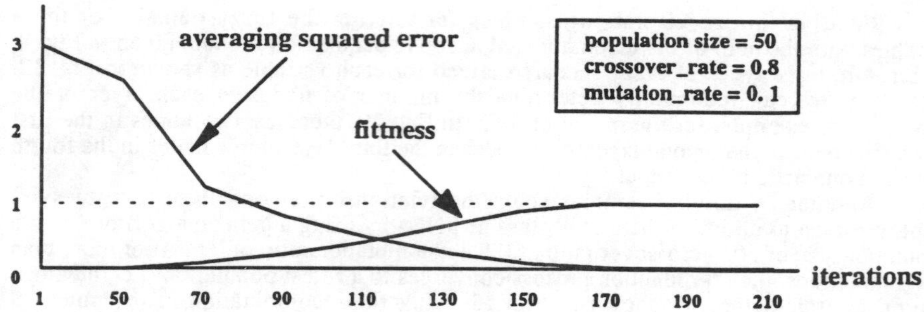

Fig. 13 The averaging squared error and the fitness of the fittest gene in a population versus iterations

Table 1: Fuzzy if-then rules on ECG learnt by the developed FNN

'Q duration'	'Q to R amplitude ratio'	'Lateral Myocardial Infarction'
LOW	LOW	NORMAL
MEDIUM	MEDIUM	SOME
HIGH	HIGH	SERIOUS

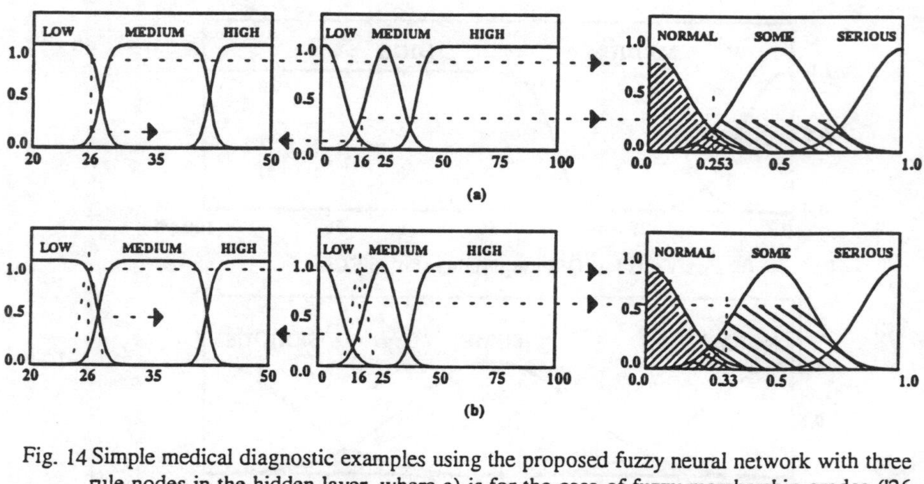

Fig. 14 Simple medical diagnostic examples using the proposed fuzzy neural network with three rule nodes in the hidden layer, where a) is for the case of fuzzy membership grades ('26 of Q duration' and '16 of Q/R amplitude ratio') as inputs obtained from a fuzzification sub-network, while b) is for the case of fuzzy sets ('*about* 26 of Q duration' and '*about* 16 of Q/R amplitude ratio') as inputs directly given by users or other fuzzy-set neural networks. In each case a crisp output can be given (e.g., 0.253 or 0.33) as the grade of confidence of the diagnostic solution by a defuzzification sub-network.

Finally, we test the developed model for different types of inputs. When a fuzzy-valued vector of inputs is given, where the 'Q duration' is 26 and the 'Q to R amplitude ratio' is 16, the model outputs a crisp value 0.253 as shown in Fig. 14(a). That is, the degree to which the disease occurs is 0.253. When a fuzzy-set vector of inputs is given, where the 'Q duration' is **about** 26 and the 'Q/R amplitude ratio' is **about** 16, the final crisp value is 0.330, as shown in Fig. 14(b), when we employed the architecture of FNNs shown in Fig. 9 together with the defuzzification sub-network shown in Fig. 11. Obviously, the model outputs different degrees of the disease in the two cases because different uncertainties of inputs are given.

It should be noted that after the development of the proposed model is finished, the membership functions (i.e., synaptic weights in Fig. 6 and Fig. 11) in this model can be further adapted in an on-line manner to the external changes in practical applications.

6. CONCLUSIONS

In this paper we have discussed issues about the adaptive knowledge processing for medical diagnosis using the **fuzzy neural approach**. First, fuzzy neural computational models were compared with conventional AI-based fuzzy expert systems. Then, an adaptive acquisition method for fuzzy membership functions which are supposed to be given in current fuzzy logic systems was proposed based on a two-step process of **adaptive fuzzy set ranking** and **function approximation**. After that, a fuzzy neuronal model with composite **fuzzy MAX-MIN neurons** using the neuro-fuzzy approach was proposed for the acquisition of experiential knowledge and the fuzzy reasoning with this knowledge, including three fuzzy neural sub-networks for adapting the fuzzification, the fuzzy reasoning and the defuzzification respectively in a fuzzy expert system.

REFERENCES

1. R.A. Collacott, *Mechanical Fault Diagnosis and Condition Monitoring*, (Chapman and Hall, London, 1977).
2. R. Davis and D.B. Lenat, *Knowledge-Based Systems in Artificial Intelligence*, (McGraw-Hill, New York, 1982).
3. M. Gaudill, *Using Neural Nets: Diagnostic Expert Nets*, **AI Expert**, (September, 1990), 43-47,.
4. R. Milne, *Strategies for Diagnosis*, **IEEE Trans. Syst., Man and Cybern., 17**, (1987), 333-339.
5. H. Ding, *Knowledge-Based Diagnosis for Complex Systems - Theory and Systems*, **Ph.D. Dissertation**, (Huazhong University of Science and Technology, China, 1990).
6. S.Z. Yang and H. Ding, *Knowledge-Based Diagnostic Reasoning*, (Qinghai University Press, Beijing, 1993).
7. B. Chu and J.A Reggia, *Modeling Diagnosis at Multiple Levels of Abstraction, Part I, Representing Causal Relations at Multiple Levels of Abstraction*, **Int. J. of Intelligent Systems, 6**, (1991), 617-644.
8. H.J. Zimmermann, *Fuzzy Set Theory and Its Applications*, Second edition, (Kluwer Academic Publishers, 1991).
9. L.A. Zadeh, *Fuzzy* Sets, **Information and Control, 8**, (1965), 338-353.
10. R.R. Yager, *Explanatory Models of Expert Systems*, **Int. J. of Man-Machine Studies, 23**, (1985), 539-549.

11. H. Ding and M.M. Gupta *Competitive and Cooperative Adaptive Reasoning with Fuzzy Causal Knowledge*, Submitted to **Int. J. of Man-Machine Studies**, (October 1993).
12. R.P Lippmann, *Introduction to Computing with Neural Nets,* **IEEE ASSP, 4**, 1987, 4-12.
13. M.M. Gupta and H. Ding H. (1993), *"Foundations of Fuzzy Neural Computations*, **J. of Intelligent and Fuzzy Systems** [In Press], 1993.
14. T. Kohonen, *Self-Organizing and Associative Memory*, (Springer-Verlag, Berlin , 1988).
15. G.G. Lorentz, *Approximation of Functions*, (Chelsea Publishing Co., NY, 1986).
16. T. Poggio and F. Girosi, *Networks for Approximation and Learning*, **Proc. of IEEE, 78, 9**, (1990), 1481-1497.
17. D.E. Goldberg, *Genetic Algorithms in Search, Optimization and Machine Learning,* (Addison-Wesley Publishing Company, Co., 1989).
18. J. Pearl, *Fusion, Propagation, and Structuring in Belief Networks*, **AI J., 29**, (1986), 241-288.

ESTIMATION OF LONG-TERM MORTALITY OF MYOCARDIAL INFARCTION USING A NEURAL NETWORK BASED ON THE ALOPEX ALGORITHM

WILLIAM J. KOSTIS, CHENG YI, EVANGELIA MICHELI-TZANAKOU
Department of Biomedical Engineering, Rutgers University
Piscataway, N.J. 08855-0909, USA

1. Introduction

Neural networks consist of groups of similar computational units and their interconnections [1]. They map input patterns encoded as vectors into output patterns. They emulate the biological structure and function of neurons and exhibit the ability to learn and generalize from previous experience, as well as to abstract the essential elements common to many inputs. These "intelligent" programs are modeled after the human nervous system and differ in this respect from other computer programs used in medical applications. They are composed of elements ("neurons") and their interconnections, and have been implemented as electronic circuit equivalents and as software. The theoretical underpinning of modeling nervous activity was explored initially by McCulloch and Pitts (1943) who demonstrated that networks of neuron-like computing elements were capable of universal computation [2]. Each element (neuron) produces an output when the weighted sum of all its inputs exceeds a threshold. Neurons are usually arranged in layers with each neuron being connected to all neurons of the next layer. The strength (weight) of each connection is modified by training.

Initially, single layer perceptrons were used to perform simple tasks, but were proven by Minsky and Pappert [3] to be theoretically unable to solve certain problems, including the exclusive-OR (XOR) function. The reason for this limitation of perceptrons is the problem of linear separability, which limits single layer networks to classification problems in which sets of points corresponding to outputs can be separated into regions by a linear equation. For the two input case, points must be separated by a straight line. For three input states, by a plane. For greater numbers of inputs (n), an n-dimensional hyperplane is generated. Increasing the number of layers, and introducing non-linear activation functions overcomes this problem. The need for non-linear activation functions originates from the fact that multilayer linear neural networks are equivalent to single layer networks, because of the associative property of matrix multiplication.

Several types of non-linear activation functions to produce the neuron's output signal have been used by different investigators. The logistic function, or "sigmoid function" is frequently used. If the input is represented by a vector **x** and the weighting function by m x n matrix, W (representing m weights for each of n neurons), the product

$$\mathrm{NET} = \mathbf{x} \bullet W \quad (1)$$

represents the algebraically weighted inputs. The NET signal is usually further processed by an activation function f to produce the output signal of the neuron. Thus, when the sigmoid function is used as an activation function, the output is given by:

$$\mathrm{OUT} = \frac{1}{1 + e^{-\mathrm{NET}}} \tag{2}$$

The hyperbolic tangent has also been used as an activation function. It is also "S" shaped and is symmetric with respect to the origin.

Rosenblatt [4] proposed the notion of training a neural network by altering the weights of the connections in order to have the network output match the desired output for any given input. These trainable networks of trainable units were named perceptrons. They have been applied widely in many fields ranging from optical character recognition to controlling autonomous land vehicles [5], [6].

There are many algorithms and activation functions that have been used in multilayer neural networks, including backpropagation, initially proposed by Werbos [7] and later popularized by Parker [8] and Rumelhart, Hinton and Williams [9]. ALOPEX is another feedback optimization algorithm, initially used for the study of single unit receptive field mappings in the visual pathway of the frog [10]. It was later used to study visual evoked potentials in the diagnosis of subjects suffering from multiple sclerosis and Alzheimer's disease [11], [12], as well as in a variety of other applications. These include: handwritten character recognition, scene analysis, object recognition, and others. In the present research, ALOPEX is used to optimize the numerical weights of the connections between neurons in a 4-layer perceptron architecture [13], [14], [15], [16].

Other methods that have been used include the informon [17], named as such because its output reflects the total information conveyed by all inputs and thus enables it to serve as an element in neural networks; the neocognitron [18], [19], is a multilayer network with modifiable and unmodifiable synapses; and the Hopfield Network that is single-layer [20]. Clark [21] has presented a thorough review of neural network modeling. An overview of recent neural network applications in the fields of computer science, robotics, neural modeling, and engineering was published by Greenwood [22] and is beyond the scope of this chapter. Neural networks have also been widely used in the medical field, especially in diagnosis.

2. Medical Applications of Neural Networks

Neural networks have been applied in several medical specialties especially in the area of diagnosis, a form of pattern recognition. Dytch and Wied [23] used artificial neural networks in quantitative pathology. The ability of neural networks to tolerate ambiguous, noisy and spurious data and their use in pattern recognition are their strengths. These authors also proposed a combination of neural networks with other non-algorithmic artificial intelligence techniques and with traditional algorithmic processing. The ability of neural networks to recognize patterns was also exploited in radiologic diagnosis [24]. Mann and Brown [25] applied artificial neural networks in the diagnosis of low back pain. Using quantified pain drawings obtained from a graphics oriented microprocessor based data acquisition system and a neural network with one hidden layer and back propagation, they were able to classify patients with low back pain to five diagnostic categories with overall reliability between 45 and 85%. This was similar to the diagnostic accuracy of low back pain experts. Other investigators have used connectionist approaches to derive criteria for weaning from respiratory support [26]. These criteria were accurate in 88.8% of trials.

A neural network with one hidden layer was used. Neural network analysis has also been used in predicting the outcome of individual breast cancer patients and in the identification of patients likely to have a recurrence [27], [28].

3. Neural Networks in Cardiovascular Disease

Active research is taking place in the use of neural networks in cardiovascular disease. They have been applied both in cardiovascular diagnosis and in the estimation of prognosis. Baxt [29] used a network consisting of 20 input units, two hidden layers of 10 units each and one output unit to make the diagnosis of acute myocardial infarction in the emergency department. Data from patient history, physical examination, and the electrocardiogram were used both by the network and physicians to make the diagnoses. The artificial neural network showed a higher diagnostic sensitivity (97.2% vs. 77.7%) and specificity (96.2% vs. 84.7%) than the physicians. Furlong and associates [30] used a neural network with 21 input nodes representing cardiac enzyme values and a single hidden layer to diagnose acute myocardial infarction. The network showed 100% sensitivity and 93% specificity in agreeing with the pathologist's interpretation of the enzyme values. The sensitivity was 92% and the specificity 67% when findings at autopsy were used as the gold standard. Neural networks have been also applied in the interpretation of the electrocardiogram where both single and multiple diagnoses can be made [31]. Yang, Devine, and Macfarlane [32] used neural networks to diagnose atrial fibrillation, a cardiac arrhythmia. The network exhibited a sensitivity of 89.9% and a specificity of 92.8%. Combination of the network with deterministic logic algorithms did not lead to appreciable diagnostic gains. Hudson, Cohen, and Deedwania [33] used an artificial neural network to categorize patients according to whether they were normal or had one, two or three vessel disease. They used demographics, electrocardiographic and exercise data as input variables, and were able to correctly classify between 85 and 90% of the subjects. Jayaweera's group [34] entered 13 clinical, exercise EKG, Thallium-201 imaging and coronary angiographic variables into a neural network to successfully predict non-fatal myocardial infarction or death [35].

In this chapter we examine the ability of neural networks in predicting the prognosis of acute myocardial infarction, six months after the event.

4. Neural Networks in Estimating the Prognosis of Acute Myocardial Infarction

Patients who survive the acute phase of a myocardial infarction (heart attack) have an increased risk of mortality persisting up to 10 years or more. Estimation of the probability of being alive at a given time is important to the patients and their physicians, and is usually ascertained by the use of statistical methods. We have employed artificial neural networks to achieve this goal.

The purpose of this investigation is to use a neural network to estimate future mortality of patients with acute myocardial infarction. The existence of a large database (Myocardial Infarction Data Acquisition System - MIDAS) that includes myocardial infarction occurring in the state of New Jersey and has long term follow-up, allows the development and testing of such a computer algorithm. Since the information included in the database does not allow the exact prediction of vital status (dead or alive) in all patients with 100% percent accuracy, the neural network should be able to categorize patients according to the probability of dying within a given period of time.

4.1. The MIDAS database

Information included in MIDAS related to future mortality was selected using the Statistical Analysis System (SAS), in order to produce ASCII data files suitable for input into the neural network.

MIDAS includes all hospital discharge records where the ICD-9 (International Classification of Diseases) code for acute myocardial infarction (410) was present in any of the diagnostic fields. Appropriate permissions were obtained from the State institutional review board (IRB) and methods for maintaining confidentiality were established and followed. The database includes many variables describing demographics, diagnosis, co-morbidity (additional diseases), complications, diagnostic and therapeutic procedures performed, discharge status, hospital and physician characteristics, insurance type, and geographic factors.

Record linkage matching procedure was used to determine if an individual who has had a myocardial infarction and is included in MIDAS was also included in the death certificate files, and therefore had died. A modified census bureau algorithm based on the SOUNDEX of the name and the birthday, written in COBOL was used. This procedure allowed verification of vital status (dead or alive) as of December 31, 1990. From these data, the vital status for up to three years can be established for all the subjects in the database.

In order to test the reliability of the diagnosis and the information contained in MIDAS, a random sample of 726 hospitalized subjects was constructed so that each record in the overall database had equal probability of being audited. Using photocopies of the medical records, the information was verified, and the electrocardiograms were read by a cardiologist. The diagnosis of acute myocardial infarction was supported by the

MIDAS variables used to train neural network

VARIABLE	TYPE	CODE
sex	BINARY	
age	ENCODED	
diabetes mellitus	BINARY	* icd 250
pulmonary disease	BINARY	icd 490.0 - 496.99
liver disease	BINARY	icd 571
chronic kidney disease	BINARY	icd 580.0 - 589.99
obesity	BINARY	icd 278
previous myocardial infarction	BINARY	icd 412
peripheral vascular disease	BINARY	icd 443.9
arrhythmia (irregular heartbeat)	BINARY	icd 426.0 - 427.0
congestive heart failure	BINARY	icd 402.9, 414.1, 425.5, 428.0, 428.1 429.3, 429.5, 429.6, 429.71, 785.01
stroke	BINARY	icd 430.0 - 438.99
hypertension	BINARY	icd 401.0 - 405.99
anemia	BINARY	icd 280.0 - 281.3, 281.9 - 282.0, 283.0 - 285.99
cancer	BINARY	icd 140.0 - 208.0
coronary angioplasty	BINARY	† cpt 36.00 - 36.05
coronary bypass surgery	BINARY	cpt 36.1 - 36.3
insurance classification	BINARY	Medicaid & Self-Pay vs. all others

* International Classification of Diseases, 9th Revision

† Current Procedural Terminology

Figure 1. MIDAS variables used to train and test the neural network. Names of variables, their type, and International Classification of Diseases (ICD-9) codes are presented.

information in the chart in 90.8% of the cases and the vital status at hospital discharge was correct in 98.8% of the cases, the gender in 99.3%, race in 98.9%, and age within one year, in 98.1%. Thus, the information in the database is fairly accurate and can be used to arrive at valid conclusions.

Of all variables included in MIDAS, only 19 were used as inputs to the neural network for this project (18 input variables and one output variable, namely 6-month mortality) (Figure 1). The arrythmia and congestive heart failure were composite variables that were set to be positive (present) if any ICD-9 codes describing arrhythmias or congestive heart failure, respectively, were present. These input variables have been associated with future mortality following acute myocardial infarction by univariate statistics.

Data were extracted from MIDAS and formatted using the Statistical Analysis System (SAS) Version 7.0 on a Hewlett Packard HP9000/835 running HP-UX. The neural network program was written in the C programming language, then compiled and executed on a Sun Microsystems SparcServer 670 running SunOS 4.1.2.

4.2. The ALOPEX algorithm

ALOPEX is a feedback optimization algorithm which was initially used for the study of visual receptive fields, visual evoked potentials and the diagnosis of subjects suffering from multiple sclerosis and Alzheimer's disease. It is used to optimize the numerical weights of the connections between neurons. The algorithm is described by the following equations:

$$w_i[n+1] = w_i[n] + r_i[n+1] + b_i[n+1] \tag{3}$$

$$b_i[n+1] = b_i[n] + \gamma \Delta w_i[n+1] \Delta R[n+1] \tag{4}$$

$$\Delta w_i[n+1] = w_i[n] - w_i[n-1] \tag{5}$$

$$\Delta R[n+1] = R[n] - R[n-1] \tag{6}$$

ALOPEX is an iterative method that unlike other optimization techniques, updates all of the parameters simultaneously at every iteration n. In Eq. 6, $W_i[n+1]$ represent the i weights of the connections at iteration [n+1], depending on the values of the weights in the previous two iterations; $b_i[n+1]$ (defined in Eq. 7) is called the bias term and it represents an historical term of the cumulative changes of all previous iterations and while $r_i[n+1]$ is a random contribution. This random value r_i is very important in that it stops the process from "getting stuck" at a local minimum or maximum. The bias term depends on what the change of the weights has been in the previous two iterations (local effect) (Eq. 5) and on what the change of the global cost function is, at the same iterations (global effect) (Eq. 6).

4.3. Conflicting cases and conflict resolution

Because the information included in the database is not sufficient to allow the exact prediction of vital status (dead or alive) in all patients with 100 percent accuracy, we developed a neural network able to categorize patients according to the probability of dying within a given period of time, rather than predicting categorically whether a patient will be dead or alive at a given time in the future.

We observed that there were many instances where two or more patients had identical input characteristics while some were dead and some alive at the end of the study period. For this reason, it is difficult to train a standard neural network. Since there is no unique output value for all input cases, the network has difficulty converging to a unique set of solutions. To alleviate this problem, we developed a conflict resolution algorithm to be applied before training. This preprocessing step takes templates with identical input vectors and averages each of their input characteristics to produce a single case (Figure 2).

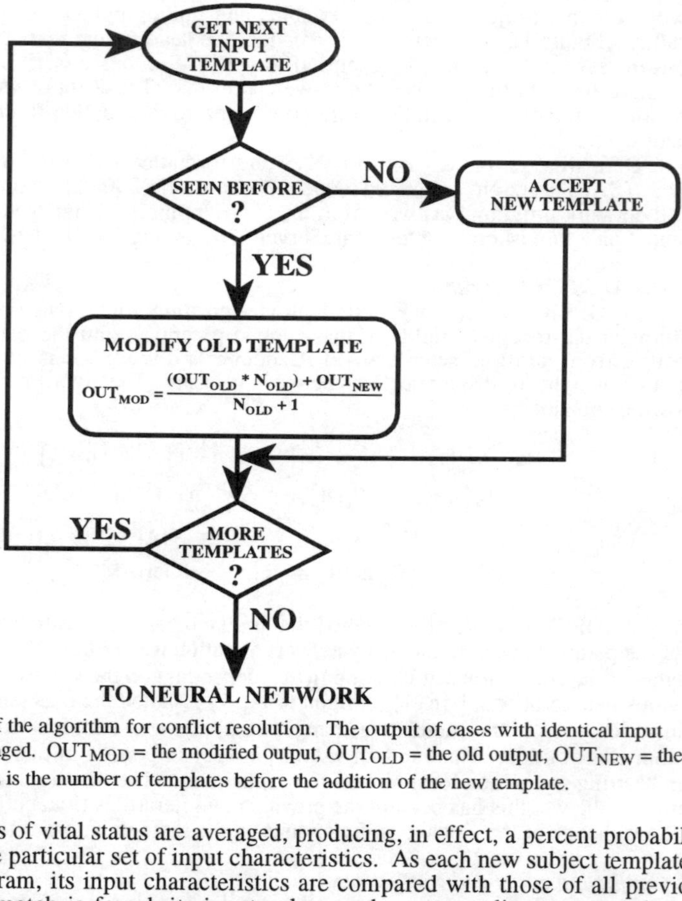

Figure 2. Flowchart of the algorithm for conflict resolution. The output of cases with identical input characteristics is averaged. OUT_{MOD} = the modified output, OUT_{OLD} = the old output, OUT_{NEW} = the new output, and N_{OLD} is the number of templates before the addition of the new template.

Their output values of vital status are averaged, producing, in effect, a percent probability of mortality for the particular set of input characteristics. As each new subject template is read into the program, its input characteristics are compared with those of all previous templates. If no match is found, its input values and corresponding output value are accepted. If a match is found, the output value is brought together with the stored output value (percent-probability of mortality, and the number of templates on which it is based), and a new output value is calculated, representing the percentage average mortality of the entire characteristic group. Thus, when two cases with identical input characteristics (i.e. both age 50, both male, etc.) are presented, and one is dead while the other is alive at six months, the program assigns 0.5 probability of death to that set of input characteristics. If another such case with identical input characteristics is later presented to the network, and this third patient is dead at six months, the program then updates the probability of death to

0.666 (2/3). This continues until all cases with this identical set of input characteristics are exhausted.

This new algorithm, using the 2-hidden layer perceptron optimized by ALOPEX (Figure 3), has converged to greater than 98% using several thousand input cases.

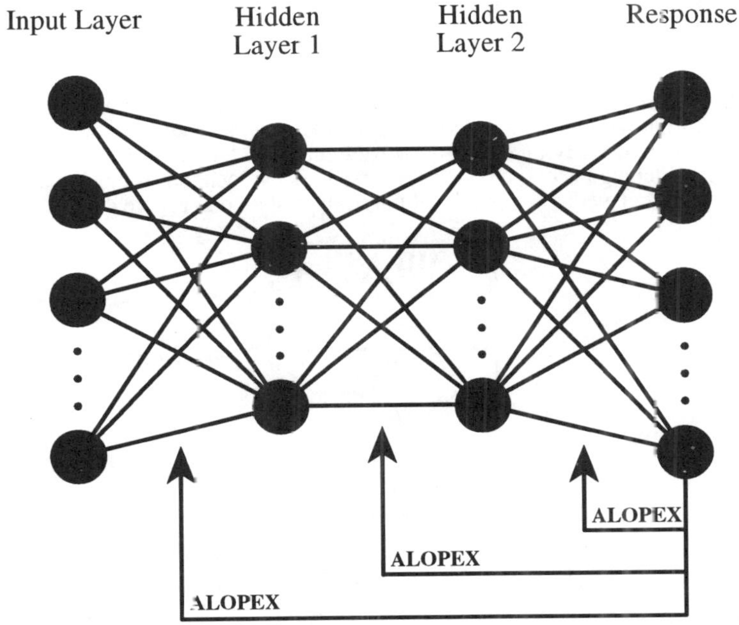

Figure 3. The neural network architecture used in this application. Two hidden layers are used, each with 20 neurons. The input layer has 21 neurons, while the output consists of 10 neurons (one for every 10% increment in probability of mortality).

In addition, 10 output nodes were used in the final layer, each corresponding to a range of percent-chance of mortality. (e.g. Node 1: 0 - 10%, Node 2: 10 - 20%, etc.). The output of the networks are designed to maximize one of ten potential output "bins," each corresponding to a decile of mortality between 0% and 100%. The output node containing the correct probability value was set to a value of 1.0, the others to 0.0. In this manner, the network should be able to provide percent-probability of mortality, and also resolve input case conflicts.

A SAS program was written to present the predicted probability of mortality, separately in patients who are dead or alive at the end of the follow-up period (Figure 4).

A different averaging scheme that was developed in hopes of both resolving the input case conflict problem, and providing a more continuous output in the prediction of mortality, was not successful. The algorithm would take groups of 10 input subjects and average each of their input characteristics to produce a single template containing the same 18 inputs, but now with a range of possible values. The output values of 6-month mortality were also averaged, producing, in effect, a percent probability of mortality for an averaged group of input characteristics. The major concerns with this approach were twofold. First, there seemed to be a convergence "ceiling" of about 90% using any number of input templates. Second, and more important, it seemed that averaging input characteristics and output values for the same group might not produce useful results. Groups larger than 10 were not used because greater numbers of people would tend to mimic the overall average mortality of the entire dataset, and thus not produce all possible percent-probability outcomes.

4.4. Results

The neural networks constructed as described above were able to be trained and evaluated according to several definitions of network response: matching the output value at every output node, identifying the correct location of which node was to contain the peak output value, matching the output value at the peak output location. A block diagram of the training, testing, and evaluation phases of the study is shown in Figure 4.

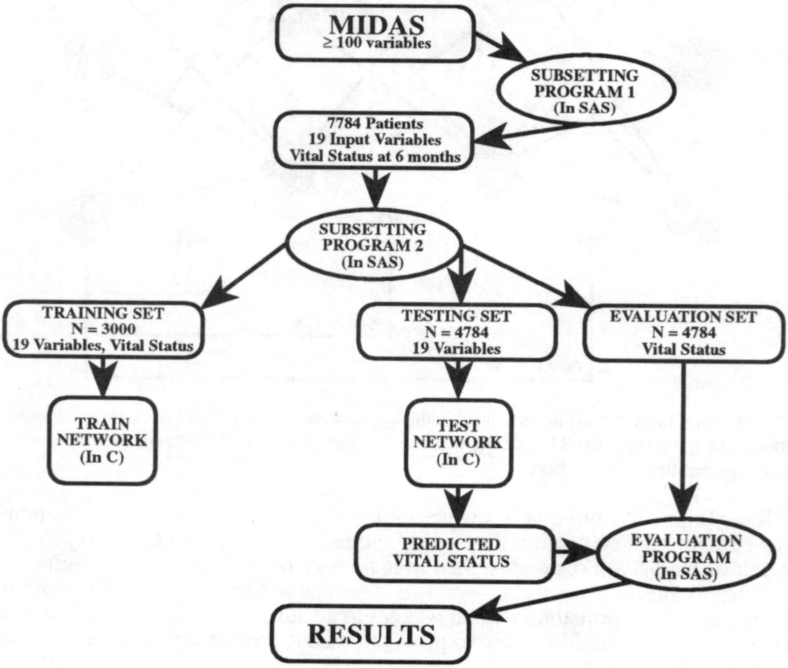

Figure 4. Flowchart of the research plan. 7784 cases from the MIDAS database were divided into a training set (N=3000) and a testing set (N=4784). Notice that the same 4784 cases used for the testing of the neural network were also assembled with their vital status for evaluation of the neural network results.

Once training was complete, the network was tested on two different datasets:

1. The 3,000 cases used to train the network.
2. 4784 new cases where vital status was not known.

A correspondence of the observed to the predicted probability of being alive at a given time was generally observed. The categorical classifications of the cases (dead or alive) yielded an overall diagnostic accuracy of 74%. A reciprocal relationship between sensitivity and specificity of the rules for determination of vital status was observed. An example of the cases categorized by the network to different probabilities of mortality versus the observed probabilities is shown in Figure 5.

To test the accuracy of the program, a SAS program was written to define measures of accuracy of assigning vital status and to study the reliability of classification of each

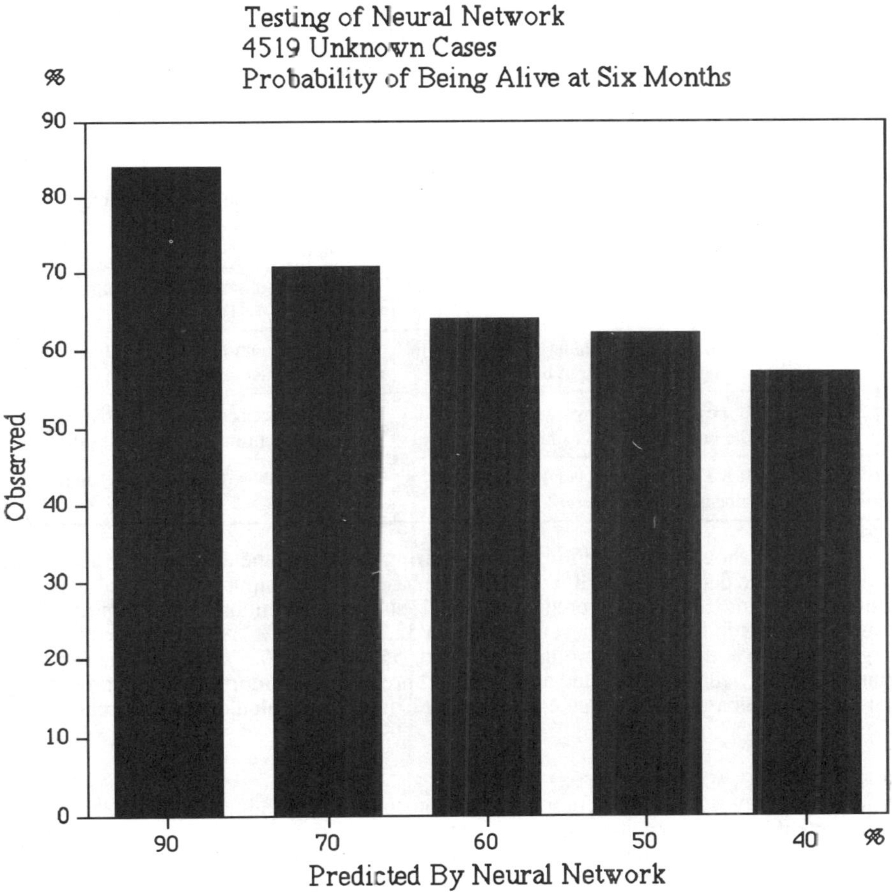

Figure 5. Histogram showing the success (or failure) of the neural network in predicting the six-month vital status of 4784 unknown cases. The probability of being alive predicted by the neural network is compared to the actual vital status. Notice that the 80% bin is omitted from the histogram since no subjects were classified by the neural network into this group.

patient in the 10 output nodes (probability bins). Eight alternate rules of assigning vital status were devised. These are shown in Table 1.

Table 1. Measures of accuracy based on eight different rules for assigning vital status.

Rule	Dead	Alive
RELY	If SUM(outputs in upper half of output bins) > SUM(lower half of output bins)	If SUM(outputs in lower half of output bins) > SUM(upper half of output bins)
RELY1	If the output with the highest value is in the upper half of the output bins.	If the output with the highest value is in the lower half of the output bins.
RELY2	If the output with the second highest value is in the upper half of the output bins.	If the output with the second highest value is in the lower half of the output bins.
RELY3	If the average of the outputs with the highest two values is in the upper half of the output bins.	If the average of the outputs with the highest two values is in the lower half of the output bins.
RELY4	If the scaled sum of all of the output bins is greater than 1.	If the scaled sum of all of the output bins is less than 1.
RELY5	If the output with the highest value is in the upper seven output bins.	If the output with the highest value is in the lower three output bins.
RELY6	If the difference between the top bin and the bottom bin (bin9 - bin0) is positive.	If the difference between the top bin and the bottom bin (bin9 - bin0) is negative.
RELY7	If MEAN(binN * (N+1)) for all output bins is greater than 1.12.	If MEAN(binN * (N+1)) for all output bins is less than 1.12.

Table 2 shows the reliabilities of categorizing patients in the dead or alive categories of eight alternate definitions (RELY to RELY 7) based on the output of the neural network. In this table, 0 indicates wrong prediction, and 1, correct prediction. The reliability of the seven predictors in the total cohort ranged from 52.7% to 65.0%. Among those alive, the range was 44.6% to 67.9%, among those dead, 55.4% to 76.7%). Figure 4 shows the relationship between the predicted and observed probability of mortality. The probability that these results are due to chance is less than 1 in 1000 as calculated by the chi-square statistic.

4.5. Discussion

Acute myocardial infarction is a common condition with high in-hospital and long term mortality. Development of methods for risk stratification for future mortality is useful in deciding whether to implement several forms of therapy, especially those with high risk or expense such as aortocoronary bypass surgery and percutaneous transluminal coronary angioplasty. Artificial neural networks can be constructed to use routinely obtainable information to classify patients to different ranges of probability for future death.

The neural networks constructed in this study to predict vital status of patients with acute myocardial infarction were able to categorize cases with fair degree of success.

Table 2. Reliabilities based on the neural network output as viewed by the eight different assignment rules (see Table 1). "1" represents correct prediction of vital status; "0" represents incorrect prediction.

Rule	Value	Frequency	Percent	Cumulative Frequency	Cumulative Percent
RELY	0	1191	26.4	1191	26.4
	1	3328	73.6	4519	100.0
RELY1	0	1243	27.5	1243	27.5
	1	3276	72.5	4519	100.0
RELY2	0	1422	31.5	1422	31.5
	1	3097	68.5	4519	100.0
RELY3	0	1174	26.0	1174	26.0
	1	3345	74.0	4519	100.0
RELY4	0	3334	73.8	3334	73.8
	1	1185	26.2	4519	100.0
RELY5	0	1580	35.0	1580	35.0
	1	2939	65.0	4519	100.0
RELY6	0	1518	33.6	1518	33.6
	1	3001	66.4	4519	100.0
RELY7	0	1175	26.0	1175	26.0
	1	3344	74.6	4519	100.0

Although their accuracy was not 100%, this probably cannot be achieved with the limited information contained in the database. On the other hand, this method of classification of patients was based on easily and cheaply obtainable information that is routinely collected on all patients who are hospitalized for heart attack. A formal comparison of the accuracy of neural networks and standard statistical techniques in prediction of mortality may ascertain the practical usefulness of neural networks in this application.

Further improvement of the performance of the networks may be obtained by additional, more exhaustive training and the use of other network architectures. This work has implemented a modification to the standard neural network methodology, i.e. conflict resolution by averaging the expected outputs corresponding to identical input cases.

5. Acknowledgements

We wish to thank Dr. Alan C. Wilson and Dr. John B. Kostis of UMDNJ-Robert Wood Johnson Medical School for access to MIDAS database and assistance with SAS programming.

6. References

1. P. J. Denning, "The Science of Computing: Neural Networks," *Am. Sci.* **80** (1992) 426-429.
2. W. S. McCulloch and W. Pitts, "A logical calculus of the ideas immanent in nervous activity (1943)," *Bull. Math. Biol.* **52(1-2)** (1990) 99-115.

3. M. Minsky and S. Pappert, Perceptrons: An Introduction to Computational Geometry (MIT Press, Cambridge, MA, 1969)
4. F. Rosenblatt, *Principles of Neurodynamics; Perceptrons and the Theory of Brain Mechanisms* (Spartan Books, Washington, 1962).
5. J. M. Zurada, *Introduction to Artificial Neural Systems* (West, St. Paul, MN, 1992).
6. D. A. Pomerleau, "ALVINN: An autonomous land vehicle in a neural network," in *Advances in Neural Information Processing Systems I*, ed. D. S. Touretzky (Morgan Kaufmann Publishers, San Mateo, CA, 1989), 305-313.
7. P. J. Werbos, *Beyond Regression: New tools for prediction and analysis in the behavioral sciences* (Harvard University Press, Boston, MA, 1977)
8. D. B. Parker, "Learning logic," Invention Report S81-64, File 1, Office of Technology Licensing, Stanford University, Stanford, CA, 1982.
9. D. E. Rumelhart, G. E. Hinton, and R. J. Williams, "Learning internal representations by error propagation," in *Parallel Distributed Processing Vol. 1*, ed. D. E. Rumelhart and J. L. McClelland (MIT Press, Cambridge, MA, 1986), 18-62.
10. E. Tzanakou, R. Michalak, and E. Harth, "The ALOPEX process: Visual receptive fields by response feedback," *Biol. Cybern.* **35(3)** (1979) 161-174.
11. J. Z. Wang and E. Micheli-Tzanakou, "The Use of the ALOPEX process in extracting normal and abnormal visual evoked potentials," IEEE-EMBS Magazine, Special Issue on DSP **9(1)** (1990) 44-46.
12. R. Iezzi Jr. and E. Micheli-Tzanakou, "2-D spatial frequency dependence of VEP's: a neural network analysis," *19th Northeast Bioeng. Conf.* (1993) 111-112.
13. E. Ciaccio and E. Micheli-Tzanakou, "A least squares algorithm with one phase weight for adaptive cancellation of noise from biomedical signals," *18th Northeast Bioeng. Conf.* (1992) 43-44.
14. E. Micheli-Tzanakou and T.S. Chon, "Image reinforcement with ALOPEX conducted on connectivity strengths using moment invariants," *IEEE Intern. Conf. on systems, man and cybernetics* (1992) 381-386.
15. E. Micheli-Tzanakou and T. J. Dasey, "Unsupervised global optimization: applications on classification of handwritten digits and on visual evoked potentials," *IEEE Intern Conf on systems, man and cybernetics* (1992) 737-744.
16. G. Friedrichs, D. Berger, and E. Micheli-Tzanakou, "Cardiovascular applications of the ALOPEX optimization technique," *J. Biomed. Eng.* **15** (1993) 73-78.
17. A. M. Utley, "The Informon: a network for adaptive pattern recognition," J Theor. Biol. **27** (1970) 31-67.
18. K. Fukushima, "Neocognitron: a self organizing neural network model for a mechanism of pattern recognition unaffected by shift in position," *Biol. Cybern.* **36** (1980) 193-202.
19. S. Deutsch, "A simplified version of Kunihiko Fukushima's neocognitron," *Biol. Cybern.* **42** (1981) 17-21.
20. J. J. Hopfield, "Neural networks and physical systems with emergent collective computational abilities," *Proc. Natl. Acad. Sci. U.S.A.* **79(8)** (1982) 2554-2558.
21. J. W. Clark, "Neural network modelling," *Phys. Med. Biol.* **36** (1991) 1259-1317.
22. D. Greenwood, "An overview of neural networks," *Behav. Sci.* **36(1)** (1991) 1-33.
23. H. E. Dytch and G. L. Wied, "Artificial neural networks and their use in quantitative pathology," *Anal. Quant. Cytol. Histol.* **12(6)** (1990) 379-393.
24. J. M. Boone, G. W. Gross, and V. Greco-Hunt, "Neural networks in radiologic diagnosis," *Invest. Radiol.* **25(9)** (1990) 1012-1016.

25. N. H. Mann and M. D. Brown, "Artificial intelligence in the diagnosis of low back pain," Orthopedic Clinics of North America **22** (1991) 303-314.
26. K. Ashutosh, H. Lee, C. K. Mohan, S. Ranka, K. Mehrotra, and C. Alexander, "Prediction criteria for successful weaning from respiratory support: statistical and connectionist analyses," *Crit. Care Med.* **20(9)** (1992) 1295-1301.
27. P. M. Ravdin and G. M. Clark, "A practical application of neural network analysis in predicting outcome of individual breast cancer patients," *Breast Cancer Res. Treat.* **22(3)** (1992) 285-293.
28. P. M. Ravdin, G. M. Clark, S. G. Hilsenbeck, M. A. Owens, et al., "A demonstration that breast cancer recurrence can be predicted by neural network analysis," *Breast Cancer Res. Treat.* **21(1)** (1992) 47-53.
29. W. G. Baxt, "Use of an artificial neural network for the diagnosis of myocardial infarction," *Ann. Intern Med.* **115** (1991) 843-848.
30. J. W. Furlong, M. E Dupuy, and J. A. Heinsimer, "Neural network analysis of serial cardiac enzyme data. A clinical application of artificial machine intelligence," *Am. J. Clin. Pathol.* **96(1)** (1991) 134-41.
31. W. R. M. Dassen, J. C. Osborne, K. Den Dulk, and R. G. A. Mulleneers, "The influence of multiple output neurons on the interpretation of the electrocardiogram using artificial neural networks," *J.A.C.C.* **21(2)** (1993) 3A.
32. T. F. Yang, B. Devine, and P.W. Macfarlane, "Combination of deterministic logic and artificial neural networks in the diagnosis of atrial fibrillation," *J.A.C.C.* **21(2)** (1993) 3A.
33. D. L. Hudson, M. E. Cohen, and P. C. Deedwania, "Diagnosis of coronary artery disease using neural networks," *J.A.C.C.* **21(2)** (1993) 6A.
34. A. R. Jayaweera, K. C. Drake, R. Abbott, and S. Kaul, "Determination of long-term outcome in patients with coronary artery disease using an artificial neural network," *J.A.C.C.* **21(2)** (1993) 7A.
35. E. Micheli-Tzanakou, C. Yi, R. Iezzi Jr., D. M. Shindler, J. B. Kostis, "Echocardiogram image analysis with neural networks," in *Imaging in Transport Processes*, ed. S. Seidman and K. Hijikata (Begell House, New York, NY, 1993), 517-524.

NEURAL NETWORK-BASED APPROACH TO OUTCOME PROGNOSIS FOR PATIENTS WITH DILATED MYOCARDIAL DISEASE

RENATO M.E. SABBATINI[1], JUAREZ ORTIZ[2] and CLÁUDIA G.M. GHEFTER[2]
[1] *Center for Biomedical Informatics, State University of Campinas, Campinas, SP;*
[2] *Centro de Cardiologia Não Invasiva, São Paulo, SP, Brazil*

1. Introduction

Elevation of left heart filling pressure and pulmonary congestion have been attributed to the disability of the left ventricle to eject blood, followed by an increase in the left ventricular volume. However, the clinical syndrome of congestive heart failure may also occur due to a decline in the left ventricular capability to receive blood during diastole. A mild degree of resistance of the left ventricle to diastolic filling may be sufficient to cause elevation of the left ventricular diastolic and pulmonary venous pressures [32]. This dysfunction has been recognized as a major health problem in the population, because *ca.* 40 % of patients with congestive heart failure of the dilated type have normal systolic function; thus presenting some kind of primary diastolic heart failure [15].

Prognosis, or prediction of the future evolution of disease, is an important step in the evaluation of patients suffering from chronic heart ailments. It can be expressed in many forms, such as quality of life, period free of symptoms, etc., but the most common type of prognosis evaluation in severe heart disease is survival within a given period, which is named outcome.

Since outcome is usually influenced by a conglomeration of abnormalities found in one or more measurement variables, multivariable pattern classification and recognition techniques represent an useful approach to quantitative prognosis. Linear discriminant analysis, multilinear regression analysis and logistic regression analysis of known patient data have been extensively used for such kinds of causal-structure analysis in medical prognosis [*e.g.* 1]. They are based on linear multidimensional models, *i.e.*, patterns are geometrically represented as points in a multidimensional Cartesian space, where its axes are measurements or predictor variables (also called as features). Classes of patients (survivors and non-survivors) are said to be linearly separable whenever the statistical method is able to find a hyperplane which more or less clearly separate their representative points into two regions of the feature space (Fig. 1A). Computations for linear statistical analysis are usually straightforward and are based on numerical matrix algebra procedures.

However, many interesting problems in medical pattern classification cannot be approached by linear methods, because separability or patient classes in feature space can be achieved only by more complex, nonlinear decision surfaces (Fig 1B). When this happens, conventional numerical algorithms for nonlinear pattern classification can be developed, but are usually very awkward and inefficient, computationally speaking. In this respect, several investigations have demonstrated that a recent new technology of Artificial Intelligence, artificial neural networks, present noticeable advantages for implementing diagnostic systems and risk stratification in outcomes research.

Artificial neural networks, a class of connectionist systems, are being increasingly used to represent and to process information by means of networks of intercon-

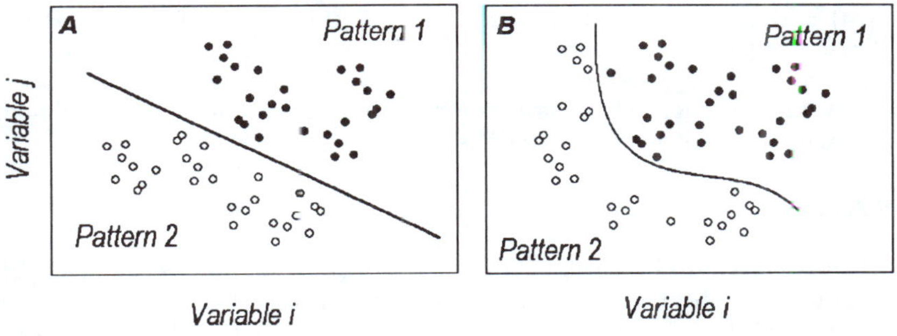

FIGURE 1

Two patterns represented in a Cartesian space (in this example, with two features only) are said to be linearly separable by a statistical method whenever a line is found that separates them into two disjoint spaces (A). In case they are separable, but not by a line or a plane, then they are said to be nonlinearly separable (B).

nected processing elements, similar to neurons. Several emerging global properties of connectionist systems, such as associative memory, distributed parallel processing, etc.; have favored its applications in a large variety of tasks involving pattern classification and recognition. Connectionist systems constitute a new and interesting paradigm for the area of Artificial Intelligence in Medicine, and have found applications in processing and interpretation of biological signals and images, decision support systems, etc. [45, 46, 50].

Artificial neural networks can be used, among other things, to find approximate maps between input and output patterns of a quantitative nature. This is achieved by exemplar-based learning, *i.e.*, by presenting to the network data about patients with known outcomes of the disease process (*e.g.*, death or survival after a given observation time). Using a proper learning algorithm, the network is able to predict outcome after reaching a minimum classification error, whenever input (predictor) variables are related in an orderly manner to outcome. It is an interesting property of a certain kind of multilayer artificial neural networks, that non-intuitive, complex nonlinear separation between patient classes can be achieved. Neural networks have an unique ability to find hidden features in input space, where none is visible by conventional statistical methods, not to mention human decision alone.

ANN models have been used so far for predicting outcome in coronary heart disease [24], critical patients under intensive care [11, 59], wound infections [23], the onset of diabetes [56], breast cancer [44] and colon cancer recurrence [12], among others. In some recent applications of medical decision making, such as diagnosis of acute myocardial infarction, ANNs have shown impressive performance in relation to conventional quantitative methods as well as to human judgment [2].

2. The Problem

Many clinical trials have been designed to detect the variables associated with favorable or unfavorable outcome in dilated myocardial disease. Previous studies have shown that several clinical and laboratory parameters could be linked with increased or reduced survival, such as ejection fraction [54, 60, 31, 39], fractional shortening [5, 26], cardiac index [9], left ventricular diameters and volumes [31, 39, 47, 54], myocardial thickness [31, 62], New York Heart Association functional class [25, 61] and ventricular arrhythmias [9, 25, 37], among others.

Despite the large number of current publications on left ventricular diastolic function [*e.g.*, 8, 32, 35, 36], there are few studies relating ventricular filling abnormalities with prognosis [7]. Thus, our clinical group has conducted a prospective study in patients with dilated myocardial disease, in order to examine the relation between echocardiographic abnormalities and the subsequent mortality rate [40]. In this study, three distinct groups of patients were studied to evaluate the influence of left ventricular filling pattern on the 12-month mortality rate: AF (atrial filling predominant pattern); N (normal or "normalized" filling pattern) and RF (rapid filling predominant pattern). A patient can be easily classified into one of these groups on basis of dynamic Doppler-echocardiographic studies of left ventricular blood flow, which shows characteristic patterns (Fig. 2). In addition, several other echocardiographic variables were measured and studied in relation to the mortality rate.

The study main finding was that subgroups NL, AF and RD exhibited distinct degrees of survival. At the 14 months follow-up, a survival rate of 89% was noted in NL, 75% in AF and 50% in RF and survival curves were markedly different. Univariate analysis of mortality showed a high one-year mortality rate associated with a mitral flow deceleration time less or equal than 140 ms (50%), a left ventricular diastolic diameter/thickness ratio larger or equal than 3.4 (35.3%) and a left atrial index larger or equal than 25 mm/m^2 (40.7%). The highest mortality rate (61.5%, p = 0.0004) was observed in patients with both increased left atrial index and decreased deceleration time. Thus, it was clearly shown that diastolic dysfunction and anatomical changes, as evaluated by

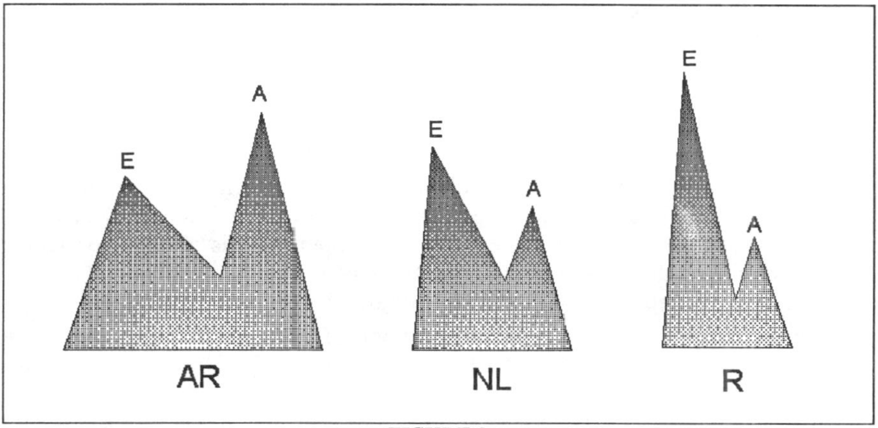

FIGURE 2

Characteristic patterns of left ventricular diastolic filling as recorded by Doppler-echocardiography. Legend: AR: atrial filling predominant pattern; NL: normal or "normalized" filling pattern; R: rapid filling predominant pattern. Labelled peaks correspond to waves E and A.

echocardiography, are reliable parameters to estimate the prognosis in dilated myocardial disease.

The aforementioned conclusions were derived using simple univariate statistical analyses, such as analysis of variance (ANOVA), χ^2 (chi-square) and Fischer's exact tests for measures of association. No attempt was made at the time of the study to explore the prognostic value of higher-order and multivariate correlations and associations between cardiac function measurements. A few previous works have used multivariate analysis, such as the Cox model [47], multiple linear regression [13] and linear discriminant analysis [62] to determine the combination of multiple prognostic factors in cardiac dilative disease, with divergent results. In the present work, we sought to determine these, by using an approach based on artificial neural network techniques for complex, nonlinear, multivariable pattern classification and recognition. The present work represents a novel and, in our view, valuable approach to medical decision making in the area of survival prognosis.

3. Aims

The present study aimed at evaluating the usefulness and accuracy of artificial neural network in a task of medical prognosis using a complex mixture of predictor variables, namely the prognosis of one-year mortality of patients with congestive heart failure of the dilated type.

4. Artificial Neural Networks

In this section, we attempt to provide the reader with a brief overview of artificial neural network (ANN) technology. Several useful, up-to-date reviews of ANN concepts and applications have been written (*e.g.*, [55]), and the reader is referred to them for detailed material on the subject of the present paper.

An artificial neural network comprises the following elements:

- processing elements, also referred to as nodes (Fig. 3), which are interconnected to each other in the form of a network. A node receives binary or continuous signals coming out from other processing elements in the network, by means of direct connections ("synapses"), or from external elements; processes these signals in some way, and sends new signals to other nodes or external elements to the network. Input signals are typically represented as a vector $A = \{a_1, a_2 \ldots a_i \ldots a_n\}$; where a_i is the signal or activity level at the ith input connection. Usually the internal connections in the network are either excitatory (positive) or inhibitory (negative), which tend to increase or decrease, respectively, the

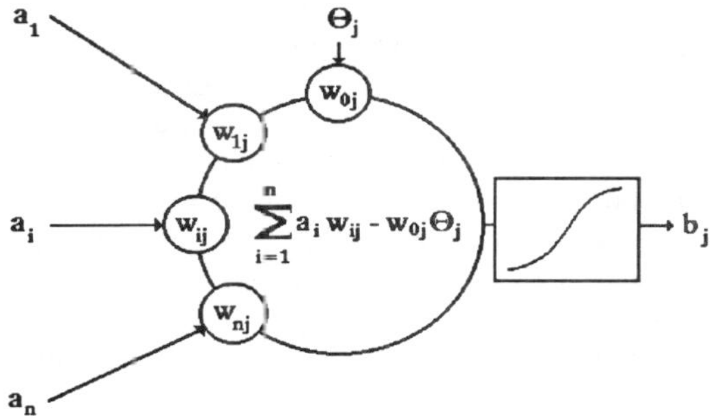

FIGURE 3 - Mathematical model for the artificial neuron

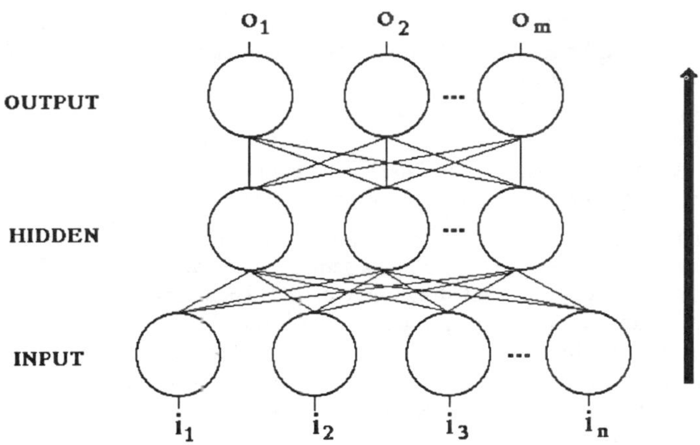

FIGURE 4 - Architecture of a multilayer perceptron

activation level of a node. Associated to each connection a_i between two nodes, there is an adjustable value or weight; thus forming another vector $W_j = \{w_{1j}, w_{2j} \ldots w_{ij} \ldots w_{nj}\}$, where w_{ij} corresponds to the connection weight between nodes a_i and b_j. The generalized node model usually includes, in addition, an extra parameter or connection Θ_j, modulated by weight $w\Theta_j$, which is called a bias. In order to calculate the output value b_j of a node, a weighted sum operation $(a_i w_{ij})$ is carried out upon all the inputs to that node, and the result is applied to an activation function, which transforms the input weighted sum to the output according to some transformation, which is usually nonlinear in character, *e.g.*, a step or the sigmoid function $(1 + e^{-x})^{-1}$. Step functions are equivalent to the firing threshold of a real neuron, while sigmoid and other nonlinear continuous functions have no equivalent in biological neurons, but have been shown to work well for formal neurons.

- an interconnection architecture, or network topology. There are several kinds of architectures: some interconnect all nodes to each other in a kind of matrix (such as that found in Hopfield nets [21], while others are formed by two or more interconnected layers of processing elements, *e.g.*, an input layer, one or more intermediate, or "hidden" layer, and an output layer (Fig. 4), such as the perceptron [48]. There are several possibilities of interconnecting layers, such as recurrent, forward or feedback connections.
- a method for storing and retrieving information from the network. The most common use of ANNs is as a pattern classifier or recognizer. For example, in a perceptron, an input vector $I = \{i_1, i_2 \ldots i_i \ldots i_n\}$ is applied to the *n* nodes of the input layer. The activation pattern processed by this layer is propagated to the successive layers, until it reaches the output layer, whereby it will produce an output vector $O = \{o_1, o_2 \ldots o_j \ldots o_m\}$. This operation corresponds to a mapping of I into O, and it may have several interesting applications:
    - In a heteroassociative network, the nature of input and output patterns is different. For example, I could be a sequence of time-ordered ECG samples, while O would represent diagnostic classes (beat-to-beat ECG interpretation). In another medical application, the input pattern could have each node associated to the presence or absence of a given symptom, while the output pattern would represent disease classes. In this way, ANNs can be used to classify patterns, interpret signals and images, perform prognostic and diagnostic tasks, etc.
    - In an autoassociative network, the input and output patterns are of the same nature. For example, I could be an array of pixels corresponding to a two-di-

mensional medical image. Each activation value in the input network would be proportional to the gray intensity level of a pixel in the array. The output layer would be also a rectangular pixel array. The network could be used to perform image manipulation tasks, such as filtering, compression, edge detection, the recovery of degraded, incomplete or blurred images, etc.

Learning is still another very important concept in the characterization of ANNs. Learning is defined as a modification performed upon the array of weights W of a network, in order to optimize an input-output mapping. Although, in simple cases, it is possible to adjust manually the weights to achieve a desired result, this task is usually so complex that is necessary to have a method to adjust weights automatically, in a self-organizing way. Thus, by means of a proper learning algorithm, the network is able to self-adjust its weights, as the learning progresses iteratively. In supervised, or directed, learning, a series of different pairs of input and output patterns, called examples, are presented to the network in the training phase. At each training cycle, the network computes an error or mismatch function between desired and obtained output, and adjusts the weights of all connections in such a way as to decrease this error. When learning is effective, the error function converges to a minimum after a suitable (finite) number of iterations through the examples. There are ANNs capable of continuous, or on-line learning, *i.e.*, after the introduction of a new, non-classifiable example, the network adapts itself quickly to the new class; but, more usually, learning is performed off-line, *i.e.*, there are separate training and classification phases, and the introduction of a new example forces a lengthy relearning.

A large number of learning algorithms has already been developed for ANNs. One of the most used is the backpropagation algorithm [49], where a small, differential quantity (*delta*) of the output error is applied retroactively to each layer in the network. There are several theorems which describe the convergence conditions of a backpropagation network. Other learning algorithms, such as Hebbian learning [4] imitate the way supposedly synapses are altered during biological learning. Supervised learning algorithms differ widely in terms of speed, efficiency and convergence, but the literature reflects continuous improvements in the underlying algorithms [27].

There are also networks capable of unsupervised learning (also called undirected learning). The training examples are presented solely at the input layer, and the network organizes itself progressively, in order to reach maximal separation between the naturally-occurring classes of examples. Thus it operates in a way similar to the classical divisive clustering algorithms found in multivariate analysis methods [22]. The Kohonen's LVQ (*Linear Vector Quantizer*) network is a good example of unsupervised learning [30], as well as all networks which work according to the principle of competitive learning, such as the ART (*Adaptive Resonance Theory*) class of networks [14].

At last, an important operational parameter of an ANN is the way learned patterns are retrieved from the network. When the network's architecture is of the feedforward kind, an input pattern is presented to the input layer. The activation pattern is propagated along the net's layers until reaching the output layers, whereby an output pattern is produced and can be retrieved. This is the way perceptrons operate, for example. On the other hand, it is also possible to have feedback retrieval, whereby the same layer is used to present and to retrieve input and output patterns, respectively. The network called BAM (*Bidirectional Associative Memory*) is a good example for this kind of network [28].

5. Materials and Methods

5.1 Study Design

The design for the present study was the following: clinical and echocardiographic data gathered from patients with myocardial disease of the dilative type and congestive heart failure, with known outcome [40], were randomly divided into two datasets of approximately the same size: a training dataset and a test dataset. Both were further subdivided, according to observed mortality 12 months after the examination, into survivors and non-survivors.

A heteroassociative multilayer feedforward perceptron (MLP) was then constructed and simulated by software in a conventional computer. Its input layer consisted of a number of nodes, each one representing the standardized value of one of the clinical and echocardiographic variables measured in the patients. Some of these nodes were binary-valued (*e.g.*, sex), while others were continuously-valued (*e.g.*, heart ejection fraction). The output layer always consisted of a single node capable of providing a continuous value between zero (representing a survivor), and one (representing a non-survivor). Thus, the output of this node could be interpreted as a non-probabilistic graded estimate of death outcome. Between the input and output layers, a "hidden" or intermediate layer of variable size (2, 5 or 10 nodes) was fully interconnected to both input and output layers (Fig. 4).

The learning procedure consisted in presenting the examples in the training dataset to the network, in the following manner:

- For each example, or patient, in the training dataset, the measured clinical and echocardiographic variables were applied to each input node in the network. The activity generated in these nodes was propagated successively to the intermediate and output layers, thus generating a given output value (the predicted estimate of death);

- The known value for the output node, *i.e.*, a zero if that specific patient had survived, or an one if he/her had died, was compared to the value predicted by the network. The difference between predicted and actual values (the classification error) was then used to compute delta and to modify the connection weights, using the backpropagation learning procedure (for the detailed equations governing this method, see [55]);
- The next example in the training dataset was then presented to the neural network, and so successively until running out of examples. This constituted a learning cycle for the network, after which a mean square classification error was computed and plotted in a learning curve, depicting error against the number of learning cycles. Additional training required the presentation of all examples in the training dataset, again. A decrease in the mean classification error was an indication that learning was taking place. Typically, several hundred learning cycles were required until the error function converged and training was stopped. Two settable parameters in the network training algorithm, called learning rate and momentum, influenced the amount of transference of classification error to connection weight modification.
- The next step was to evaluate the trained network's classification performance. If training converged well, typically the classification accuracy was close to 100 % when the same training data were used for testing. However, when data from the separate testing dataset were used, performance was usually lower. As described below, several performance indexes were computed after the test (specificity, sensitivity, predictivity and the ROC curve), since accuracy alone is not descriptive enough of the overall network performance [33].

Several experiments were done using different number of input variables, different number of hidden nodes and different learning rates; and its results were compared in terms of the calculated performance indexes.

In the following sections we describe in more detail the methods used in the study.

5.2 Patients

Ninety-five consecutive patients with left ventricular dilated myocardial disease were studied echocardiographically. Inclusion criteria were: 1) clinical diagnosis of congestive heart failure; 2) echocardiographic demonstration of left ventricular dilation and 3) diffuse impairment of myocardial contractility. Patients with arrhythmias and heart failure resulted from primary valvular disease were excluded. The time of examination in relation to the onset of extant disease was not controlled. At the echocardiographic examination and during the follow-up period, treatment was determined solely by the patients' cardiologists, according to their own criteria. Drug therapy was not homogeneous and included digitalis, diuretics, vasodilators, and antiarrhythmics.

5.3 Evaluation of Myocardial Function

M-mode and Doppler echocardiographic examinations were performed using a commercially available Aloka SSD 870 ultrasound system (Japan), with 2.5 MHz and/or 3.5 MHz transducers. The following measurements were taken, according to the *American Society of Echocardiography* recommendations:

AO	Mean aortic diameter in mm
LAD	Left atrial diameter in mm
LVSD	Left ventricular systolic diameter in mm
LVDD	Left ventricular diastolic diameter in mm
PWTh	Left ventricular posterior wall myocardial thickness in mm
IVSTh	Interventricular septum diastolic myocardial thickness in mm
LVDDTh	Left ventricular diastolic diameter/thickness ratio
MEPSS	Mitral valve E point-septal separation in mm
MVFV	Mitral valve flow velocity, in ml/s. It was obtained by pulsed Doppler examination with the sample volume size standardized in 3 mm and positioned inside the left ventricle, at the level of the mitral valve leaflet tips.
MVDT	Mitral valve flow deceleration time, in ms. It was calculated by measuring the time from the peak filling velocity (E wave) to an extension of the rate decline of the velocity to baseline [36].
HR	Heart rate in beats/min

The following variables were also calculated:

BSA	Body surface area in m^2. It was calculated according the following formula: $BSA = W^{0.425} \times H^{0.725} \times 0.007184$ where: W = weight in kilograms and H = height in centimeters.

LADI	left atrial diameter index (the ratio LAD/BSA) in mm/m^2
LVSI	left ventricular systolic diameter index (the ratio LVSD/BSA) in mm/m^2
LVDI	left ventricular diastolic diameter index (the ratio LVDD/BSA) in mm/m^2
LVM	Left ventricular mass in grams. It was calculated using the following formula: $LVM = [(LVDD + PWTh + IVSTh)^3 - (LVDD)^3] \times 1.05 - 14$ where: LVDD = left ventricular diastolic diameter; PWTh = posterior wall diastolic thickness; IVSTh = interventricular septum diastolic thickness.
LVFS	Left ventricular fractional shortening, in percent
LVEF	Left ventricular ejection fraction, in percent. Calculated according to the following formula: $LVEF = (EDV-ESV)/EDV$ where: EDV - left ventricular end diastolic volume; ESV - left ventricular end systolic volume. Left ventricular volumes were calculated by the Teicholzs' method.
CI	Cardiac index in ml/m^2. Calculated by the formula: $CI = (EDV-ESV)/BSA$ where: EDV - left ventricular end diastolic volume; ESV - left ventricular end systolic volume; BSA - body surface area.
FLOW	Left ventricular filling pattern. It was classified for each patient by examining the dynamic blood flow obtained by Doppler-echocardiography, according to the following three types (Fig. 2): 0) normal or "normalized"; 1) restrictive, or rapid filling predominant pattern; 3) - atrial filling predominant pattern
MI	Mitral valve incompetence. It was searched, and quantified when present, in all patients, by color flow mapping and pulsed Doppler. It was coded according to the following three types: 0) absent; 1) minimal; 2) mild; 3) moderate; 4) severe.

The following data were obtained by patient interview at the time of the initial examination:

AGE	Age in years
SEX	Sex (coded: 1 for males, 2 for females)
W	Weight in kg
H	Height in cm

NYHA0 New York Heart Association functional class. It was ranked according to the severity of symptoms reported during a complete history and physical examination was taken for each patient (coded: 1) Class I; 20 Class II; 3) Class III; 4) Class I).

ET Basic presumed underlying etiology was classified according to the following types: 1) Chagas' disease, 2) Systemic arterial hypertension; 3) Coronary insufficiency; 4) Idiopathic cardiomyopathic disease; 5) Myocarditis; 6) Alcoholis; 7) Diabetes

During the follow-up period, information regarding survival or circumstances of death of the patients were obtained by letter or phone interview. This produced the prognostic variable:

OUTCOME Outcome after a 12-month observation period:
Coded: 0 - survivor, 1 - non survivor.

For deceased patients, the following variable was also recorded:

LOS Length of survival, in months.

5.4 Data Preparation

Including all input clinical, measured and calculated echocardiographic variables and the output variable (survival within 12 months), a matrix of 95 patients by 29 variables was obtained and manually keyed into a relational database disk file in a microcomputer (dBASE III+ , Ashton-Tate Inc., USA) and thoroughly verified for errors and inconsistencies. Following this, the full data matrix was analyzed statistically using the EPI-INFO 5.0 system (developed by the Centers for Disease Control and Prevention, Atlanta, GA, USA):

- Frequencies, means and standard deviations for each variable;
- χ^2 measures of association between categorical variables, such as sex, mitral incompetence, etiology, flow pattern, NYHA index and 12-month mortality;
- ANOVA or Student-t tests of significance of differences between survivor and non-survivor groups for all scalar variables;
- Linear correlations and regressions between selected scalar variables;
- Scattergrams between selected scalar variables and column diagrams between all scalar variables and patient group (survivors/non-survivors).

In addition a linear discriminant analysis (LDA) was performed with the full dataset of scalar variables, in order to evaluate its separability power upon the original patient data, as well as to further point out the linear predictive power of individual variables.

The results of this analysis were used to derive an overall picture of data association and causal structure; and to guide the selection of input variables to the neural network.

Finally, the full relational database was divided randomly into a training database (45 cases with 8 deaths) and a testing database (50 cases with 7 deaths) and each one converted to the ASCII sequential datasets required by the neural network and linear discriminant analysis programs, as described below. For the LDA analysis, only scalar variables were used, and where appropriate, BSA-corrected indexes only. For use by the neural network, all input variables were automatically standardized into the interval [0,1]. The maximum and minimum values used for standardizing each variable were obtained from the univariate data analysis of the full dataset. Categorical variables, when binary (such as SEX), were allocated to a single node and standardized. When the variable was multinomial (*e.g.*, etiology), it was allocated to a suite of binary nodes, each one bearing a [0| 1] value for each possible alternative (*e.g.* ET1, ET2, ET3, etc.)

After extensive experimentation with several network configurations, which is reported elsewhere [53], we have centered our investigation on the prognostic ability of ANNs in dilative heart disease with the following configurations:

- Three-layer feedforward perceptron with the "vanilla" back-propagation learning rule;
- Input variables: two sets of variables were investigated (Table 1): the first one (COMPLETE) included almost all recorded variables, with 29 nodes for 18 variables. The second set (REDUCED) included only the 11 most significant variables, which were indicated by the univariate and LDA statistical analysis; giving 13 input nodes;
- Number of hidden nodes: 2, 5 or 10;
- One output node (survival/death);
- Transfer function: sigmoid. Internal thresholds of 0.0, learning rate of 1.0 to 1.5, and momentum of 0.0.
- Weight initialization: randomized in the range [-0.5,+ 0.5]. Method of presentation of examples during training: randomized. Method of weight updating: continuous.

TABLE 1
Outcome prognosis of dilative myocardial disease
List of input variables

VARIABLE				ANALYSIS SET		
Code	Name	Type[1]	Unit	LDA[2]	Complete Set ANN[3]	Reduced Set ANN
AGE	Age	S	years	x	x	x
AO	Diameter of Aorta	S	mm	x		
CI	Cardiac Index	S	ml/m^2	x	x	
ET	Etiology	C	1-6		x	
FLOW	Mitral Valve Flow Pattern	C	1-3		x	x
HR	Heart Rate	S	bpm	x	x	
IVSTh	Intraventricular Septum Thickness	S	mm	x	x	x
LADI	Left Atrial Index	S	mm/m^2	x	x	x
LVDDTh	Left Ventricular Diameter /Thickness Ratio	S	--	x	x	x
LVDI	Left Ventricular Diastolic Diameter Index	S	mm/m^2	x	x	x
LVEF	Left Ventricular Ejection Fraction	S	%	x	x	
LVM	Left Ventricular Mass	S	g	x	x	
LVSI	Left Ventricular Systolic Diameter Index	S	mm/m^2	x	x	x
MEPSS	Mitral E-IV Septum Separation	S	mm	x	x	x
MI	Mitral Valve Insufficiency	C	0-4		x	
MVDT	Mitral Flow Deceleration Time	S	ms	x	x	x
NYHA0	Initial NYHA Index	O	1-4		x	
PWTh	Left Ventricular Posterior Wall Thickness	S	mm	x	x	x
SEX	Sex	C	1-2		x	

[1] Type - S = scalar, C = categorical, O = ordinal
[2] LDA - Linear Discriminant Analysis
[3] ANN - Artificial Neural Network

5.5 Hardware and Software

Processing was entirely carried out in a 80486-based microcomputer with 33 MHz clock, 8 Mb RAM memory, 200 Mb hard disk storage and 1 Mb color Super VGA video display. Computer software especially developed by one of the authors (R.M.E.S.) for neural network projects in Medicine [51], and used for this research, were:

- LINDISCR - A linear discriminant analysis package for two groups, adapted from the FORTRAN version in [42]. A ROC curve analysis module was incorporated to it by the author. Developed in Turbo BASIC® 1.1 (Borland Inc., USA):
- NEURONET - A complete program for simulation of multilayer, feedforward ANNs. Implemented paradigms are: two-layer perceptron with delta rule learning; three-layer backpropagation, and linear vector quantizer (with supervised and unsupervised learning). It allows data standardization, extensive parameter setting, analysis of learning curves, analysis of network performance using test statistics, etc. Developed in Turbo BASIC. The software's throughput was around 10.000 connections per second.

5.6 Evaluation of ANN Performance

Evaluation of ANN performance was carried out using the original training dataset for each network, as well as its complementary test dataset, containing patient data which were not used for training the network. Thus, test datasets containing the reduced and the complete set of variables used by NEURONET. The procedure was the following: first, the file containing the trained network model was loaded by NEURONET into memory. Then, the file containing either the training or the test datasets were read and automatically classified by the network. For each patient in these datasets, the program compared actual with predicted outcome, generating a file of comparative results. Finally, this file was analyzed and the following test parameters were computed, on the basis of a 2 x 2 contingency table constructed from expected/obtained statistics (Fig. 5): accuracy, sensitivity, specificity, positive predictivity and negative predictivity.

Generally, for any given medical decision making task, such as the prognosis of binary outcomes or the determination of diagnostic test results, sensitivity and specificity vary in opposite directions, *i.e.*, when the test is too sensitive to positives, it tends to generate too many false positives. Therefore, specificity decreases, because the number of true negatives decreases. The opposite happens when the test has a low

		ACTUAL OUTCOME		
		Death	Survival	
PREDICTION	Death	A True Positives	B False Positives	Positive Predictivity: B/(A+ B)
	Survival	C False Negatives	D True Negatives	Negative Predictivity: D/(C+ D)
		Sensitivity: A/(A+ C)	Specificity: D/(D+ B)	Accuracy: (A+ D)/ (A+ B+ C+ D)

FIGURE 5 - Calculation of test performance statistics

sensitivity: specificity decreases, due to a large number of false negatives, on the expense of a higher sensitivity. In consequence, a perfect decision method (100 % sensitivity and specificity) is rarely achieved, and a balance must be stricken. Since the output of the ANN and LDA analysis were graded, *i.e.*, a number in the inclusive continuous range [0,1] was produced for each test record, it was necessary to define a cutoff point in order to count the number of true and false predictions to build the 2 x 2 contingency table. Since this definition is essentially arbitrary, the best procedure is to study the effect of different cutoff points upon the performance statistics. Thus, the following cutoff points were used for the ANN: 0.005, 0.01, 0.02, 0.05, 0.1, 0.2, 0.3, 0.4, 0.5, 0.6, 0.7, 0.8, 0.9, 0.98, 0.99 and 0.995. For each cutoff point, sensitivity and specificity were calculated and plotted one against the other in a bidimensional line graph, producing a curve called ROC, or *Receiver Operating Characteristic* [3]. A perfect ROC curve would be a horizontal line at the top (100 % sensitivity) all the way up to 100 % specificity and then down to the horizontal axis. Curves below this level denote less than perfect decision methods, but any ROC curve above the diagonal going from [0,0] to [100,100] in the graph (which marks the predictions where sensitivity is equal to specificity), can be considered a good one. The area under the ROC curve (AUC) is another measure which is usually employed two compare different ROC curves [17]. In the present context, the AUC can be interpreted as the probability that, given two individuals, one who died and one who didn't, the calculated prediction will be the largest for the individual who will die.

The final problem is, given a ROC curve, what is the best cutoff point to be adopted ? A simple way to do this is by using a measure called efficiency: which is the arithmetic mean of sensitivity and specificity. The χ^2 statistics derived from the 2 x 2 contingency table is also used as an indicator of the best mix of sensitivity and specificity along a ROC curve.

Another comparative measure of network performance was the mean error of classification, calculated by averaging all the absolute differences between expected and predicted value for each test record.

6. Results

The patient group was composed of 57 males (with 47 survivors) and 38 females (with 33 survivors), from 13 to 86 years old (mean 51.25 and standard deviation of 15.27). Observed overall 12-month mortality rate was 15.8 %. Presumed etiologies were distributed, in descending order of prevalence, into: idiopathic cardiomyopathic disease (46.3%), systemic arterial hypertension (23.2 %), Chagas' disease (13.7 %), coronary insufficiency (12.6 %) and other cardiomyopathic diseases, including due to diabetes and alcoholism (4.2 %). The majority of patients had minimal or no mitral valve impairment (77.9 %). For non-survivors, time of survival ranged from 23 to 367 days, with a mean of 166.07 days and standard deviation of 123.07 days.

6.1 Association Statistics

Univariate statistical analysis of the study variables resulted in the following (Tables 2 and 3):

Scalar variables significantly associated with 12-month mortality were: age (AGE), left ventricular diastolic diameter/thickness ratio (LVDDTh), mitral E-point to intraventricular septum separation (MEPSS), left ventricular diastolic measurements (LVDD and LVDI), left ventricular systolic measurements (LVSD and LVSI), left atrial diastolic diameter (LAD) and index (LADI) -- all directly proportional to death risk; left ventricular fractional shortening (LVFS), mitral flow deceleration time (MVDT) and left ventricular ejection fraction (LVEF) -- all inversely proportional to death risk. The variables not associated with death risk were: interventricular septum thickness (IVSTh), left ventricular posterior wall thickness (PWTh), heart rate (HR), diameter of aorta (AO), left ventricular mass (LVM) and cardiac index (CI). Furthermore, all categorical variables, such as sex, degree of mitral valve insufficiency (MI),

TABLE 2
Outcome prognosis of dilative myocardial disease
Univariate analysis of association - scalar variables

VARIABLE			SURVIVAL		DEATH		STATISTICS		
	Name	Unit	Mean	S.D.	Mean	S.D.	Diff.	F	p
AGE	Age	years	50.10	14.73	56.87	17.36	-6.67	2.44	0.1173
AO	Diameter of Aorta	mm	32.20	4.57	32.60	3.91	-0.40	0.10	0.7499
IVSTh	IV Septum Thickness	mm	9.27	1.33	8.87	1.19	0.48	1.23	0.2702
PWTh	Poster. Wall Thickness	mm	8.91	1.29	8.40	1.18	0.51	2.06	0.1511
LVDDTh	LV Diameter/Thickness		3.71	0.69	4.20	0.54	-0.49	6.49	0.0120
LVFS	LV Fraction. Shortening	%	19.07	4.96	14.48	3.31	4.60	11.81	0.0012
MEPSS	Mitral E-IV Septum Separ.	mm	23.37	6.36	26.73	5.23	-3.36	3.70	0.0542
MVDT	Mitral Flow Deceleration	ms	183.16	57.92	157.40	51.61	25.76	2.58	0.1077
HR	Heart Rate	bpm	78.56	14.16	86.93	19.47	-8.37	3.89	0.0485
LVDI	LV Diastolic Index	mm/m^2	38.31	5.84	42.52	6.13	-4.21	6.47	0.0121
LVSI	LV Systolic Index	mm/m^2	31.08	5.51	36.59	5.85	-5.52	12.42	0.0010
LADI	Left Atrial Index	mm/m^2	24.27	4.20	28.83	4.04	-4.56	15.04	0.0004
LVM	LV Mass	g	326.67	88.86	364.40	141.61	-37.73	1.85	0.1739
LVEF	Ejection Fraction	%	38.10	8.69	29.74	6.16	8.36	12.62	0.0009
CI	Cardiac Index	ml/m^2	49.29	14.25	48.91	18.71	0.38	0.01	0.9270

SD - Standard Deviation; Diff. - Difference between means; F - F-ratio statistics; p - two-tailed probability

disease etiology (ET), type of mitral flow (FLOW) and NYHA index were not significantly associated with death risk. Several of the significant variables were statistically correlated to a larger or lesser degree, but only left ventricular fractional shortening (LVFS) was removed from the variable set because it had a linear correlation of 1.0 with left ventricular ejection fraction (LVEF).

A separate ANOVA analysis relating the left ventricular filling pattern (FLOW) to echocardiographic scalar variables had the following results (Table 4): a restrictive filling pattern was significantly associated to a decreased mitral flow deceleration time (MVDT), as expected from its own definition, increased systolic left ventricular index (LVSI) and left atrial index (LADI), decreased left ventricular fractional shortening (LVFS) and ejection fraction (LVEF). On the other hand, the atrial filling predominant

TABLE 3
Outcome prognosis of dilative myocardial disease
Univariate analysis of association - categorical variables

			SURVIVAL	DEATH	STATISTICS	
Variable	Name	Meaning	%	%	χ^2	p
SEX	Sex	1 Male	58.75	66.67	0.33	0.5657
		2 Female	41.25	33.33		
ET	Etiology	1 Chagas	11.25	26.67	5.57	0.3499
		2 Hypertension	25.00	13.33		
		3 Coronaries	13.75	6.67		
		4 Idiopathic	46.25	46.67		
		5 Myocarditis	1.25	6.67		
		6 Alcoholism	1.00	0.00		
		7 Diabetes	1.00	0.00		
MI	Mitral Insuff.	0 No	15.00	6.67	4.93	0.2949
		1 Minimal	66.25	53.33		
		2 Mild	11.25	26.67		
		3 Moderate	6.25	6.67		
		4 Severe	1.25	6.67		
FLOW	Ventr.Flow	1 Normal	46.25	26.67	2.93	0.2310
		2 Restrictive	31.25	53.33		
		3 Atrial Dominant	22.50	20.00		
NYHA0	Initial NYHA	I	30.00	13.33	3.92	0.2698
		II	35.00	26.67		
		III	20.00	40.00		
		IV	15.00	20.00		

p = two-tailed probability

pattern was associated only with a highly increased mitral flow deceleration time (MVDT), as it is expected from its own definition.

The results are generally compatible with the literature, and demonstrate that high risk cardiac patients have notable anatomic alterations, namely hypertrophy of the heart, characterized by enlarged left atrium and ventricle, and a disproportionately enlarged ventricular cavity. Functionally, they seem to present a filling dysfunction in left ventricular diastole, which leads to a lower cardiac output (as evidenced by the ejection fraction measurement). The observed anatomical and functional alterations are most severe in the group of patients characterized by a restrictive ventricular filling pattern.

A good indication of the variability of causal factors acting in this sample of patients is that time of survival was not statistically associated to any other variable, scalar or categorical.

6.2 Linear Discriminant Analysis

The linear discriminant analysis resulted in the following (Table 5): as judged from the final discriminant weights, the most important variable was the left ventricular systolic index (LVSI). Other important variables were: left ventricular posterior wall thickness (LPWTh), left ventricular diastolic diameter/thickness ratio (LVDDTh), left ventricular diastolic index (LVSI) and left ventricular ejection fraction (LVEF).

The linear discriminant analysis was not efficient enough for separating survivors from non-survivors on the basis of input scalar variables. The distributions of the discriminant function for both patient groups overlapped considerably (Fig. 6), and

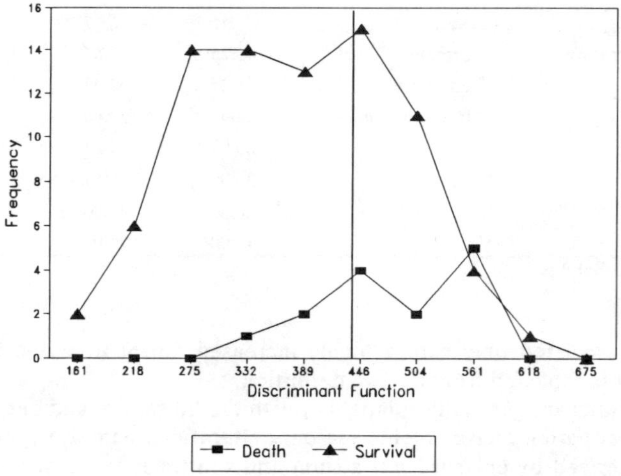

FIGURE 6 - Distribution of the linear discriminant function

TABLE 5
Prognosis of Dilative Myocardial Disease: Results of Linear Discriminant Analysis

Variable	Name	Discriminant Coefficient
AGE	Age	0.0595
IVSTh	Intraventricular Septum Thickness	-0.7998
PWTh	LV Posterior Wall Thickness	-2.1362
LVDDTh	LV Diastolic Diameter/Thickness Ratio	1.3513
MEPSS	Mitral E-IV Septum Separation	0.0719
MVDT	Mitral Valve Flow Deceleration Time	0.0098
HR	Heart Rate	0.0910
LVDI	LV Diastolic Diameter Index	-1.2668
VLSI	LV Systolic Diameter Index	17.5586
LADI	Left Atrial Index	0.5296
LVM	Left Ventricular Mass	-0.0762
LVEF	Left Ventricular Ejection Fraction	-2.4943
CI	Cardiac Index	-0.0320

Mean for discriminant function (Death): 495.85
Mean for discriminant function (Survival): 380.72
Difference between means (Mahalanobis Distance): 115.13
Cutoff point of discriminant function: 438.28 z: -5.36
F ratio : 142.40 df: 13/93

accuracy at the ideal cutoff value was only 67,4 %, with a sensitivity of 66.7 % and an specificity of 67.5 %. The weakest point of the LDA solution was positive predictivity which was only 27,8 % (*i.e.*, LDA predicted far more deaths than actually occurred in the patient sample), while negative predictivity (91,5 %) was excellent. These results show that a statistical linear model is not able to perform class separation in multidimensional space, and that a nonlinear approach is justified.

6.3 Artificial Neural Networks

Results are summarized in Table 6 and in Figures 7 to 14. In the following discussion, ANN configurations are denoted by three numbers, meaning the number of nodes in the input, hidden and output layers, respectively (for example, 13-5-1).

All networks trained to convergence within 3,000 training cycles, and many of them were able to converge to acceptable mean error just below 1,000 cycles. Global

TABLE 6
Prognosis of Dilative Myocardial Disease
Comparative Results of Classification Performance

Method	Dataset	Accuracy	Sensitivity	Especificity	Positive Predictivity	Negative Predictivity
Linear Discriminant Analysis	Full Set	67.37	66.67	67.50	27.78	91.53
Heuristics Rule by Clinician	Full Set	82.00	46.67	88.75	43.75	89.87
Heuristics Rule by Program	Full Set	91.50	46.67	100.00	100.00	90.90
Neural Network 13-2-1	Training Set	95.60	75.00	100.00	100.00	94.87
	Test Set	88.00	42.90	95.30	60.00	91.10
Neural Network 13-5-1	Training Set	100.00	100.00	100.00	100.00	100.00
	Test Set	90.00	71.42	93.00	62.50	95.24
Neural Network 13-10-1	Training Set	93.33	75.00	97.33	85.70	94.70
	Test Set	88.00	28.60	97.70	50.00	89.10
Neural Network 29-2-1	Training Set	97.80	87.50	100.00	100.00	97.40
	Test Set	72.00	42.90	82.20	33.33	84.60
Neural Network 29-5-1	Training Set	100.00	100.00	100.00	100.00	100.00
	Test Set	80.00	42.90	86.00	33.33	90.20
Neural Network 29-10-1	Training Set	100.00	100.00	100.00	100.00	100.00
	Test Set	72.40	42.86	76.74	23.08	89.19

mean squared error (RMS) was below 0.01 in all cases, reaching up to 0.004 for the best cases. The distribution of network output gave evidence that the solutions converged to the near proximity of 0 and 1 in all cases (Fig. 7). The test power statistics varied considerably with the cutoff point, as evidenced by the χ^2 statistic for each calculated 2 x 2 contingency table, and peak performance was correlated with peak χ^2.

All networks were able to predict outcome (Table 6, Figure 8), with accuracy ranging from 93.33 % (net 13-10-1) to 100 % (several nets), for the training dataset; and ranging from 72 % (net 29-2-1) to 90 % (net 13-5-1). In general, the networks with the reduced set of variables (11 variables) fared better than those with the full set of variables (18 variables); and within each of these two groups of ANNs, those with the intermediate number of hidden nodes had the best performance. Differences were not large, however, except for the best network (13-5-1), with 11 variables and five hidden node, which yielded 90 % accuracy, 71,4 % sensibility and 93 % specificity. The worst

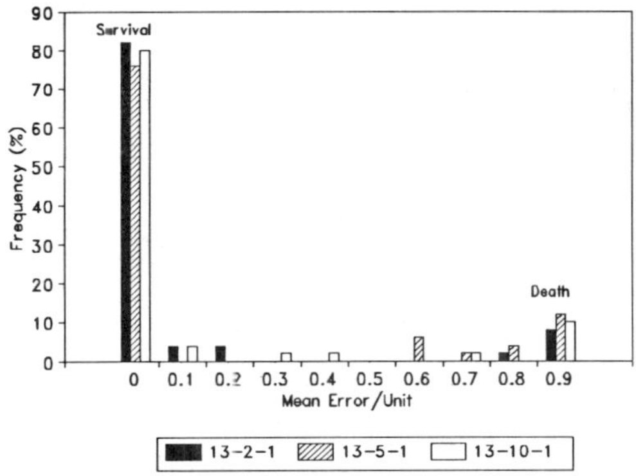

FIGURE 7 - Distribution of outputs for three trained ANNs

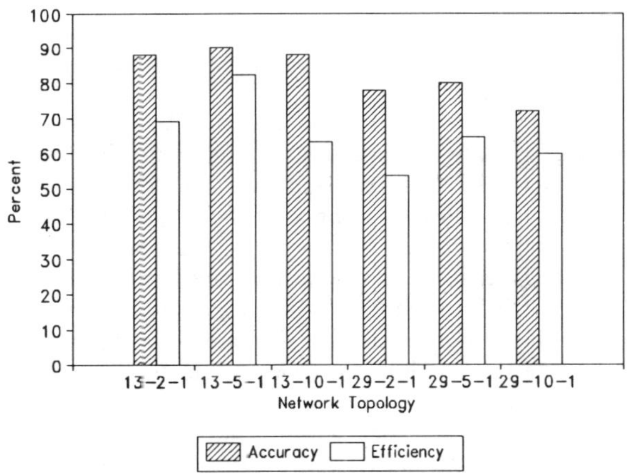

FIGURE 8 - Accuracies and efficiencies of neural networks

parameter for all networks was always sensitivity, denoting a relative inability to predict correctly the number of non-survivals.

Unfortunately, the comparison between the ROC curves for the several neural networks was not conclusive. When analyzed individually they were consistent with data resulting from univariate performance statistics, and a comparison could be made with other decision making techniques, thus demonstrating that nonlinear neural networks provided more powerful separation of outcome classes, particularly in relation to linear discriminant analysis. However, when several ROC curves were plotted or their AUC (area under the curve) was calculated, the resulting picture was quite confusing, because the ROC curves overlapped considerably, rendering quantitative comparisons meaningless.

6.4 Contribution of Individual Variables

One of the major criticisms of ANNs it's the difficulty of identifying the contributions of input variables to the decision, particularly in multilayer networks, where the large number of connections and nonlinear combinations of inputs obscure the rôle of individual input variables. In fact, the perceptron's topology dictates that the output (*e.g.*, prognostic estimate of survival) is a simultaneous functions of all inputs. In a two-layer perceptron, output can be interpreted as a linear combination of inputs. In contrast, there is no easy mathematical formula resulting from the operation of a three-layer perceptron [22].

However, an approximate measure of the contribution of each input variable to the output node can be derived by a simple expedient, following a suggestion by Harrison [20]. Maintaining all inputs constant (*e.g.*, equal to zero), except one of them (which is set to one, for example), the trained network is propagated with this artificial example and the output is evaluated. The larger it is in relation to the output obtained with all inputs equal to zero, the larger will be the impact of that particular input variable upon the output. This parameter, which we call the *Relative Output Magnitude*, can be negative or positive, highlighting the direction of contribution.

An example of this technique (which has been incorporated into the NEURONET program) is shown for the network 13-5-1 (Fig. 9). It is easy to see that variables age (AGE), interventricular septum thickness (IVSTh), mitral E-point to intraventricular septum separation (MEPSS), left ventricular diastolic index (LVDI), left ventricular systolic index (LVSI), left atrial diastolic index (LADI) and mitral flow deceleration time (MVDT), have a significant impact upon output; while left ventricular diastolic diameter/thickness ratio (LVDDTh), ejection fraction (LVEF) and left ventricular posterior wall thickness (PWTh) have negligible effect. Mean absolute

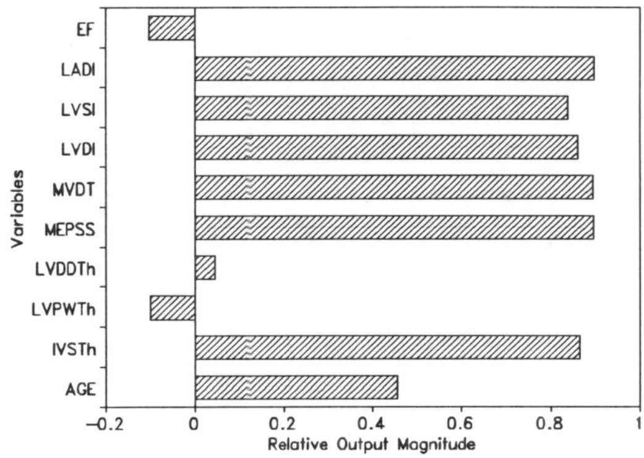

FIGURE 9 - Contribution of input variables to output

output magnitude with all variables set to zero was 0.103 in this case. With a few exceptions, these are the associations which were present in the previous univariate and LDA analyses. The technique seems to be useful for discovering the approximate mapping obtained iteratively by the network's learning procedure.

6.5 Repeatability of ANN Solutions

In order to evaluate the repeatability of ANN solutions, one of the networks (13-2-1) was retrained 15 times, always departing from a randomized set of weights and with randomized presentation of examples. Training was limited to 1,500 epochs maximum, with a learning rate of 1.5. Figre 10 shows the resulting learning curves, Figure 12 shows a comparative display of the contribution of individual variables, and Figure 11, a bidimensional plot of the values of the two connection weights from the hidden layer to the output node, for each repetition.

The ANN reached a different solution every time it was ran, which gives evidence about the complexity of the solution space, and that there is no single hypersurface which is able to separate outcome classes. However, these solutions were not random, *i.e.*, as one can observe in the weight space plot (Fig. 11), the networks that were able to learn (global error of 0.0764 ± 0.005), have solutions falling into four

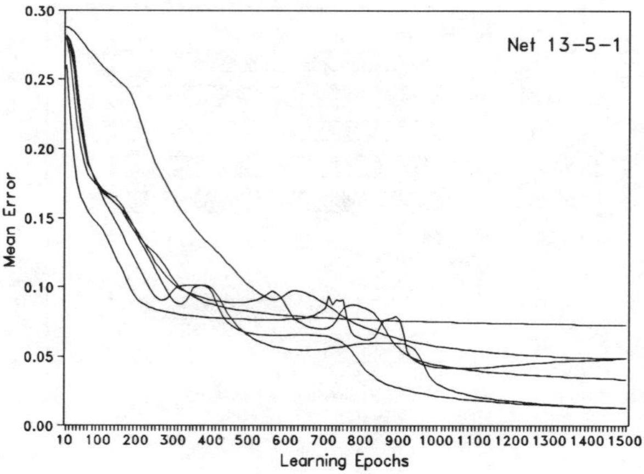

FIGURE 10 - Effect of repeated training of the same network

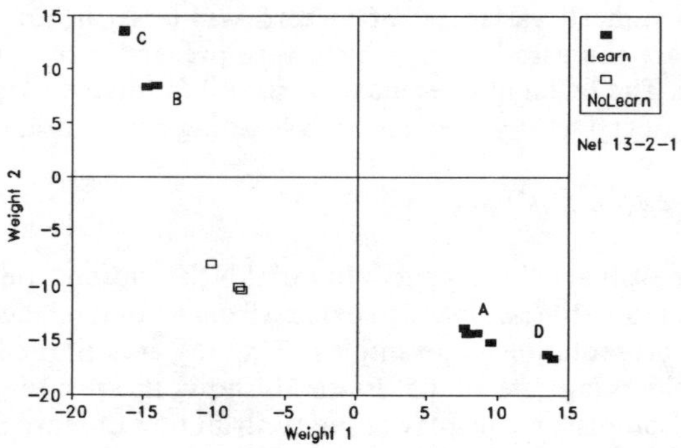

FIGURE 11

Effect of the repetition of training of the same neural network (13-2-1). The weights of the connections from the two intermediate nodes to the output node are placed in each axis of the graph. Each final solution reached by a repetition is shown as a point in bidimensional space. The solutions which converged can be grouped in four distinct clusters (A, B, C, D), depicted as filled squares, while networks which were unable to learn generated another separate cluster (open squares) distinct groups, which we have called A, B, C and D (in fact, these four groups could be coalesced into two separate quadrants of the graph), while the networks which were not able to learn (global error of 0.1218 ± 0.0002), fell into another completely different region of the weight space.

The same regularity could be observed in the profile of contribution of individual variables. Three distinct profiles were found for ANNs which learned, named Q, R and T (Fig. 12). Profiles R and T were quite similar, with a high positive contribution from variables age (AGE), diameter/thickness ratio (LVDDTh), mitral E-IV septum separation (MEPSS), mitral flow deceleration time (MFDT) and left atrial diameter index (LADI). The only differences between profiles R and T were variables LV diastolic diameter index (LVDI) and LV systolic diameter index (LVSI), with no contribution to profile R and a high contribution to profile T. The profile Q seems to represent a "wrong" solution, since it goes against all other analyses, i.e., LVSI and LVDI show negative contributions. However, when performance of the ANN solution patterns Q, R, T was tested, no significant differences emerged (the same accuracy of

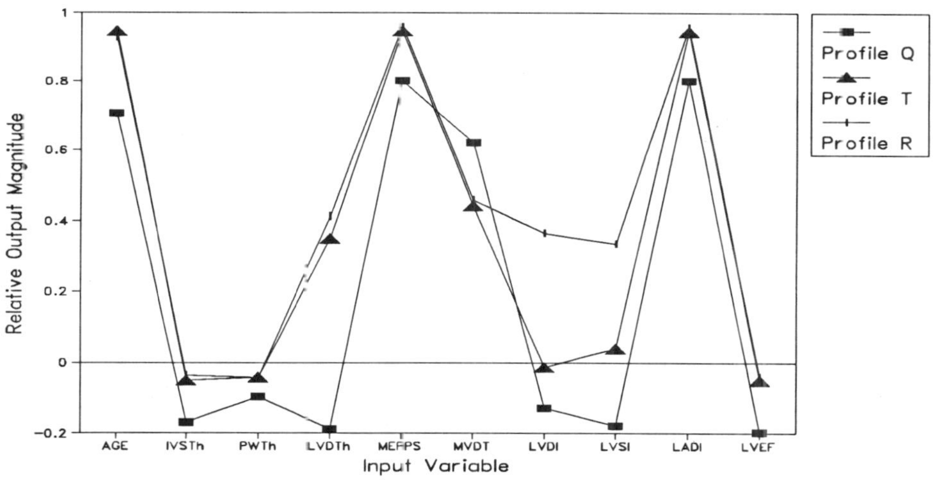

FIGURE 12

Comparison between the profiles of individual input variable contribution to output variable. Abscissa: name of the variable (see Table 1); Ordinate: relative output magnitude with single input= 1 (see text for details)

86 %, sensitivity of 42.9 % and specificity of 93 % for profiles R and T, at a cutoff point of 0.7). Profile Q, which seemed to be wrong, actually had a slightly higher performance (accuracy of 88 %, sensitivity of 42.9 and specificity of 95.3 %, also at cutoff point of 0.7).

The profile of the ANNs that were unable to learn (repetitions no. 9, 12 and 15) was totally different from Q, R and T, as expected, and is not shown in the graph. A surprising result is that there was no relation between patterns A, B, C and D (location in weight space) and Q, R and T (input contribution profile), as one would expect.

6.6 Comparison with Heuristic Methods

An interesting proposition would be to compare the results of ANN classification with those resulting from clinical judgment and conventional heuristics-based programs. We have done this by estimating the classification accuracy of heuristic rules

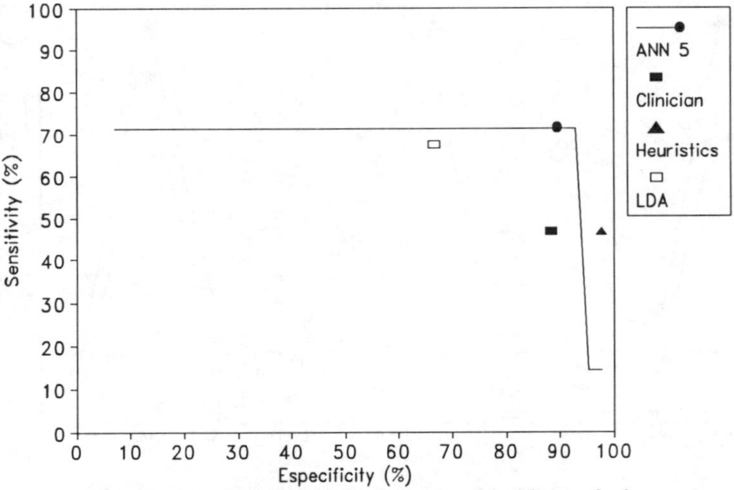

FIGURE 13 - Classification performance of decision methods

The line represents the ROC curve for best configuration of neural networks (REDUCED set of variables, number of nodes in the hidden layer equal to 5). The filled circle shows the best combined performance tests achieved. For the sake of comparison with other methods, the best performances are shown as isolated points for logical rules produced by a clinician, by an automatic induction program and for linear discriminant analysis (LDA).

derived previously by a group of experienced physicians for the present dataset [40], as well as by a commercially-available program for automatic induction, KnowledgeSEEKER® (First Mark Technol. Ltd., USA). The rule produced by the clinicians was:

```
IF MVDT less or equal than 140 ms AND
   LADI larger or equal than 25 mm/m2 AND
   LVDDTh larger or equal than 3.4
THEN OUTCOME = Death
```

When applied to the full dataset, this deterministic rule yielded an accuracy of 82 %, a sensitivity of 46.7 % and an specificity of 88 % (Table 6). Using the rule, actual mortality rate was 10.1 % in the low risk group versus 43.8 % in the high risk group (statistically significant, χ^2= 11.31, df= 1 and p= 0.00077). The decision rule formulated by physicians has unexpected characteristics, because it ignores other variables with a higher univariate association with survival.

The method of automatic induction used by KnowledgeSEEKER is rule derivation by successively dichotomizing the dataset with decision points aimed at maximizing differences in mortality rates (this is the essence of machine learning programs such as ID3, the *Interactive Dichotomizer 3* [43]). The following decision rule was produced for the full database:

```
IF LADI larger or equal than 28.571 AND
   HR larger or equal than 75 AND
   LVEF less or equal than 31.121
THEN OUTCOME=Death (100 %)
```

Note that this rule, besides being quite different from the rule produced by the clinicians, is also surprising, because it uses a variable (HR - heart rate), which was not found to be significantly associated to outcome neither in the univariate analysis nor in any of the multivariate LDA or ANN models. The rule achieved an accuracy of 91.5 %, a sensitivity of 46.7 % and an specificity of 100.0 % (Table 6). Using this criterion, actual mortality was 10 % for the low risk group and 100 % for the high risk group (statistically significant, χ^2= 40.3, df= 1 and p less than 0.000001), which is better than human judgment.

While both heuristic solutions have good to excellent accuracies and specificities, which are similar to those obtained by neural networks, sensitivities are unacceptable low for good clinical decision support (46.7 %). Furthermore, they were derived in knowledge of the full dataset, so the comparison with ANN, which had much more stringent criteria of test performance, cannot be made with fairness. In fact, all ANNs with 5 and 10 hidden nodes tested in the present study had accuracies, sensitivities and specificities of 100 % when trained with the full dataset. Even when tested with the separate test dataset, ANN's ROC curves lie above the point of performance of heuristic rules (Fig. 13).

7. Discussion

In analyzing the performance of neural networks, linear discriminant analysis and heuristic rules in outcome prognosis of dilative myocardial disease, it is clear that all the methods systematically predicted more deaths than actually occurred. Considering all 95 patients in the training and testing datasets, the best ANN had only five erroneous predictions: three false positives (patients no. 19, 26 and 38; the latter died within 24 months) and two false negatives (patients no. 44 and 48). Since the number of non-survivors is considerably smaller than of survivors, the impact of three errors is large, leading to a low positive predictivity for all neural networks tested in the study. A highly inflated false-positive error is also observed for the linear discriminant analysis, which, in consequence, had a very low positive predictivity (27.8 %). Simple heuristic rules derived by clinical expertise or automatic induction also suffered from the same problem, *i.e.*, high specificities and low to medium sensitivities.

This result could be explained by the fact that patients underwent uncontrolled therapeutic intervention after the initial examination. Assuming that therapy has been conducted effectively for most of the patients, it is reasonable to expect that many of them who were predicted to die, did not. Therefore, adding therapeutic variables to the predictor variables could lead to an improvement in decision specificity. Another difficulty is typical of diseases where the proportions of outcomes differ too much (in the present study, 10.5 % of non survivors versus 84.2 % of survivors, within 12 months). In this situation, it is harder to build a model where the lowest risk should be predicted with the same accuracy as the highest one.

The ANNs performance in the prognosis of outcome for patients with dilated myocardial disease can be rated as very good, considering that: 1) the time of measurement of variables was not fixed in relation to the onset of disease; 2) a large number of input variables was associated with outcome; 3) input variables presented a large variability across patients of the same outcome class; 4) the number of training examples was too low in relation to problem dimensionality; and 5) subsequent therapeutic intervention was not controlled or accounted for. A near optimal combination of high sensitivity and specificity was achieved with the 13-5-1 network, which was the decision method that outperformed all others. We have support, therefore, to propose that artificial neural networks are valid and reliable tools to carry out quantitative medical decision making in the area of prognosis of cardiac diseases.

The results show also some puzzling aspects of using neural networks for decision making. First, the networks with the largest number of hidden elements are not necessarily the best. Second, extreme numbers of input variables (large or small) do not lead to better predictions. Third, learning curves show sudden jumps and falls and other irregular or chaotic features which are not easy to explain. Another point of interest is that we are forcing the network to learn to output a binary number in response to a highly graded input. This is not the case of linear discriminant analysis or other multivariate analysis techniques, which provide a graded output. Surprisingly, the network learns this task quite well, judging from the distribution of outputs (Fig.8). Only about 2 % to 8 % of the outcome predictions fell into intermediate ranges (from 0.3 to 0.8), showing a "fuzzy" prognosis.

This mathematical expression used for calculation the weight modification during learning corresponds to the derivative of the sigmoid activation function, and it has a serious problem when the output (oj) is close to 0 or 1, as is the present case: the oj(1-oj) term becomes very small and learning progresses very slowly. Even so, we have been able to train our networks within a reasonable number of epochs. Solutions to this problem have been proposed (*e.g.*, [10]), but were not tried here.

What are ANNs representing after its learning converges to a low classification error ? In order to interpret this, one must remember that the multidimensional "data landscape" is very complex and "noisy", i.e, there are many sources of variation in the input variables. The ANN tries to learn a nonlinear mathematical function which will be able to separate exemplars, as sharply as possible, into the two groups which the supervisor is indicating. A major consideration, then, is whether the ANN has learned to represent a particular model of the data (a phenomenon called "memorization"), or it has learned a generic model ("generalization"). The solution to this, of course, is to test the model with novel data: theoretically, a poor performance indicates that the ANN has memorized, while a good one indicates that the ANN has been able to generalize. A good convergence of the learning curve alone cannot provide an estimation of generalization: it only gives a clue whether the ANN was able to fit well a discrimination function to the training data. If we interpret the combination of all possible weights as a multidimensional surface, backpropagation is a local gradient-seeking procedure, which suffers from the well-known problems for this kind of algorithm, *i.e.*; it will not guarantee to find a global minimum in the error surface. Thus, good convergence, in fact, might represent overfitting to data (memorization), only. Several improvements to the backpropagation algorithm have been proposed in order to provide better and speedier solutions, such as the use of other gradient-seeking methods, memory of error evolution, adaptive or decoupled learning rates, other error metrics and transfer functions, etc. [34, 55]; which were not been tried here.

The path to achieve a good generalization is not an easy one for neural networks, and it requires extensive experimentation with several configurations. The experiment which compared the classification solutions achieved by retraining several times the same ANN configuration has clearly demonstrated that nonlinear networks are able to memorize quite different solutions, even with a small hidden layer. They even have almost equal performances. The three most influent factors for achieving generalization seem to be: 1) the size of the hidden layer: it creates a kind of "bandwidth" effect for the feature classificator. A small number of hidden nodes impedes both generalization and memorization, while a large number facilitates memorization at the expense of generalization; 2) the number and type of input variables: a large number of variables creates a difficult landscape for the ANN to separate, because several of them do not bear any relation to prognosis (and we do not know which ones). On the other hand, a small number of input variables removes some of the higher-order associations between variables which have prognostic value (also unknown *a priori*). This, again, is a dilemma which must be solved by careful experimentation; 3) the number and variability of training exemplars. In some way, the final weight configuration in the neural network reflects the statistical distribution of cases in the population. Thus, the law of large numbers apply to the design of the training and test datasets. Large variability in data and a large number of input variables require a large size for both datasets, so that a sufficient number of all extant variants of patterns be present for training and testing.

In the present work, we have found that the best network contained five hidden nodes and a reduced set of variables. Unfortunately, the number of cases available for training and testing was not large, and some of the classification inaccuracies may stem from this. One should be aware that the performance statistics (accuracy, sensitivity, specificity, etc.) become very unstable and unreliable when the number of cases is small in any given class, *i.e.*, one false-negative or false-positive error has a disproportionately large impact upon them. Thus, generalization seems to have been achieved, but larger sample sizes would provide a firmer ground for this statement.

The essence of the heuristical approach to Artificial Intelligence is to find the most economical decision strategies, in terms of production rules, it attempts to perform a sharp reduction in the dimensionality of the feature space. Thus, it ignores the "*gestalt*" present in the predictor variables, *i.e.*, the overall multidimensional picture which ANNs and other mathematical classification methods are able to consider. This seems to be the key to ANN's success in dealing with complex pattern classification tasks such as those exemplified in the present paper. However, it is widely acknowledged that ANNs, unable as they are to provide logical explanations to the end-user for its decisions, meet higher user unacceptance rates than heuristics-based programs, and utmost care should be taken when determining the validity of neural-based decision-making tools [18].

In the present study, we have noticed that expert clinicians have a strong tendency to reason in terms of simple, easy-to-remember rules for making prognosis for individual patients, and that they use them a lot to "justify" their own prescience. Moreover, the black-box nature of neural networks and the need to use a computer to apply their decisions to everyday prognostic problems will surely preclude their wider use in Medicine for a time to come [19]. In this context, ANNs could be more useful if used to extract the dominant rules which are able to achieve highest classification performances. Work along these lines is already taking place [38], and hybrid decision support systems, which combine ANN's and logical reasoning in many different ways seem to have an interesting future for medical applications [6, 23].

Another important lesson extracted from the study was that accuracy alone is not a good indicator of performance for medical decision making tools. Due to the disproportion of outcome rates in the population, specificity and sensitivity tend to assume rather disparate values, usually lower than the overall accuracy rate. When this happens (see, for example, the performance of the neural networks with 10 hidden nodes, which had good accuracy, but a very poor sensitivity), the overall ANN performance is impaired. Unfortunately, many papers on the use of ANNs in medical decision making do not calculate or explicitly publish the full set of test performance statistics; thus marring their conclusions as well as rendering impossible an adequate evaluation of its usefulness. The ROC curve seems to be the best solution for completely describing performance of decision methods and for making statistically valid comparisons between them (although, according to some authors [3], the area under the ROC curve is not a good comparative measure when one the curves to be compared do not lie completely above or below the other, as we have observed in the present study).

In conclusion, artificial neural networks have proved to be a good device for implementing medical decision making in the area of outcome prognosis, because: 1) the so-called "gold standard" (a definitive decision for outcome in the training and test datasets) exists and is clear-cut. It is also avoids problematic procedures of appraisal by human experts; 2) the field has a tradition of using quantitative analysis and graded estimates of outcome, thus making the entrée of ANNs an easily acceptable one; 2) the complex nonlinear mixture of predictor variables is always present, and cannot be solved satisfactorily with conventional linear multivariate statistical analysis. Recent work has combined ANN technology with conventional statistical estimators, such as logistic regression and log-likelihood analysis [57], with promising results. A final advantage of ANNs is that the prognostic model derived by them is closely dependent upon the casuistics gathered in a particular institution or geographical area. In consequence, it will perform better than "global" indices (such as the well known APACHE index, which is widely used for outcome prognosis of critical patients [29]).

From the clinical point of view, the work shows that echocardiography may be considered an excellent tool to diagnose and evaluate the prognosis of dilated myocardial disease [36], despite the recommendation by some authors that other invasive and non-invasive diagnostic studies should be carried out in order to better evaluate important variables in the disease's natural history [47]. It is clear that many other potentially important variables for prognosis in dilative heart disease were not collected in the present work, such as angiographic and hemodynamic parameters [31, 62], myocardial thallium perfusion studies [9], myocardial biopsy [41, 58], electrocardiographic signals [37] and cardiovascular stress testing [13]. Perhaps, adding them to the study would improve prognosis (and ANN technology would made this easy to do), but this is uncertain, as evidenced by the results of using ANNs with all input variables. Anyway, we are convinced that many uncontrolled variables, such as therapeutic intervention and individual organic predisposition will make impossible to achieve higher prognostic performances than those reported here. However, further studies with a larger number of patients are required to better understand the mechanisms involved in systolic and diastolic functional changes affecting the prognosis of patients with dilated myocardial disease.

8. Acknowledgments

The authors gratefully acknowledge the helpful assistance given during the work by the following persons: Afonso Y. Matsumoto, MD, Carlos E. Suaide Silva, MD and Odila T.U. Nakano, MD., all from the *Centro de Cardiologia Não Invasiva*, São Paulo, Brazil; and Paulo M. Carvalho-Júnior, MD, Paulo Felipe Jr., MD, Jaime O. Ilha, MD, MSc and Goytá F. Villela Jr., MD, all from the *Center for Biomedical Informatics, State University of Campinas*, Brazil.

9. References

1. Avanzolini, G.; Barbini, P.; Gnudi, G. - Unsupervised learning and discriminant analysis applied to identification of high risk postoperative cardiac patients. *Int. J. Bio-Med. Comput.*, 25 (1990) 207-221.
2. Baxt, W.G. - Use of an artificial neural network for the diagnosis of myocardial infarction. *Ann.Intern. Med.*, 115 (1991) 843-848.
3. Beck, J.R.; Schultz, E.K. - The use of relative operating characteristic (ROC) curves in test performance evaluation. Arch. Path. Lab. Med. 110 (1986) 13-20.

4. Brown, T.H.; Kairiss, E.W.; Keenan, C.L. - Hebbian synapses - biophysical mechanisms and algorithms. *Ann. Rev. Neurol.*, **13** (1990) 475-511.
5. Caso, P.; Cioppa, C.; Musto, B.; De Leva, F.; Vitale, D.; Calabro, R. - Aspetti clinici della cardiomiopatia dilatativa in età pediatrica. *Cardiologia*, **35** (1990) 839-44.
6. Cios, K.J.; Liu, N. - A machine learning method for generation of a neural network architecture: a continuous ID3 algorithm. *IEEE Trans. Neural Networks*, **3** (1992) 280-291.
7. Clements, I.P.; Brown, M.L.; Zinsmeister, A.R.; Gibbons, R.J. - Influence of left ventricular filling on symptoms and survival in patients with decreased left ventricular systolic function. *Am. J. Cardiol.*, **67** (1991) 1245-50.
8. DeMaria, A.N.; Wisenbaugh, T.W.; Smith, M.D. et al. - Doppler echocardiographic evaluation of diastolic dysfunction. *Circulation*, **84** (suppl I) (1991). I 288-95.
9. Doi, Y.L.; Chikamori, T.; Tukata, J.; Yonezawa, Y.; Poloniecki, J.D.; Ozawa, T.; McKenna, W.J. - Prognostic value of thallium-201 perfusion defects in idiopathic dilated cardiomyopathy. *Am. J. Cardiol.*, **67** (1991) 188-93.
10. Fahlman, S.E. - Faster learning variations on back-propagation: an empirical study, in: *Proceed. (1988) Connectionist Models Summer School*, ed. Touretzky, R (Morgan Kauffman, New York, 1989).
11. Felipe Jr., P.; Sabbatini, R.M.E.; Carvalho-Júnior, P.; Beseggio, R.E.; Terzi, R.G.G. - Outcome prediction for critical patients under intensive care, using backpropagation neural networks. *Anais I Fórum Nacional de Ciência e Tecnologia em Saúde*, (1992) p. 344-47.
12. Ferrer Salvans, P.; Alonso Valles, L.; Osorio Gullon, A.; Suarez Menendez, M.; Vilaplana Birba, J.; Rubio Garcia, R.; Valino Blanco, J. - An empirical comparison ofbackpropagation and multivariate discriminant analysis to the prediction ofcolon cancer recurrence after surgical treatment. *International Neural Network Conference. Proceed. INNC 90 Paris*, (Kluwer, Dordrecht, 1990) **1**: 348.
13. Griffin, B.P.; Shah, P.K.; Ferguson, J.; Rubin, S.A. - Incremental prognostic value of exercise hemodynamic variables in chronic congestive heart failure secondary to coronary artery disease or to dilated cardiomyopathy. *Am. J. Cardiol.*, **67** (1991) 848-853.
14. Grossberg, S. - *The Adaptive Brain*. (Elsevier, New York, 1986).
15. Grossman, W. - Diastolic dysfunction in congestive heart failure. *New England J. Med.*, **325** (1991) 1557-1564.
16. Grossman, W.; McLaurin, L.P.; Rolett, E.L. - Alterations in left ventricular relaxation and diastolic compliance in congestive cardiomyopathy. *Cardiovasc. Res.*, **13** (1979) 514-22.

17. Hanley, J.A.; McNeil, R.J. - The meaning and use of the area under receiver operating characteristic (ROC) curve. *Radiology*, **143** (1982) 29-36.
18. Hart, A.; Wyatt J. - Connectionist models in medicine: an investigation of their potential. In: Hunter, J.; Cookson, J.; Wyatt, J. (Eds.) *Proceedings of Artificial Intelligence in Medicine Europe.* Heidelberg: Springer-Verlag, Lecture Notes in Medical Informatics, **38** (1990): 115-124.
19. Hart, A.; Wyatt, J. - Evaluating black-boxes as medical decision aids: issues arising from a study of neural networks. *Medical Informatics*, **15** (1990) 229-36.
20. Harrison, R.F.; Marshall, S.J.; Kennedy, R.L. - The early diagnosis of heart attacks: a neurocomputational approach. *Proceed. Internat. Joint Conf. Neural Networks*, **1** (1991) 1-5.
21. Hopfield, J.J. - Neural networks and physical systems with emergent collective computational abilities. *Proc. Nat. Acad. Sci. USA*, **79** (1982) 2554-2558.
22. Huang, W.Y. & Lippman, R.P. - Comparisons between neural nets and conventional classifiers. *Proc. 1st. International Neural Networks Conference*. (IEEE Press, New York, 1987) p. 485.
23. Hudson, D.L.; Cohen, M.E.; Lammers, R.K. - Use of a hybrid expert system to predict wound infections. In: *Proceed. 7th World Congress Medical Informatics*, ed. K.C. Lun; Degoulet, P.; Piemme, T.E.; Rienhoff, O. (North-Holland, Amsterdam, 1992) p. 546-551.
24. Jayaweers, A.; Drake, K.C.; Abbott, R.; Kaul, S. - Determination of long-term outcome in patients with coronary artery disease using an artificial neural network. *J. Amer. Coll. Cardiol.*, **21**(1993) 7A.
25. Keogh, A.M.; Baron, D.W.; Hickie, J.B. - Prognostic guides in patients with idiopathic or ischemic cardiomyopathy assessed for cardiac transplantation. *Am. J. Cardiol.*, **65** (1990) 903-8.
26. Kimball, T.R.; Daniels, S.R.; Meyer, R.A.; Scharwtz, D.C.; Kaplan, S. - Left ventricular mass in childhood dilated cardiomyopathy: a possible predictor for selection of patients for cardiac transplantation. *Am. Heart J.* **122** (1991) 126-31.
27. Kinser, W.; Indrayanto, A.; Langi, A. - A study of backpropagation, counterpropagation and adaptive resonance theory neural network models. *Proceed. 12th. Ann. Conf. IEEE Engineer. Med. Biol. Soc.*, (IEEE Press, New York, 1990).
28. Kosko, B. - Bidirectional associative memories. *IEEE Trans. Syst. Man, Cybern.*, **SMC-18** (1988) 42-60.
29. Knaus, W. A.; Draper, E. A.; Wagner, D.; Zimmerman, J. E. - APACHE II: A severity of disease classification system. *Critical Care Medicine*, **13** (1985) 818 - 829.
30. Kohonen, T. - *Self-Organization and Associative Memory.* (Springer-Verlag, Berlin, 1984).

31. Kuroda, T.; Shiina, A.; Suzuki, O.; Fujita, T.; Noda, T.; Tsuchyia, M.; Yaginuma, T.; Hosoda, S. - Prediction of prognosis of patients with idiopathic dilated cardiomyopathy: a comparison of echocardiography with cardiac catheterization. *Jap. J. Med.*, **28** (1989) 180-8.
32. Lorell, B.H. - Significance of diastolic dysfunction of the heart. *Annu. Rev. Med.*, **42** (1991) 411-36.
33. Meistrell, M.L.; Spackman, K.A. - Evaluation of neural network performance by receiver operating characteristic (ROC) analysis: examples from the biotechnology domain. *Comput. Methods Programs. Biomed.* **32** (1990)73-80.
34. Minai, A.A.; Williams, R.D. - Fast backpropagation with adaptive decoupled momentum. In: Soucek, B. (Ed.) - *Fast Learning and Invariant Object Recognition.* (Wiley, New York, 1992) p. 9-26.
35. Nishimura, R.A.; Housmans, P.R.; Hatle, L.K.; *et al.* - Assessment of diastolic function of the heart: background and current applications of doppler echocardiography. Part I. Physiologic and pathophysiologic features. *Mayo Clin. Proc.*, **64** (1989) 71-81.
36. Nishimura, R.A.; Abel, M.D.; Hatle, L.K.; *et al.* - Assessment of diastolic function of the heart: background and current applications of doppler echocardiography. Part II. Clinical studies. *Mayo Clin. Proc.*, **64**:181-204, (1989).
37. Ohnishi, Y.; Ynoue, T.; Fukuzaki, H. - Value of the signal-averaged electrocardiogram as a predictor of sudden death in myocardial infarction and dilated cardiomyopathy. *Jap. Circ. J.*, **54** (1990) 127-36.
38. Omlin, C.W.; Giles, C.L.; Miller, C.B. - Heuristics for the extraction of rules from discrete-time recurrent neural networks. *Proceed. Int. Joint Conf. Neural Networks.* (IEEE Press, New York, 1992) **1**: 33-38.
39. Ortiz, J.; Matsumoto, A.Y.; Silva, C.E.S. - O ecocardiograma na avaliação prognóstica da insuficiência cardíaca. *Arq. Bras. Cardiol.*, **51** (1988) 89-91.
40. Ortiz, J.; Matsumoto, A.Y.; Ghefter, C.G.M.; Silva, C.E.S; Durazzo, A.E.; Barretto, A.C.P.; Nanda, N.C. - Prognosis in dilated myocardial disease: influence of diastolic dysfunction and anatomical changes. *Echocard.*, **10** (1993) 1-7.
41. Otsuka, H. - Factors to determine the survival of idiopathic dilated cardiomyopathy: selecting candidates for cardiac transplantation. *Nippon Kyobu Geka Gakkai Zasshi*, **37** (1989) 318-25
42. Overall, J.E.; Klett, C.J. - *Applied Multivariate Analysis.* (McGraw-Hill, New York, 1972).
43. Quinlan, J.R. - Semi-autonomous acquisition of pattern-based knowledge. In: ed. Michie, D *Introductory Readings in Expert Systems.* (Gordon & Breach, London, 1982).

44. Ravdin, P.M.; Clark, G.M. - A practical application of neural network analysis for predicting outcome of individual breast cancer patients. *Breast Cancer Res. Treat.*, **22** (1992) 285-93.
45. Reggia, J.A.; Sutton III, G.G. - Self-processing networks and their biomedical implications. *Proc. IEEE*, **76** (1988) 580-92.
46. Reggia, J.A. - Neural computation in Medicine. *Artif. Intellig. Med.*, **5** (1993) 143-57.
47. Romeo, F.; Pelliccia, F.; Cianfrocca, C.; Gallo, P.; Barilla, F.; Cristofani, R.; Reale, A. - Determinants of end-stage idiopathic dilated cardiomyopathy: a multivariate analysis of 104 patients. *Clin. Cardiol.*, **12**, (1989) 387-92.
48. Rosenblatt, F. - The perceptron: a probabilistic model for information storage and organization in the brain. *Psychol. Rev.*, **65** (1958) 368-408.
49. Rumelhart, D.E.; Hinton, G.E.; Williams, R.J. - Learning internal representation by back-propagating errors. *Nature*, **323** (1986) 533-6.
50. Sabbatini, R.M.E. - Applications of connectionist systems in Biomedicine. *Proceed. 7th World Congress on Medical Informatics* (North Holland, Amsterdam, 1992), p. 418-426.
51. Sabbatini, R.M.E.; Carvalho-Júnior, P.M.; Freitas, N.C.; Felipe Jr., P. - NEURONET: a connexionist shell system for automatic pattern classification in Biomedicine. *Anais I Forum Nacional de Ciência e Tecnologia em Saúde*, (1992).
53. Sabbatini, R.M.E. - *Artificial Neural Networks in Medical Decision Making.* . Associate Professorship Dissertation (Chair of Medical Informatics, Faculty of Medical Sciences of the State University of Campinas, Campinas, Brazil, 1993).
54. Sachs, R.N.; Vuong, P.; Fischbein, C.; Nitenberg, A.; Palski, D.; Fischbein, L.; Beaudet, B.; Dievart, F.; Lanfranchi, J. - Etude des facteurs prognostiques des cardiomyopathies dilatées. *Ann. Med. Interne. Paris* **140** (1989) 683-6.
55. Simpson, P.K. - *Artificial Neural Systems: Foundations, Paradigms, Applications and Implementations.* (Pergamon Press, London, 1990).
56. Smith, J.W.; Everhart, J.E.; Dickson, W.C.; Knowler, W.C.; Johannes, R.S. - Using the ADAP learning algorithm to forecast the onset of diabetes mellitus. *Proc. 12th. Ann. Symp. Comput. Appl. Med. Care.* (IEEE Press, New York, 1988), p. 261-265.
57. Spackman, K.A. - Combining logistic regression and neural networks to create predictive models. *Proceedings of the 16th Annual Symposium on Computer Applications in Medical Care* (AMIA, Washington, 1992).
58. Tanganelli, P.; Di Lenarda, A.; Bianciardi, G.; Salvi, A.; Silvestri, F.; Mestroni, L.; Camerini, F. - Correlation between histomorphometric findings on endomyocardial biopsy and clinical findings in idiopathic dilated cardiomyopathy. *Am. J. Cardiol.*, **64** (1989) 504-506.

59. Tu, J.V.; Guerriere, M.R.J. - Use of a neural network as a predictive instrument of lenght of stay in the intensive care unit following cardiac surgery. *Proceed. 16th. Annu. Symp. Comput. Appl. Med. Care*, (AMIA: Washington, 1992).
60. Unverferth, D.V.; Magorien, R.D.; Moeschberger, M.L.; *et al.* - Factors influencing the one year mortality of dilated cardiomyopathy. *Am. J. Cardiol.*, **54** (1984) 147-52.
61. Varani, E.; Magelli, C.; Bassein, L.; Truncellito, L.; Ribani, M.A.; Rubino, I.; Fini, M.; Ferretti, R.M.; Magnani, B. - Caratteristiche cliniche e fattori prognostici dello scompenso cardiaco cronico secondario a miocardiopatia dilatativa primitiva ed a cardiopatia ischemica. *G. Ital. Cardiol.*, **19** (1989) 1-6.
62. Zanchetta, M.; Pedon, L.; Carlon, R.; Franceschetto, L.; Maiolino, P. - Cardiomiopatia dilatativa. Analisi discriminante multivariata dei principali indici emodinamico-angiografici. *G. Ital. Cardiol.*, **20** (1990) 15-9.

IMPLEMENTATION OF STATISTICAL PATTERN RECOGNITION FOR CONGESTIVE HEART FAILURE

Edward A. Patrick
The Patrick Institute
7939 Bar Harbor Drive
Cincinnati, Ohio 45255, USA

1. INTRODUCTION

Herein we present the deliberations leading to developing a system which provides continuous quality improvement (CQI) for patients whose presentations look like congestive heart failure (CHF). Discipline begins with the Statistical Pattern Recognition (SPR) model which can capture **a priori knowledge** (i.e. expert knowledge) and training data (fresh knowledge) to produce **a posteriori knowledge.** Usefulness is enhanced through facility to store cases, provide a differential diagnosis, recommended next findings to affect the process, provide for outcome analysis (OA) and provide for **individualized outcome analysis**^{tm} (IOA).

OA is a facility synthesized from a population of cases to predict an outcome B given a condition A where both B and A are characteristic of the cases. On the other hand, IOA is the facility to predict an outcome B for any new patient's presentation no matter how different that presentation is from any previously seen case in the population.

From the practical standpoint, emergency medicine physicians, critical care physicians, cardiologists, and others may feel that the diagnosis and treatment of congestive heart failure (classical CHF) is straightforward. After all, only a small percentage, for example those with pulmonary edema or associated cardiogenic shock, require invasive monitoring. So why do we need to further reason with respect to CHF, especially by using SPR?

In answering this question we are first mindful of a popular definition of congestive heart failure: **decrease in myocardial contractility such that the cardiac output (CO) is inadequate for the body's needs, manifest with fluid retention.** Realize that discussion and emphasis from a clinical viewpoint may differ from that of a physiologic/anatomic viewpoint or molecular-biologic viewpoint because clinically we are faced with making a diagnosis and providing treatment to achieve the best process.

Through deliberation, which includes literature review, we identify clinical problems which do not meet the classical CHF definition, but which "may look like CHF clinically." Foremost among these problems are **high output failure** such as hyperthyroid, non cardiogenic pulmonary edema (CARDS), pneumonia, chronic obstructive pulmonary disease (COPD), ischemic heart disease including myocardial infarction, septic shock, and nephrotic syndrome. Thus any clinical consideration of CHF mandates considering problems that may look like CHF clinically. Now we proceed to develop appropriate categories and subcategories by studying an article suggested by the editors - "Diastolic Dysfunction in Congestive Heart Failure," by Grossman [1]. Grossman divides CHF into **systolic failure** - with passive backup of blood into the pulmonary and systemic venous beds and **diastolic failure** - increased resistance to left and right ventricular inflow.

An alternative (second) subdivision of CHF discussed by Hurst, Schlant, Rackley, Sonnenblock, and Wenger [2] and Stapczynski [3] and The Merck Manual [4] is **Left heart failure (LHF), Right heart failure (RHF)**, or both **LHF + RHF**. Symptoms and signs of LHF consist of increased pressure and congestion in pulmonary veins and capillaries; and symptoms and signs of RHF consist of increased pressure and congestion in systemic veins and capillaries. Yet a third subdivision of CHF is **forward failure** vs **backward failure** (The Merck Manual [4]). Forward failure implies that most of the patient's signs & symptoms result from low cardiac output - easy fatigability, weakness, confusion, and shock. Backward failure implies that most of the patient's signs & symptoms result from increased venous pressure behind the failing ventricle(s), for example as in mitral stenosis or tricuspid stenosis.

These subdivisions of CHF guide our approach, **based on SPR (Patrick, Ullman, Dasarathy), whereby clinical syndromes are captured as clusters (subcategories) of presentations in a hyperspace defined by a feature list**. Clusters provide an "attachment" for strategies (treatments), updatability, CQI including cost, and disease process. Mathematically, a subcategory (cluster) is described by the subcategory conditional probability density function (SCCPDF) - the ultimate collection of patient presentations; and subcategories are collected into categories.

2. THE SPR APPROACH TO CHF

Thus we will develop and expand a list of subcategories and collect them together into categories. A natural feature list is developed with some features **significant** for each subcategory (and remaining features **insignificant** for that subcategory). The approach was named Statistical Pattern Recognition [SPR] in Ullman's book review in Nature 1973 [6]; the reviewed book was Fundamentals of Pattern Recognition by Patrick [5]. A **normal category** later was defined as having all insignificant features [7].

The discovery of subcategories can involve unsupervised learning type 1 [5] and characterization of two subcategories active at the same time, i.e. a complex class [8,7], can involve unsupervised learning type 2 (see Appendix B). SPR provides facility to capture case presentations into subcategories and complex subcategories.

There is ad-hoc evidence that some physicians do not warm-up to the SPR approach, possibly because it is a new way of thinking. Many physicians seem adverse to organized approaches to diagnosis. Some physicians may accept decision trees; and we note that rule based expert systems implement decision trees. On the other hand, ultimate performance and analysis will be achieved by the SPR approach to which a decision tree is an approximation. Physician reluctance to embrace organized decision making approaches may be because: (1) it is difficult to remember them; (2) it is unnatural to embrace them; (3) it is difficult to communicate with them; (4) they just aren't necessary. Nevertheless it seems fundamental: process a set of findings (features) to provide a differential diagnosis of CHF with strategies, and indicate additional features to "sharpen" the differential diagnosis (CQI); also, capture new subcategories and complexes of these subcategories.

3. AN INSTRUMENT TO IMPLEMENT THE SPR APPROACH TO CHF

The implementation of SPR has been likened to a modern implementation of the scientific method. For twenty eight years we have been developing methods and software (Patrick 1965-1993 [5,7-15]) which can capture an application of SPR such as CHF. The software, called Consult^R is the integration of Consult-I^R whose subcategories (clusters) are trained with a priori knowledge (expert knowledge) and Consult Learning System^R (CLS) which is trained with hard data. The SPR facility for decision making and facility to update a priori knowledge with hard data is described theoretically in Appendix A and Appendix B.

Consult-I^R and CLS share the same feature list and can share the same category space. All possible patterns of a category, which could be generated, are represented naturally by the clusters in Consult-I^R. In SPR terminology, the subcategory generator mathematically is called the subcategory conditional probability density function (SCCPDF) (see Appendix B).

The integration of CLS with Consult-I^R provides true updating of a priori (expert) knowledge by hard data to produce a posteriori knowledge. This is accomplished in part when CLS creates hard data clusters to integrate with Consult-I^R's expert clusters.

Advanced SPR methods in Consult-I^R provide for **"cloning" existing clusters with the findings to produce new clusters either with or without supervision.** These methods include the production of new clusters to define "complex classes" which are required when multiple subcategories are needed to explain the findings.

Continuous Quality Improvement (CQI) results in part from the recommendation of additional features, for which feature values will be selected. Such feature selection is accomplished by comparing the probability density of significant features of a cluster within a category with the insignificant features of the normal cluster. In general, CQI results because a new model is created which includes new training records.

For comparison purposes, the clusters in both Consult-I^R and CLS are analogous to the middle-layer nodes in a conventional neural net. But CLS does not form clusters (middle layer nodes) until the findings are presented. An advantage is that the findings provide a great deal of "correlation" information to assist in local probability density estimation. The upshot is the formation of a virtual cluster, or just the potential from a cluster. This is an extension of the Generalized K-nearest neighbor decision rule (Patrick and Fischer 1969,1970 [12,13], Patrick 1972,1979,1990 [5,14,15], Dasarathy 1991 [16]); and in comparison it is like a conventional neural net with a virtual middle layer cluster [15].

The SPR methods, developed mathematically, attempt to describe the reasoning as pragmatic as possible. To this end, these mathematics will coincide with an actual working Consult^R subsystem which can be used in clinical practice to diagnose and treat CHF. **The system's performance can be expected to improve through updating the expert knowledge clusters, cloning with the findings to produce new expert knowledge clusters, updating hard data clusters, or just storing new patterns of patient cases.**

4. THE CHF SUBSYSTEM IN CONSULT[R]

Our perception is that diagnosis, treatment, and CQI for CHF is based on a model. We do not attempt to define the model that physicians use to view CHF. Their model may use visual images, auditory images, or kinesthetic images (feelings). Our model is that of Statistical Pattern Recognition (SPR); and only time may or may not show how this model is regarded by physicians. We do know that it is beneficial for diagnosis, CQI, OA, and IOA.

In the **beginning there was hyperspace**[tm] is a concept we developed [7] to describe categories, features, treatments, and outcomes as respective dimensions of a hyperspace. As a practical matter, categories are diseases, features are findings (signs, symptoms, and laboratory tests); and treatments also can be findings. Mathematically, the feature values of a feature are a set identical to a set of categories or a set of outcomes. Realizing this for design leads to enormous flexibility in a system which learns from hard data.

Augmenting the model with time yields a process or time series. At an instance in time t_1, a frame results consisting of processing findings to produce a differential diagnosis with actions. These actions are incorporated with the findings at time t_2 to produce a new differential diagnosis with new actions. Each of these frames is in the hyperspace originally defined and a resulting process lies in an expanded hyperspace defined by the union of original hyperspaces and called the **process space** (Patrick 1979).

What is interesting for CQI is that each such process lies in the process space. Capturing these processes allows retaining knowledge of "good" and "bad" processes. The processes themselves cluster into process categories. When such a system is appropriately trained it is possible to predict the process category with a minimum subset of findings - such as one or a few of the time frames. This could avert following a "bad" process given early or minimal information about the process. For instance, examples of processes experienced at one hospital could be used avert a costly experience at another hospital.

For the model to be complete it is important that at each time frame facility exist to learn without a teacher. Both learning without a teacher type 1 and learning without a teacher type 2 (Appendix B) is required. Learning without a teacher type 1 is the process of learning clusters when necessary to achieve optimum performance. But learning without a teacher type 2 is required to discover and form complex classes at each frame. New actions associated with the new complex classes can be devised at each frame. The sophisticated nature of these processes will be important in terms of their outcomes. Outcomes are defined in terms of ejection fraction, respiratory rate, length of stay in the hospital, cost, etc.

5. CATEGORIES, FEATURE LIST, AND SIGNIFICANT FEATURES

We spur on our study of using SPR to describe CHF by designing a Consult^R subsystem based on the classical description of CHF, with extensions. It is soon apparent by using the system that for practical reasons the subsystem should be extended to embrace many subcategories that look like CHF.

Starting with the first version of the subsystem, the foremost characterization of CHF is Right Ventricular Failure (RVF) vs Left Ventricular Failure (LVF). Additional characterization is based on precipitating cause, presence or absence of pulmonary edema and presence or absence of peripheral edema & ascites. In addition there are subsets of significant features for CHF in general, non-cardiogenic pulmonary edema, hyperthyroidism, septic shock, arteriovenous fistula, Paget's disease, cirrhosis, nephrotic syndrome, protein-losing enteropathy, inferior vena cava obstruction, and mesenteric or hepatic venous obstruction.

The objective is to define categories with subcategories, be mindful of strategies for the subcategories, and create a feature list. Some features should be type 0 and others type 1 (see Appendix B). A type 0 feature has feature values which are mutually exclusive while a type 1 feature has features which are embedded binary type 0 features.

Traditionally the literature distinguishes between Left Heart Failure (LHF) and Right Heart Failure (RHF) (one of the three models mentioned in the Introduction) and alludes to the most common cause of RHF as being LHF. This is one of the reasons to define the category LHF + RHF. In our first list of categories, subcategories are listed under categories in a way suggested by the literature; but the presentation needs to be updated by clinical experience. For example, within the Consult-I^R module a complex cluster can be created by an operation called **cloning**, implementing the new theorem on a posteriori probability (Patrick 1983, 1986 [8,7]), **which views two existing clusters as classes and forms a new subcategory.** A **cloning** operation also can from a complex subcategory for LVH + RVH using two existing clusters in LVH and RVH respectively viewed as subclasses.

What is the difference between Bayes theorem and the theorem by Patrick (Appendix B) as applied to the previous example? **Bayes theorem has no provision for discovering and combining the significant and insignificant features of a subcategory of LVH with the significant and insignificant features of a subcategory of RVH to form a complex subcate-**

gory. That is, Patrick's theorem accomplishes this by using a Normal category to define insignificant features, models for existence of complex classes, and the "glue" to form a complex class. This facility to use a priori knowledge is fundamental to Patrick's theorem and absent in Bayes theorem.

Neither Patrick's theorem nor Bayes theorem are complete until the frameworks for estimating the category conditional probability density functions (CCPDF's) and subcategory conditional probability density functions (SCCPDF's) are developed. This is accomplished in Consult^R.

6. THE PATIENT PROCESS

The time course of a patient, corresponding to multiple exacerbations of CHF, describes a sequence of sets of findings, differential rankings, and treatments. This describes a sequence of different patient states [14] called a process. This process can be stored in Consult^R within a new subsystem called a **process subsystem.** The categories of the process subsystem correspond to different clusters of paths that the patient can take. The dimensionality of this process subsystem obviously is a multiple E of the original CHF subsystem where E is the number of exacerbations recorded.

The CLS module in the Consult^R process system can store patient paths. In the usual way, the CLS module in Consult^R can provide outcome analysis and individualized outcome analysis on the processes of the patients. This facility is useful to study processes in congestive heart failure.

7. THE INITIAL CONSULT^R SUBSYSTEM FOR CHF

The categories with subcategories defined in the first Consult-I^R module are shown in Table 1; and the feature list shared by both modules, Consult-I^R and CLS, is shown in Table 2. Table 3 shows the parameters for the subsystem. Each subcategory is characterized by a SCCPDF which uses features from the feature list. For any given subcategory, only some of the features from the feature list are significant with the rest insignificant for that subcategory.

This subsystem undoubtedly has value when the scope of the patient's problem is known limited to CHF or certain related problems. For example it has application in studying the patient presentations for OA, and IOA; and it may have application for integration in certain medical equipment.

The subsystem's usefulness in clinical practice for diagnosis, treatment, and CQI is limited by the frustration of not having subcategories other than CHF or closely related problems. For this reason we turn attention to an expanded subsystem that includes subcategories discussed thus far.

8. THE EXTENDED CONSULT^R SUBSYSTEM FOR CHF

Clinical practice has guided our experience in developing Consult^R for cardiac problems. A subsystem called **Chest** began with a focus on cardiac ischemia, i.e. Myocardial infarction vs Ischemia - Non MI. Experience resulted in its natural expansion to include additional subcategories. The subcategories dealing with CHF are identical to those in the previously discussed smaller subsystem. The size of this extended subsystem is illustrated in Table 4 which shows there now are 77 features and 142 trained subcategories. These subcategories are grouped into 28 categories.

The expanded subsystem includes the major ways that a patient can present: as CHF or pneumonia with rales, as ischemic heart disease with chest pain, as an abnormality on chest X-ray such as cardiomegaly, alveolar infiltrate, a pleural effusion, or a pulmonary nodule.

9. CREATING COMPLEX CLASSES THROUGH CLONING

It is not practical to anticipate or store the SSCPDF's for all possible complex subclasses; and for this reason a system build on Patrick's theorem rather than Bayes theorem is desired (see Appendix B). For example we may wish to create a complex of a subcategory CHF with a subcategory of pulmonary infiltrate due to a collagen vascular disease. Another example is that we might want to create a complex of a subcategory RHF associated with mitral stenosis 'AND' a subcategory Permeability Pulmonary Edema caused by aspirin ingestion. This is illustrated in Section 10.

The desirability to create such complex subclasses is discovered while using the Consult^R instrument in actual practice. One simply finds that when such a complex is discovered in clinical practice it is desirable to preserve and store the clinical presentation concerned. This storage can be as a new subcategory in the Consult-I^R module or as a training example in CLS. In either situation the existence of this case in storage can assist a later diagnosis or IOA for a prospective patient, possibly by a different physician.

10. USING CONSULT^R

When the findings are directed into Consult-I^R, the CCPDF is evaluated at the findings for the category as the **fuzzy set maximum** over the SCCPDF's at the findings for that category (see Appendix A). Then the ranked **a posteriori probabilities or likelihoods** of the categories are displayed. This can be followed by a ranking of the subcategories within each category.

Alternatively, the findings can be directed into the CLS module for ranked decisions based on hard data. The method of computing a posteriori probability densities is that of local probability density estimation as previously described. In effect, the "cluster potential" for each category is evaluated at the findings.

Finally, the findings can be directed to the integration of the two modules where CCPDF's are computed using both the Consult-I^R expert knowledge clusters and the CLS hard data lusters. This indeed is the true spirit of SPR.

When the findings are directed into the Consult-I^R module, CQI results when the system suggests those feature values significant for the leading categories which are not in the current findings. The user then can affect the process immediately by soliciting the new findings and appending them to the old findings for a new decision.

The CLS module when trained is able to perform both outcome analysis (OA) and Individualized Outcome Analysis^{tm} (IOA). For OA, the system can compute p(B|A) for any outcome event B and condition event A; and these events can be defined as the 'AND' of any of the features with the internal 'OR' of any of the feature values. IOA results because the system can perform a similar computation for any new findings A not stored as the training.

CLS implements the Leave-one-out decision rule (Patrick 1972 [5]) which allows CLS to perform self evaluation of its ability to separate categories and subcategories in hyperspace.

Table 1: Categories and Subcategories - Preliminary

I LVF (Left Ventricular Failure) or Systolic Failure
- Hypertension
- Coronary artery disease - ischemia or MI
- Aortic stenosis - volume pressure overload
- Mitral regurgitation - volume pressure overload
- Dilated (congestive) cardiomyopathy
- Acute Aortic Regurgitation
- Chronic Aortic Regurgitation

II RVF (Right Ventricular Failure) or Diastolic Dysfunction
- Pulmonary artery hypertension
- Mitral stenosis
- Tricuspid valve disease
- Cardiomyopathy - restrictive
- Cardiomyopathy - infiltrative
- Myocarditis - viral or idiopathic
- Congenital heart disease (CHD) Secondary to LHF
- Hypertropic cardiomyopathy
- Acute pericarditis
- Constrictive pericardial disease

III LVF + RVF (Left Ventricular Failure & Right Ventricular Failure)
- LVF + RVF

IV Elevated Cardiac Output
- Hyperthyroidism
- Septic shock - early
- Septic shock - late
- Arteriovenous fistula
- Paget's disease

V Non Heart Failure Edema
- COPD
- Ascites
- Pulmonary emboli

VI Permeability Pulmonary Edema - ARDS
- Pulmonary edema, drug
- Permeability pulmonary edema - drowning

VII Normal
- Normal subcategory

Table 2: Features - Preliminary (tp is type)

tp	#	
0	1	Edema in the lungs - rales 1 Yes 2 No
0	2	Edema dependent areas - feet, ankles, pretibial 1 Yes 2 No
1	3	Sensation of shortness of breath (SOB) 1 Can be flat without sensation of SOB 2 When upright - dyspnea 3 Exertional 4 When supine - dyspnea 5 When recumbent - rapid onset: orthopnea 6 Paroxysmal nocturnal dyspnea
0	4	Ascites 1 Yes 2 No
1	5	Onset 1 Gradual 2 12-72 hours after an injury 3 After discontinuation of medication - diuretic 4 After increased sodium ingestion 5 After physical exertion 6 Sudden
0	6	Blood pressure (relative to patient's baseline) 1 Increased 2 Normal 3 Decreased
0	7	Temperature 1 Increased 2 Normal 3 Decreased
0	8	Tachycardia out of proportion to temperature elevation 1 Yes 2 No

0 9 Respiration
- 1 Normal
- 2 Tachypnea
- 3 Cheyne - Stokes

0 10 Pulmonary edema fluid
- 1 None detected
- 2 Rusty tinged or brownish sputum
- 3 Frothy, pink sputum
- 4 Edema fluid-to-plasma ratio of total protein > 0.6

1 11 Symptoms
- 1 Chest pain
- 2 Palpitations
- 3 Syncope
- 4 Myalgia and rigors
- 5 Dysphagia
- 6 Nocturia
- 7 Abdominal discomfort
- 8 Anorexia
- 9 Chronic productive cough

1 12 Signs
- 1 Cyanosis
- 2 Diaphoresis
- 3 Systolic murmur
- 4 Diastolic murmur
- 5 Holosystolic murmur
- 6 S3 or S4 heart sound
- 7 Pulsas alterans (alternating weak or strong pulse)
- 8 Jugular venous distension (JVD)
- 9 Hepatic tenderness and/or enlargement
- 10 Pulsatile liver
- 11 Pericardial friction rub
- 12 Confusion
- 13 Agitation
- 14 Abdominal percussion - shifting dullness; fluid wave

1 13 Heart Sounds
- 1 Increase in the normal splitting of two components of S2
- 2 Pulmonary ejection click
- 3 Early diastolic blow left 2nd, 3rd space (Graham-Steel)
- 4 Mid diastolic rumble (Austin-Flint murmur)

1 14 Drug History
- 1 Beta-adrenergic antagonist
- 2 Calcium channel antagonist
- 3 Heroin abuse
- 4 Methadone
- 5 Paraquat
- 6 Ethchlorvynol
- 7 Aspirin

1 15 Injury or suspected associated condition
- 1 Liquid aspiration: gastric, fresh water, salt water
- 2 Inhalation: smoke, corrosive, (CL2,NH3, SO2, NO2, Phosgene)
- 3 Bacterial shock
- 4 Other shock
- 5 Bacterial or viral pneumonia
- 6 History of recent chest trauma
- 7 Pulmonary thromboembolism
- 8 Disseminated intravascular coagulation
- 9 Thrombotic thrombocytopenic purpura
- 10 Pulmonary contusion
- 11 Multiple transfusions
- 12 Eclampsia
- 13 Reexpansion of collapsed lung
- 14 Tumor lysis
- 15 Radiation

1 16 Other condition
- 1 Hyperthyroidism
- 2 Coronary artery disease
- 3 Aortic valve disease
- 4 Mitral valve disease
- 5 Tricuspid valve disease
- 6 Family history of sudden cardiac death
- 7 Arteriovenous fistula
- 8 Paget's disease
- 9 Nephrotic syndrome
- 10 Inferior vena cava obstruction
- 11 Mesenteric or hepatic venous obstruction
- 12 Nephrotic syndrome
- 13 Alcoholism
- 14 Chronic active hepatitis

```
1   17 Electrocardiogram
       1 Atrial fibrillation
       2 Nonspecific ST/T changes
       3 Acute myocardial ischemia
       4 Acute myocardial infarction
       5 Left ventricular hypertrophy
       6 Left atrial enlargement
       7 Poor R wave progression
       8 Right ventricular hypertrophy

1   18 Chest X-ray
       1 Patchy alveolar infiltrate
       2 Alveolar infiltrate in butterfly pattern
       3 Enlarged cardiac silhouette
       4 Biventricular enlargement
       5 Pulmonary venous hypertension: enlarged hila
       6 Pulmonary venous hypertension: "cephalization of
         flow"
       7 Straightening of left heart boarder
       8 Kerley B lines at the bases
       9 Hyperinflation

1   19 Echocardiography
       1 Decreased ejection fraction
       2 Increased systolic volume
       3 Increased diastolic volume
       4 Ventricular enlargement
       5 Atrial enlargement
       6 Septal hypertrophy
       7 Reduced LV end-diastolic dimensions
       8 Systolic anterior motion of the mitral valve
       9 Pericardial effusion

1   20 Laboratory
       1 SGOT increased
       2 Prothrombin time increased
       3 Abdominal ultrasound: fluid
       4 Serum albumin decreased

0   21 PAWP
       1 < 12
       2 12 - 18
       3 19 - 25
       4 > 25
```

0 22 Blood gases
1 PaO2 significantly decreased for the patient
2 Respiratory alkalosis
3 Metabolic alkalosis
4 Respiratory acidosis
5 Metabolic acidosis

Table 3: Consult Parameters for CHF Subsystem - Preliminary

It was reasonable to develop the first version of Consult for CHF with the following parameters:

Maximum # of categories -	Mmax	= 20
# of categories used -	M	= 7
Maximum # of subcategories per category -	K	= 15
Maximum # of features -	L	= 30
Number of features used -	F	= 22
Maximum # of records in CLS	n	--

As clinical experience was gained with the CHF subsystem, it was integrated into a more general subsystem called CHEST. In this CHEST subsystem there were 28 categories with a total number of trained subcategories equal 142:

Table 4: Consult Parameters for CHEST Subsystem

The expanded CHEST subsystem has the following parameters:

Maximum # of categories -	Mmax	= 35
# of categories used -	M	= 28
Maximum # of subcategories per category -	K	= 15
# of subcategories trained		**= 142**
Maximum # of features -	L	= 80
Number of features used -	F	= 77
Maximum # of records in CLS	n	--

This is the subsystem used to process an actual patient as illustrations in what follows. When a new subcategory is created through cloning, the number (which would appear above) of trained subcategories increases.

11. ILLUSTRATIONS

A series of illustrations using the Consult^R instrument will demonstrate much of what has been discussed. The illustrations are for a patient **who presented with the following findings the first time he was seen in the Emergency Department:**

```
1  AGE
 4  51 - 60 YEARS
2  2 TEMPERATURE: 3 PULSE: 4 BLOOD PRESSURE: 5 SEX
 3  Normal
3  PULSE
 2  Normal
4  BLOOD PRESSURE
 2  Normal
33 HEART & LUNG SOUNDS
 10 Diastolic murmur (including Austin Flint & Grahm Steel)        T
36 CARDIOPULMONARY SIGNS
 1  Edema ( feet, ankles, pretibial )                               T
 6  Hepatomegaly                                                    T
 8  JV Distension                                                   T
43 Cardiopulmonary History
 2  Mitral valve disease                                            T


        Do you want to make inferences using these Findings: Y(Yes), N(No)
```

Figure 1: Findings

The Consult-I^R differential diagnosis, which follows, shows the highest ranked diagnosis in the differential is Right Ventricular Failure - Diastolic failure. The significant feature values are diastolic murmur, edema (peripheral), hepatomegaly, JV distension, and a history of mitral valve disease. Physicians would not have difficulty recognizing this as CHF; but they may not recognize it specifically as RHF. This is one of the first advantages of using Consult^R. Rather than store the case, we proceed directly to rank the subcategories of the leading category.

Do you want to store this decision as a permanent record (Y/N)?

E : a posteriori probabilities with Equal priors
L : Likelihoods (normalized)
U : A posteriori probabilities with Unequal a priori probabilities

Category Aposteriori probabilities - equal priors:
Top 10 Categories

Category	Probability
3 RVF - Diastolic Failure	0.205916
16 LVF (Left Ventricular Failure) - Systolic Failure	0.102958
2 CARDIAC CHEST PAIN	0.098416
5 VALVULAR HEART DISEASE	0.051479
14 FUNGAL PNEUMONIA	0.042178
7 OBSTRUCTIVE PULMONARY DISEASE	0.033310
11 MUSCULOSKELETAL CHEST PAIN or PSYCHIATRIC CHEST PAIN	0.033310
18 TRANSUDATIVE PLEURAL EFFUSION - NON CHF	0.033310
22 PULMONARY NODULE: CHEST WALL, PLEURAL, VASCULAR	0.031796
20 PULMONARY NODULE - NON NEOPLASTIC	0.031147

Figure 2: Consult-I[R]'s Ranked Differential Diagnosis

The subcategories of this category, Right Heart Failure (RHF), are ranked within a **subsubsystem** (subsystem within the subsystem). This ranking, output from the Consult[R] instrument, provides (with RVF, Mitral Stenosis) as leading subcategory:

Category: 3 RVF - Diastolic Failure

Subcategory:

Subcategory	Probability
9 RVF, Mitral Stenosis	.5390285
1 RVF Secondary to LVF	.1179125
8 RVF, Cor Pulmonale / Pulmonary Hypertension	.1105429
2 RVF, Hypertropic cardiomyopathy	6.737856E-02
6 RVF, Restrictive cardiomyopathy	6.737856E-02
3 RVF, Myocarditis - viral or idiopathic	5.143631E-02
4 RVF, Acute Pericarditis	4.632275E-02

Press Return

Figure 3: Ranked Subcategories (clusters) for Leading Category

This shows that the leading subcategory (cluster) corresponds to Right Heart Failure associated with Mitral Stenosis. Next, **the same patient several months later presented with modified findings as shown in Figures 4 and 5 which follow:**

```
1  AGE
 4  51 - 60 YEARS
2  2 TEMPERATURE: 3 PULSE: 4 BLOOD PRESSURE: 5 SEX
 2  Increased but <= 106
3  PULSE
 1  Tachycardia
6  RESPIRATORY PATTERN
 1  Tachypnea
 2  Kussmual Respiration (rapid deep respiration)
7  ACID BASE (quick entry)
 4  Respiratory Alkalosis                                        T
13 LEVEL OF CONSCIOUSNESS
 2  Confused
33 HEART & LUNG SOUNDS
 1  Rales ( Crackles )                                           T
36 CARDIOPULMONARY SIGNS
 1  Edema ( feet, ankles, pretibial )                            T
 6  Hepatomegaly                                                 T
43 Cardiopulmonary History
                    Press RETURN key to continue
```

Figure 4 Findings for Second Presentation of Same Patient

```
 2  Mitral valve disease                                         T
50 DRUGS
 5  ASA                                                          T




        Do you want to make inferences using these Findings: Y(Yes), N(No)
```

Figure 5 Findings Continued

When these new findings are entered into the Consult[R] instrument, a new differential diagnosis for the patient shows categories 17 and 13 respectively as the leading categories:

```
                    Consult-I POST DECISION MENU
Program 7b          Subsystem:CHEST   .
 O : Observe Leading Subcategories &/OR Their Strategies (Actions) (9)
 E : Explanation of Category & Subcategory Decisions & Quality Assurance (8)
 I : Input Findings - Consult (6)           P : Print differential decisions
 R : Rerun - Pre Decision Menu (7)          S : Store Findings Menu (10)
 M : Main Consult menu                      T : Train with this Test Case
                                                            Select option
   Category          Aposteriori probabilities - equal priors:
 Top  10  Categories

17 PERMEABILITY PULMONARY EDEMA - ARDS                                0.586165
13 ATYPICAL PNEUMONIA                                                 0.044340
21 PULMONARY NODULE - NEOPLASTIC                                      0.040492
3  RVF - Diastolic Failure                                            0.032779
12 BACTERIAL PNEUMONIA                                                0.032779
20 Elevated Cardiac Output                                            0.032779
19 EXUDATIVE PLEURAL EFFUSION ( NON PNEUMONIA & NON NEOPLA            0.028923
20 PULMONARY NODULE - NON NEOPLASTIC                                  0.023130
14 FUNGAL PNEUMONIA                                                   0.021692
16 LVF (Left Ventricular Failure) - Systolic Failure                  0.021210
```

Figure 6: Differential Diagnosis for Second Presentation of Same Patient

Now, at the time of the second presentation, the patient has a leading diagnosis of Permeability Pulmonary Edema - ARDS. When the Consult instrument is asked to rank the subcategories within this category, **ARDS secondary to aspirin ingestion** is the leading subcategory of the leading category. It turns out that this indeed is the correct diagnosis.

But what happened to the diagnosis of RVF which was present at the time the patient was first seen? Is it possible it is still present?

```
  Category: 17
PERMEABILITY PULMONARY EDEMA - ARDS
  Subcategory:
 11  Salicylate-induced Noncardiogenic Pulmonary Edema          .8172043
 8   ARDS FOLLOWING SEPSIS SYNDROME                             9.139787E-02
 9   ARDS - O2 TOXICITY, PANCREATITIS, ASPIRATION, BURN, FAT E 4.569894E-02
 1   PUL. EDEMA, DRUG: HEROIN, METHADONE, ASA, PARAQUAT, ETHCH 1.142473E-02
 2   PERMEABILITY PULMONARY EDEMA - DROWNING                    5.712367E-03
 3   PUL. EDEMA, INHALATION: SMOKE, CL2, NH3, SO2, NO2, PHOSGE 5.712367E-03
 4   PUL. EDEMA: HIGH ALTITUDE                                  5.712367E-03
 5   PUL. EDEMA: ECLAMPSIA                                      5.712367E-03
 6   PUL. EDEMA: HEAD TRAUMA, MULTIPLE TRAUMA, PULMONARY CONTU 5.712367E-03
 7   PUL. EDEMA: MULTIPLE TRANSFUSIONS                          5.712367E-03




        Press Return
```

Figure 7: Leading Subcategory for Second Presentation

We have withheld from Consult^R those findings reflecting the patient's chronic Right Heart Failure (features 31,35,8,62). Now we add these earlier findings to the new findings to obtain the more nearly complete set of findings shown below:

```
 1  AGE
  4  51 - 60 YEARS
 2  2 TEMPERATURE: 3 PULSE: 4 BLOOD PRESSURE: 5 SEX
  2  Increased but <= 106
 3  PULSE
  1  Tachycardia
 6  RESPIRATORY PATTERN
  1  Tachypnea
  2  Kussmual Respiration (rapid deep respiration)
 7  ACID BASE (quick entry)
  4  Respiratory Alkalosis                                           T
 13 LEVEL OF CONSCIOUSNESS
  2  Confused
 31 SPECIFIC EKG CHANGES & ARRHYTHMIAS
  18 P pulmonale                                                     T
 33 HEART & LUNG SOUNDS
  1  Rales ( Crackles )                                              T
  10 Diastolic murmur (including Austin Flint & Grahm Steel)         T
 35 CARDIOPULMONARY SYMPTOMS
                    Press RETURN key to continue
```

Figure 8: Findings for Second Presentation

```
 5  Dyspnea at Rest                                                   T
 6  Exertional Dyspnea                                                T
36 CARDIOPULMONARY SIGNS
 1  Edema ( feet, ankles, pretibial )                                 T
 6  Hepatomegaly                                                      T
 8  JV Distension                                                     T
43 Cardiopulmonary History
 2  Mitral valve disease                                              T
50 DRUGS
 5  ASA                                                               T
62 Chest X-ray: Other
 8  Straightening of left heart boarder - left atrial hypertrophy     T


        Do you want to make inferences using these Findings: Y(Yes), N(No)
```

Figure 9: Second Set of Findings Continued

Entry of this set of findings into Consult-I^R results in the differential diagnosis,

```
    Do you want to store this decision as a permanent record (Y/N)?

    E : a posteriori probabilities with Equal priors
    L : Likelihoods (normalized)
    U : A posteriori probabilities with Unequal a priori probabilities

  Category             Aposteriori probabilities - equal priors:
 Top  10  Categories

17 PERMEABILITY PULMONARY EDEMA - ARDS                          0.294574
3  RVF - Diastolic Failure                                      0.263566
4  PULMONARY EMBOLISM                                           0.055233
20 PULMONARY NODULE - NON NEOPLASTIC                            0.046512
16 LVF (Left Ventricular Failure) - Systolic Failure            0.042636
5  VALVULAR HEART DISEASE                                       0.032946
28 Elevated Cardiac Output                                      0.032946
2  CARDIAC CHEST PAIN                                           0.029070
13 ATYPICAL PNEUMONIA                                           0.022287
14 FUNGAL PNEUMONIA                                             0.021802
```

Figure 10: Differential Diagnosis with Complete Findings which reflects the patient's chronic condition plus the new condition due to aspirin ingestion.

Now the leading two categories are Permeability Pulmonary Edema - ARDS, and RVF - Diastolic Failure. **We ask, could both of these categories be present for the Patient? With a Bayes Theorem framework the answer is "no" because the categories are mutually exclusive in a Bayes framework.**

With a Patrick's Theorem framework these two leading categories are viewed as two categories (only classes) within respective classes, Class 17 and Class 3. Since classes can occur together, it is possible that the intersection of Class 17 AND Class 3 includes a complex class corresponding to RHF associated with mitral stenosis AND Permeability Pulmonary Edema caused by ASA. More precisely there is a complex subcategory of the subcategory 11 of category 17 with subcategory 9 of category 3.

It is reasonable for there to be a complex subcategory because the patient's right heart failure associated with mitral stenosis isn't going to go away just because the patient later takes too much ASA and develops ARDS.

One of the options at the Consult-I^{R} Post Decision Menu is facility to automatically create complex classes or to clone a new subcategory from an existing category and the new findings. We now will illustrate how to form a complex class by selecting the option causing branch to what is called the "cloning menu". There complex classes can be formed with or without supervision:

```
                                  (R)
Program 5              C O N S U L T - I                        CHEST
                      C L O N I N G   M E N U

S : Supervised Training of a Category (cluster modification)
U : Unsupervised Training of a Category (cluster modification)
C : Complex Class from two Existing Categories - Patrick's Theorem

P : Subcategory probabilities (clusters) - Review
R : Ranked Decisions (Categories & Subcategories)
D : Display previous findings
N : Normal Category & Subcategory


M : Main Consult Menu (4)
B : Back to Consult-I Post Decision Menu - Rerun after Training

                                                      Select option
```

Figure 11: Consult-I^{R} Display for Forming a Complex Class

A model, as discussed in Appendix B, can be used to automatically detect a complex class and then form it by Unsupervised Learning type 2. Alternatively, if the user of the Consult^{R} instrument feels that this does indeed represent a complex class, then they can elect to form a new complex subcategory through supervised learning. Still, Patrick's theorem is in effect.

Selecting (C) at the previously displayed menu results in a description of the method of forming a complex class;

and this is followed by options to use either a supervised or unsupervised method. It practice, the experienced user likely will elect to use a supervised option where the user actually is the teacher.

```
A Complex class (category) is about to be created from two existing
categories. These existing categories are now viewed as classes.
Whereas categories are mutually exclusive, classes need not be.
Patrick's theorem provides that existing classes can be combined to
create a complex class which is mutually exclusive of the existing
categories.

The Complex class can be inserted as a cluster in an existing category;
or a new category of Complex Classes can be formatted in the utility. If
that is desired, exit to the Consult Utilities before running this program.

              Previous Test Case Utilized with:

 S : Supervised
 U : Unsupervised (not yet available)
 X : Exit

              Select :
```

Figure 12: Ready to Form a Complex Class with Supervision

We select (S) and then acknowledge the two categories, along with their subcategories, that are to be used to "clone" to produce a complex subclass. **The resulting complex subclass will have significant features which include significant features from class 17 and significant features from class 3**. This is possible because each SSCPDF has both significant and insignificant features; and the insignificant features are facilitated by the Normal category/subcategory defined using insignificant features.

The pair of selected category/subcategories to be used to form a complex subcategory are shown next:

```
The two existing categories, with subcategories, now are specified:


Input # of First Existing Category : 17
Input its Sub Category #: 11

Input # of Second Existing Category : 3
Input its Sub Category #: 9


Input the # of the category to receive the Complex class cluster:
```

Figure 13 Selection of Subcategories to Form Complex Sub categories

The Consult^R instrument asks where the new complex subcategory should be store; and we elect to store it with category 3 at available subcategory slot 12:

```
 3  : RVF - Diastolic Failure
For Category  3  there are  15  Cluster Slots
and  7 are trained; available Slots for the new complex cluster are:

                  Slot:  5
                  Slot:  7
                  Slot:  10
                  Slot:  11
                  Slot:  12
                  Slot:  13
                  Slot:  14
                  Slot:  15

          Input Cluster Slot # for Clone: 12
```

Figure 14: Storing the new complex subclass

We proceed to train by creating and storing the new subcategory:

```
   Feature values in the Findings Direct Combining the significant
   features of the two existing category clusters.

 P : Proceed

 X : Exit

                  Select :

                  Ready to Combine Class: 17 , Subclass  11
                  with Class: 3 , Subclass 9  and place
                  as Category: 3 , Subcategory 12

                  (X) Exit, (T) Train
```

Figure 15: Cloning Ready to Proceed

The new complex subcategory is created and stored as shown below in subcategory slot 12 of the category RVF - Diastolic Failure:

```
Category:                                       Apriori Category Probability:
 3    RVF - Diastolic Failure                                              10

Subcategory:                                 Apriori Subcategory Probability:

 1    RVF Secondary to LVF                                                 10
 2    RVF, Hypertropic cardiomyopathy                                      10
 3    RVF, Myocarditis - viral or idiopathic                               10
 4    RVF, Acute Pericarditis                                              10
 5    RVF, Constrictive pericarditis                                       0
 6    RVF, Restrictive cardiomyopathy                                      10
 7                                                                         0
 8    RVF, Cor Pulmonale / Pulmonary Hypertension                          10
 9    RVF, Mitral Stenosis                                                 10
 10   RVF, Tricuspid valve disease                                         0
 11                                                                        0
 12   Cloned Cat. 17,Sub.: 11 & Cat. 3,Sub.: 9  05-06-1993                 10
 13                                                                        0
 14                                                                        0
 15                                                                        0
(E) Edit Above, (T) Train Subcategory, (X) Exit, Return for next Category
```

Figure 16: Creation and Storage of New Complex Subcategory

This new subcategory now resides within Consult-I^R; and this experience can be used to recognize the next patient who presents with a similar complex of findings. If the findings now are entered into the Consult^R instrument which has been updated by the new subcategory, we expect that the findings will be "closer" to the new complex subcategory than any other subcategory. The findings were again processed and category 3 was the highest ranked category; and as expected, the highest ranked subcategory indeed is the new complex subcategory:

```
 Category: 3  RVF - Diastolic Failure

 Subcategory:
12  Cloned Cat. 17,Sub.: 11 & Cat. 3,Sub.: 9  05-06-1993      .986353
 9  RVF, Mitral Stenosis                                      .0103977
 8  RVF, Cor Pulmonale / Pulmonary Hypertension               9.747842E-04
 3  RVF, Myocarditis - viral or idiopathic                    6.49856E-04
 4  RVF, Acute Pericarditis                                   6.49856E-04
 1  RVF Secondary to LVF                                      3.24928E-04
 2  RVF, Hypertropic cardiomyopathy                           3.24928E-04
 6  RVF, Restrictive cardiomyopathy                           3.24928E-04




          Press Return
```

Figure 17: Consult-I^R Ranks Complex Subcategory Highest

The two (E=2) successive presentations for the patient represent a **process** over time as previously discussed. At each presentation the patient's findings and differential diagnosis can be stored. At the second presentation, the formation of a complex class causes a change in category space through the creation of a new subcategory through **concept formation.**

Clearly the discovery of processes using the Consult^R instrument can become more and more complex depending on the objectives.

Appendix A

A. KNOWLEDGE BASE STRUCTURE IN CONSULT-I^R and CLS

A.1. Categories, Subcategories, Features and Feature Values

Categories, subcategories and features form the basis for a knowledge base structure as follows:

$$\textit{Categories}: \tau_i,\ i=1,2,\ldots,M$$

$$\textit{Subcategories}: \tau_{ik},\ \begin{matrix} i=1,2,\ldots,I; \\ k=1,2,\ldots,V \end{matrix}$$

But the feature values are random variables and described by a multidimensional subcategory conditional probability density function (SCCPDF). Thus there are many possible patterns for each subcategory; and a particular pattern occurs with probability prescribed by the SCCPDF.

A.2. Subcategory Conditional Probability Density Function

$$\textit{sccpdf.}: p(\underline{x} \mid \tau_{ik})$$

The SCCPDF is said to belong to a family of functions, each member of the family having the same structure and characterized by a set of fixed but unknown parameters, $\underline{b}_{ik}$. A family of functions which is quite general, and distribution free, is the multinomial family. Each point in the feature space, whether candidate sample or training record, is in the domain of each SCCPDF. A set of regions or "bins" can be constructed as mutually exclusive combinations of the feature values. The union of these regions or "bins" form a cover in the mathematical sense. For each bin (i.e. in each bin) is a probability p indexed by the L feature values. If there are L features and each feature has V values, then there R^V bin probabilities, in general a prohibitive number. We certainly are not proposing to estimate all these bin probabilities.

A.3. Patterns as Rules

Each pattern $\underline{x}$ "falls" in one of the previously described bins and can be thought of as a rule in the sense of a rule-based expert system. But the design objective for Consult-I^R and CLS is a classification system(s) or outcome predicting system(s) with a probabilistic foundation. This design objective is not achieved by rule-based systems.

Rule-based expert systems can be thought of as constructing "pointers" to the bins in our knowledge base construction for the purpose of search or deterministic classification. A rule-base system, if modified to grasp the statistical nature of the classification problem, would have to utilize the structures just discussed.

Patterns in effect are examples of rules used to estimate the parameters characterizing the SCCPDF's.

A.4. Neural Net Structure

Neural nets utilize parametric structures; and the parameters include the weights (connecting the nodes) which are estimated from the training examples. Neural net structures provide another method for engineering SCCPDF's. The weights and links between layers provide a mathematical structure, such as a three layer network where nodes in the middle layer correspond to SCCPDF's and nodes in the output layer correspond to CCPDF's.

Using a little ingenuity, it can be shown why <u>CLS is not a conventional three layer neural net</u>. Let there be a single node in the middle layer for the single cluster to be estimated. Each of the n training records can be thought of as a link between the findings (first layer) and this middle layer node. The weight of the link is the "correlation" between the findings and the training record concerned. With this view, the number of links between the first layer and the node in the middle layer grows with n.

On the other hand, CLS can be implemented as a new neural net structure (Patrick 1990) which is different from classical neural nets. What is different about the CLS neural net is that the training samples are themselves part of the new, unique neural net structure.

A.5. Category: Union of Subcategories

In Consult-I^R, the multidimensional statistical dependencies among features is intentionally limited in constructing the SCCPDF. The design objective is to achieve extensive multidimensional statistical dependency among the features through the construction of the CCPDF - it is made a mixture or fusion of SCCPDF's.

There are several advantages to keeping the structure of the SCCPDF simplistic:

(1) ease of user training with expert knowledge.
(2) allows a more nearly distribution free representation for the CCPDF.
(3) statistical dependencies can be achieved by increasing the number of subcategories.
(4) affords a particular advantage for implementing Patrick's theorem to *clone* subcategories thus producing complex subclasses or complex classes.

With this model, the features of the SCCPDF are statistically independent:

$$p(x|\tau_{ik},b_{ik}) = \prod_{j=1}^{L} p(x_j|\tau_{ik},b_{ikj}) * P_{ik} \qquad (5)$$

$$k=1,2,\ldots,K_i$$

Thus the CCPDF is constructed as a function of these subcategory condition probability density functions. One such function used in Consult-I^R is as follows:

$$p(x|\tau_i,b_i) = \underset{k}{Max}\{\prod_{j=1}^{L} p(x_j|\tau_{ik},b_{ikj})\}. \qquad (5)$$

This function for the CCPDF has statistically dependent features even though the individual sccpdf's on the right hand side have statistically independent features.

A.6. Concept of a Column or Fuzzy Rule

In practice and during training, the expression in Eq. 1a is viewed as a "column" because it is stored as a column of rows of numbers. Each row is a set of up to L probabilities, one probability for each feature value. The practical interpretation of a column is that it is a cluster of presentations (subcategory) of a category; and there can be as many clusters as needed. The column contains a rule-like structure, IF_ AND IF_ ....AND IF_ THEN_; but more generally, it is a fuzzy rule because the _ is selected from a row with probabilities.

A.7. Type 0 and Type 1 Features

Two fundamental types of features used in Consult-I^R and CLS are now described. A type 0 feature has values which are mutually exclusive. A pattern can have only one value of a type 0 feature. The set of values with the corresponding set of probabilities for a type 0 feature is a fuzzy set. A type 1 feature is a set of V binary features with values of T (true or 1) and F (false or 2). Each pattern has a value for each feature in a Type 1 feature. Various operations are possible with respect to the embedded features in a Type 1 feature; for example, at decision making time when multiple embedded features in a type 1 feature are provided feature values, the maximum probability for these selected features can be taken (a type 3 feature).

A.8. Unavailable Feature Value vs. Missing Feature

If a pattern were observed and one or more of the features are without specified feature values, these are referred to as *unavailable feature values*. Patterns with unavailable feature values usually arise in training examples for CLS and not in Consult-I^R.

On the other hand, at decision making time when a vector $\underline{x}$ is presented for decision making, certain of its V feature values may not be specified. These features are referred to as *missing* features.

Thus missing features are a property of the findings to be recognized while unavailable feature values are a property of training samples.

APPENDIX B. DECISION MAKING AND UNSUPERVISED LEARNING

B.1. Introduction

Bayes theorem is very well known but often misunderstood. It is valuable as the inspiration for learning in SPR but its structure is incomplete. Bayes theorem (Patrick 1972,1979,1986,1990) is incomplete because it simply relates the a posteriori probability of an event B to the a priori probability of event B after given another event A (a condition):

$$p(B|A) = p(A|B)*p(B) / p(A)$$

This iterative relationship inspires many methods in SPR such as *reproducing probability density functions*, the *iterative estimation of parameters*, *a posteriori decisions* vs *maximum likelihood decisions*, and even *local probability density estimation at a focus*.

Another horizon that Bayes theorem provides is that of *relativity*: when M mutually exclusive and exhaustive events B_i, i=1,2,....,M, are defined in a decision space, and the a posteriori probabilities of each event is calculated given the condition A, the ranked a posteriori probabilities are *relative* to each other. This suggests that decision making is "relative". It is relative to the specific categories in the decision space.

Bayes theorem does not provide the methods and structure for learning $p(A|B_i)$, which incites the CCPDF. Another limitation of Bayes theorem is that it requires that the events B_i be mutually exclusive.

In the 1960's Patrick developed SPR methods as extensions of Bayes theorem, which includes methods for engineering the CCPDF's. Discussions in references (Patrick) concern engineering of CCPDF's and SSCPDF's. Parameters characterizing these functions can be estimated by recursive formulas.

In the 1980's a new theorem named *Patrick's theorem* by Fattu, was formulated where, like in Bayes theorem, there are mutually exclusive *categories* but also there are *classes* which need not be mutually exclusive. The structure of the theorem provides for important processes such as *cloning* existing categories with the findings to produce a new category called a *complex class*. Cloning is discussed in more detail later in Section B.10.

B.2. Bayes Theorem

Two fundamental approaches to probability theory are the *classical probability approach theory* and the *relative frequency approach*. The classical approach is based in part on set theory, a review of which may be helpful. For our purposes we proceed as follows:

Let

$$B_1, B_2, \ldots, B_M \qquad (1)$$

be M mutually exclusive and exhaustive sets, and A another set. Applying the three axioms of probability theory [3], we obtain

$$p(B_i|A) = \frac{p(A|B_i) * p(B_i)}{\sum_{i=1}^{M} p(A|B_i) * p(B_i)}, i=1,2,\ldots,M \qquad (2)$$

The feature values of the selected *category feature* defines the categories or classes. Since a Type 1 feature can have multiple values (classes), it can be used in CLS to define a *complex class* - a category with multiple classes active at the same time. For example, the category feature may deal with complications taken one at a time; and multiple complications (two complications at a time) is a complex class.

B.3. Bayes Framework used in Consult-I^R

For Consult-I^R, Eq. 2 applies where the event A is the findings $\underline{x}$, and events B_i are the categories. The expression in the numerator of the right hand side of Eq. 2 is the CCPDF multiplied by the a priori category probability; and the term in the denominator of the right hand side of Eq. 2 is the total probability (i.e., the sum of terms in the numerator). The CCPDF is further engineered using the SCCPDF's. The terms $p(B_i)$ are *a priori category probabilities* and the left hand side of Eq. 2 defines *a posteriori category probability*. No learning from examples is provided at this point.

B.4. Modification of Bayes Framework to Incorporate Learning

The ith CCPDF is said to be from a family of functions characterized by a set of *fixed but unknown parameters*, $\underline{b}_i$; and each CCPDF is denoted

$$p(x|\tau_i, b_i).$$

Given supervised training samples from the ith category,

$$\underline{X}n_i = \{\underline{x}_i\},\ i=1,2,\ldots,n_i,$$

an iterative expression for the fixed but unknown parameters is

$$p(b_i|Xn_i,\tau_i) = \frac{p(x|\tau_i,b_i)*p(b_i|X(n-1)_i,\tau_i)}{\int[\text{numerator}]\,db_i}. \qquad (3)$$

This is the iterative learning equation for learning the fixed but unknown parameters characterizing the CCPDF. It further can be shown that

$$p(x|\tau_i) = \int p(x|\tau_i, b_i) * (b_i|Xn_i)\, db_i. \qquad (4)$$

B.5. Bayes Framework Applied to CLS

Equation 2 for Bayes Theorem also applies to CLS, but there are important differences between Consult-I^R and CLS. CLS has two modes of operation - the *inference mode* and the *classification mode* or *multiple category mode*. The classification mode of CLS is devised to be compatible with Consult-I^R. The inference mode is discussed next.

B.6. Inference Mode in CLS

In the inference mode, the user defines an *outcome event* B as a logical 'AND' of any of the features, and within each feature a logical 'OR' of any of its feature values. A *condition event* A is defined in a similar way. Then, utilizing training samples, the CLS computes

$$p(B|A) = \frac{p(A,B)}{p(A)} = \frac{p(A|B)\,p(B)}{p(A)}. \qquad (5)$$

Use of training samples $\underline{X}_n$ is made explicit by rewriting Eq. 5 as follows:

$$p(B|A,X_n) = \frac{p(B,A|X_n)}{p(A|X_n)}. \qquad (6)$$

Definition of events A and B dictate that (B,A)+($\bar{B}$,A) equals the entire feature space; and Eq. 6 defines a *reproducing binomial probability density with central limit theorem properties*.

B.7. SPR Option - __New Definition of Relative Frequency__

A new development, first published in 1986 (Patrick, Fattu [7]) is an outgrowth of the *Patrick-Fischer generalized k-nearest neighbor rule* and is a significant departure from the classical implementation of Eq. 6. In this new approach events A, B and (A,B) are defined just as before. Event A is considered a focus $\underline{x}$ and the n training samples, now called *candidate samples* $\underline{x}_c$ (which satisfy event B) are "brought to the *focus*.

With classical statistics (classical option in CLS), a candidate sample $\underline{x}_c$ contributes a relative frequency of 1 if it is at the focus and relative frequency of 0 if not at the focus; there is no in-between. With the SPR option in CLS, probability density estimated in lower dimensional space of dimension d (d<L) provides the *probability that the sample "could have been at the focus.* This is represented mathematically by the following equations:

$$p(A,B|X_n) = \frac{1}{n}\sum_{c=1}^{n} p^d(x,x_c,B) \qquad (7a)$$

$$p(A|X_n) = \frac{1}{n}\sum_{c=1}^{n} p^d(x,x_c) \qquad (7b)$$

The SPR option is selected at decision making time to utilize this method.

B.8. Decision Making Mode for CLS

CLS has a *classification mode* whereby any feature can be used as a category feature which means that the feature values of that feature index categories in the category space. The remaining features are used to describe the findings A. In this mode there is not just outcome pair

$$B, \overline{B} \ ,$$

but there are M mutually exclusive outcomes (where M is the number of feature values),

$$B_i, \ i=1,2,\ldots,M.$$

Because the outcomes must be mutually exclusive, features selected as category features "usually" are type 0 features. Alternatively, an advanced procedure in CLS allows selection of type 1 features as category features where mutually exclusive complex classes are constructed from the feature values. This involves the use of Patrick's Theorem and the feature values are called classes. An *only-class*, a category, is the event of a single class. A *complex class*, also a category, is the event of any two classes together; these complex classes are mutually exclusive of only-classes. In this way categories are constructed from the values of a type 1 feature which are mutually exclusive.

Similar to Eq. 6, the a posteriori probability for the M categories, when in the decision making mode, is

$$p(B_i|A,X_n) = \frac{p(A|X_n,B_i) * p(B_i)}{p(A|X_n)}, \qquad A=X. \qquad (8)$$

B.9. Classification Mode for CLS with SPR Option

Just as was done for the inference mode, an alternative to the classical approach to statistics in the classification mode is the *SPR option* whereby candidate samples are brought to the focus using estimated probability densities in lower dimensional spaces. In this mode,

$$p(B_i|x,X_n) = \frac{p(x|B_i,X_n) * p(B_i)}{\sum_{i=1}^{M} [numerator_{\ i}]} \qquad (9a)$$

where

$$p(x|B_i,X_n) = (\frac{1}{n}) \sum_{c=1}^{n} p^d(x,x_c|B_i) \qquad (9b)$$

B.10. Patrick's Theorem

B.10.1. Introduction

By the nature of the model used in deriving Bayes Theorem, categories are mutually exclusive. Thus when ranked a posteriori probabilities are provided as output by Consult-I^R, only one of these categories is the true category. The ranked a posteriori probabilities are the probabilities that the respective categories are the *true category*.

Replace the word category with the word class for sake of discussion in the rest of this section. In practice, one is tempted to take, for example, the leading two a posteriori classes as two classes active at the same time; and indeed in some cases that is the true situation. We refer to these two classes active at the same time as a complex class. In the framework of Patrick's theorem, this *complex class* is a category which is mutually exclusive of only one class (a category) or only the other class (a category).

We thus refer to these latter categories as *only classes*. Within the framework of Patrick's theorem, classes are not necessarily mutually exclusive while categories are mutually exclusive. In general, complex classes can be formed from only classes or classes by *concept formation*.

The formation of complex classes by concept formation is, in general, a difficult problem in unsupervised learning. The previous example where the leading two classes in Consult's output are taken as a complex class presupposes a model for the complex class as discussed elsewhere (Patrick and Fattu 1986).

When a type 1 feature is used as a category feature in CLS, complex class CCPDF's actually can be learned as dis-

cussed elsewhere (Patrick and Fattu 1986).

B.10.2. Patrick's Theorem and Complex Classes

i. Definitions

In this subsection the following notation is used:

w_i : class

w^*_i : only class (only class w_i) - a category

W^*_{ij} : complex class - a category

ii. Assumptions

Patrick's theorem is presented in detail in Patrick and Fattu 1986 [7] and Patrick 1983 [8]. Herein assumptions are made to specialize the theorem to *cloning* applications. It is assumed that any class is influenced by at most one other class than that class. Accordingly, the relationship between any two classes is as follows:

$$w_i = w^*_i + W^*_{ij} \quad (10.1a)$$

$$w_j = w^*_j + W^*_{ji} \quad (10.1b)$$

The classes are not mutually exclusive while the categories are mutually exclusive.

iii. Significant and Insignificant Features

It is assumed that the features $\underline{x}$ can be divided into a subset $\underline{x}_i$ *significant* for the ith only class and another subset $\underline{x}_j$ *significant* for the jth only class. Also, training is assumed to take place for *only classes* (categories) and not classes.

iv. CCPDF's, ccpdf's, the Normal or Reference Category, and Insignificant Features

The category conditional probability density function

and class conditional probability density function were defined in previous sections. In this section we will incorporate the class probabilities and category probabilities into the definitions for convenience.

A special category called the *Normal* or *Reference* category is defined as that category with *insignificant features*; i.e., the p.d.f. for each feature is uniform or neutral with respect to the other categories. The CCPDF for the normal category over features $\underline{x}$ for category W^*_n is defined,

$$p(\underline{x}, W^*_n) \quad . \qquad (10.2)$$

This function also applies to any subset of features in the feature list.

v. Factoring the CCPDF into significant and insignificant parts

The CCPDF for the only class w^*_i thus can be factored into a *significant part* and an *insignificant part*. Denoting the significant part with the subscript I, we obtain

$$p(\underline{x},w^*_i) = p(\underline{x}_i,w^*_i)*p_I(\underline{x}_j,w^*_i) \qquad (10.3)$$

where the later part of the right hand side is insignificant for the ith only class and

$$\underline{x} = [\underline{x}_i, \underline{x}_j] \ .$$

vi. Deriving the CCPDF for a Complex Class in terms of Trained CCPDF's for Only-classes

It is natural to train only classes and occasionally complex classes; although it is not natural to train classes. Thus we assume that the above expression (10.3) for only class, CCPDF's are available.

Usually it is not practical to provide for all possible complex classes in the rudimentary design of a subsystem; therefore a method is needed, possibly without a teacher, to learn the CCPDF for a complex class from the CCPDF's of only classes and the findings. The method ideally would be suggested when a criteria indicates a complex class is probable.

Applying Eq. 10.1a to the partitioned <u>findings</u> we obtain

$$p(\underline{x}_i, \underline{x}_j, w_i) =$$

$$p(\underline{x}_i, \underline{x}_j, w^*_i) + p(\underline{x}_i, \underline{x}_j, W^*_i) \quad (10.4)$$

and it follows that

$$p(\underline{x}_i, \underline{x}_j, W^*_{ij}) =$$

$$(1/2)*[\ p(\underline{x}_i, \underline{x}_j, w_i) - p(\underline{x}_i, \underline{x}_j, w^*_i) + p(\underline{x}_j, \underline{x}_i, w_j) - p(\underline{x}_j, \underline{x}_i, w^*_j)\ ] \quad (10.5)$$

Next we use the assumption of Eq. 10.3 to obtain

$$p(\underline{x}_i, \underline{x}_j, , w_i) =$$

$$p(\underline{x}_i, w^*_i)*p(\underline{x}_j, w^*_j) + p(\underline{x}_i, w^*_i)*p_I(\underline{x}_j, w^*_j)$$

and a similar expression when i and j are reversed.

Substituting these expressions into Eq. 10.5

$$p(\underline{x}_i, \underline{x}_j, W^*_{ij}) =$$

$$p(\underline{x}_i, w^*_i) * p(\underline{x}_j, w^*_j) \quad (10.6)$$

Thus Eq. 10.6 is the expression for computing the CCPDF for a complex class from the CCPDF's of only classes.

vii. Suspecting a Complex Class

When should Eq. 10.6 be invoked and a complex class probability computed? Suppose that for two only classes i and j the probabilities are 0.5 and 0.5 respectively; it is reasonable to suspect a complex class. From Eq. 10.3, this suggests examination of the only class probabilities,

$$p(\underline{x}, w^*_i) = p(\underline{x}_i, w^*_i)*p_I(\underline{x}_j, w^*_i) > T$$
$$p(\underline{x}, w^*_i) = p(\underline{x}_i, w^*_i)*p_I(\underline{x}_j, w^*_i) > T \quad (10.7)$$

and if greater than some threshold T, then suspect a complex class and compute Ex. 10.6. This process depends on the ability to identify significant and insignificant features for the only classes; and then the complex class must be characterized by the significant features.

viii. Cloning with the Findings to Produce a Complex Class

In practice, on occasion the <u>user may assert</u> that the findings are from a complex class; and in this eventuality it may be desirable to *clone* the complex class from the two highest ranking only classes (or other only classes chosen by the user) and the findings. Compared with the unsupervised creation of a complex class (discussed in the previous section), the cloning is partly supervised.
Eq. 10.6 still applies but the subsets $\underline{x}_i$ and $\underline{x}_j$ would be determined as those which are significant for the two respective only classes. A feature in this context is significant if it is in the findings and significant for the only class. Incidentally, this is the method used in Consult-I^R in the *explanation* of its decisions.

ix. Unsupervised Learning of Complex Subcategories

The same methods previously discussed to create complex classes can be applied to the subcategories of a single category to produce complex subcategories. Creation of a complex subcategory may well make it easier to recognize a category. Likewise, two subcategories can be cloned with the findings to produce a complex subcategory.

B.11. <u>Basic Unsupervised Learning</u> - <u>Bayes</u>

B.11.1 Early History

Unsupervised learning is precisely defined mathematically in Statistical Pattern Recognition for the Bayes framework. As previously discussed, this framework does not provide for multiple classes active at the same time. Patrick and associates defined a group of unsupervised learning problems based on the Bayes framework. We may consider that the problems addressed using cloning and Patrick's theorem provide an extension to this group of problems.

B.11.2 Definition Within Bayes Framework

Unsupervised learning, also called *learning without a teacher*, can be practically stated as follows: suppose you are given n samples of a single random variable. You can construct a histogram to approximate the underlying probability density function of the random variable; but suppose that there are two or more sub populations in this sample. Can you learn the number of sub populations, the sub population relative frequencies, and the individual probability density functions of these sub populations ? The answer is yes; but there is a necessary and sufficient condition (Patrick 1972).

From an engineering standpoint, unsupervised learning was defined and researched in the early 1960's. Patrick preferred to use the phrase *unsupervised estimation* because the problem has its foundation in statistics and feeling that the word "learning" implied something human-like that wasn't really the case. From a practical standpoint, solutions to the unsupervised learning problem can involve *clustering approaches*. In fact the early application of unsupervised estimation or clustering was considered by Pearson in 1894 [17] and 1902 [18]. Pearson "clustered" a species of animals into one category he felt was becoming extinct and another category he felt was going to survive. The application concerned the study of evolution.

B.11.3 Mathematical Notation

A picture, waveform, data, or pattern to be classified is denoted by an L dimensional column vector $\underline{x}$ after *feature extraction*,

$$\underline{x} = [\, x_1, x_2, \ldots\ldots, x_L] \ . \tag{1}$$

A sequence of n vectors or patterns is denoted

$$\underline{x}_n = \{\underline{x}_s\}_{s=1}^{n} \tag{2}$$

The vector $\underline{x}$ has a *probability distribution* $F(\underline{x})$, also called the *mixture probability distribution*. There are M categories $?_i$, i=1,2,...,M and M *category conditional probability distribution functions* (CCPDF's),

$$F(\underline{x}|\tau_i)$$

and M *a priori category probabilities* $P_{\underline{i}}$, also called *mixing* parameters.

The mixture pdf is expressed in terms of CCPDF's and mixing parameters as,

$$F(\underline{x}) = \sum_{i=1}^{M} F(\underline{x} \mid \tau_i) * P_i \qquad (3)$$

The classic problem of unsupervised learning *(ie unsupervised estimation or clustering) is, given the left had side of Eq 3, how do we learn (ie estimate) the number of categories M, their mixing parameters, and the CCPDF's themselves? When is the solution unique?*

B.11.4 Family of CCPDF's and Unsupervised Learning Type I

The classical unsupervised learning problem will be called unsupervised learning Type 1 (USLI); and it is distinguished from the newer form of unsupervised learning Type 2 (USLII) based on Patrick's Theorem.

A necessary and sufficient condition for there to exist an unique solution to USLI is that the family of CCPDF's be linearly independent [5]. This mathematical requirement is translated into the engineering requirement that there must be a sufficient amount of a priori problem knowledge to solve the problem.

In practice we define a family of CCPDF's where the ith CCPDF is characterized by a set of fixed but unknown parameters $\underline{b}_i$:

$$\{F(\underline{x} \mid \tau_i, \underline{b}_i)\}$$

B.11.5 Estimating Parameters in Unsupervised Learning Type 1

An iterative estimator for the fixed but unknown parameters in USLI was discovered by Patrick and Hancock [10]. Patrick defined a class of USLI problems, elaborated on in 1968 [11] and later by Patrick and Liporace, and Patrick and Costello.

The USLI estimator is instructive. An estimator for the set of fixed but unknown parameters illustrates the foundation of the problem in that there is no provision for using knowledge of one category in helping to estimate another category. The learning samples $\underline{x}_s$ are statistically independent and identically distributed according to the mixture CCPDF. As knowledge is learned about the categories in the mixture, there is no provision for learned knowledge of one category to directly help in learning about another category. The structure of each ccpdf is known by definition *of the family.*

In USLI there is no provision for knowledge about one or more categories to help in forming the concept of a new category.

B.11.6 Training to Learn the Clusters

The basic problem of learning the clusters or subcategories of a category is an unsupervised learning problem. That is, where best in feature space should the clusters (subcategories) be placed (and shaped) to represent a category?

Consult^R *can avoid the unsupervised learning type 1 problem by using supervised learning to engineer subcategories of categories. The Outcome Advisor & CLS ingeniously wait for the findings (focus), having stored training samples, and then estimate the CCPDF at the focus. Unsupervised learning or clustering takes place at the focus for these systems but* <u>*it is unnecessary to exhibit or declare the actual clusters*</u>.

B.12 <u>Individualized Diagnosis, Prescription, and Outcome Analysis</u>

B.12.1 Dependent and Independent Events Instead of Just Variables

Independent Event

The CLS module in Consult is not limited to defining a single variable (i.e. feature) as the independent variable. Any subset of the features as a set of multivariables can be defined as a dependent event denoted A.

Dependent Event(s)

The dependent event is either an event B, *defined as 'AND' of any set of features with 'OR' of the feature values; or the dependent event is defined* B_i *- corresponding to the feature values of a* category *feature. The set of* B_i *are called categories.*

The computation of $P(B|A)$ *is defined the* Inference mode *of CLS while ranked computations of* $p(B_i|A)$ *is defined* the classification mode *of CLS.* $p(B_i|A)$ *is an a posteriori probability which involves both the likelihood* $p(A|B_i)$ *of category* B_i *and the a priori category probability* $p(B_i)$. *Ranked classifications of the categories are provided by CLS both as ranked a posteriori probabilities and as ranked likelihoods. Note that a posteriori category probabilities involve the incidence of the category in the population.*

B.12.2 Relationship Between A posterior probability and Likelihood

The relationship between the a posteriori probability $p(B_i|A)$ and the likelihood $p(A|B_i)$ is

$$p(B_i|A) = \frac{p(B_i,A)}{p(A)} = \frac{p(A|B_i)*p(B_i)}{\sum_{j=1,2,\ldots M} [p(A|B_j)*p(B_j)]} \quad (1)$$

$$p(A|B_i) = \frac{p(B_i,A)}{p(B)} \quad (2)$$

It is important to state that the likelihood $p(A|B_i)$ is an expression of how "close" the findings A is to category B_i, as measured by probability, compared with that for other possible A's; and the likelihood is not affected by the a priori category probability or p(A). The likelihood $p(A|B_i)$ measures the relative closeness of each of the specific A relative to the other possible A's for the category B_i. In general the sum total of the likelihoods, summed over the categories, is not one.

Alternatively, a posteriori probability $p(B_i|A)$ compensates for incidence of the category B_i in the population as well as the incidence of the event A in the population (over all the categories). The a posteriori probability $p(B_i|A)$ is a measure of how "close" category B_i is to the findings A. This "closeness measure" is relative - relative to the probabilities for the other categories. This is in contrast with the lack of relativity across categories for the likelihood. For example if A is B_i, a particular category, and $p(A|B_i)$ high for this category, a low a priori category probability $p(B_i)$ can turn this likelihood probability into a low a posteriori probability $p(B_i|A)$ per Eq. 1. The practical upshot of this is that even if A "looks like" category B_i in terms of "closeness" within the category as reflected by the likelihood, A may not be classified as from that category if that category has a relatively low incidence in the population - because the category does not look like A.
Thus A "may not look like" category B_i in that $p(A|B_i)$ is relatively low for that A but not necessarily for other A's; but low incidence of A for the total population over all categories, i.e. low p(A), drives up the a posteriori as per equation 3.1 for a posteriori probability. Put another way, a low $p(A|B_i)$ in this situation 'probably' is because A has low incidence in the population across all the categories,

not just within category B_i.

Ultimately, "closeness" of a category B_i to findings A is defined with relative frequencies of A, B_i, and (A,B_i) at the findings A. But CLS with the SPR option utilizes a new definition of relative frequency to define the closeness measure - a scientific breakthrough.

References

[1] W. Grossman, Diastolic Dysfunction in Congestive Heart Failure, New England Journal of Medicine, ***324** (22), 1991, 1557-1564.*

[2] J.W. Hurst, R.C. Schlant, C.E. Rackley, E.H. Sonnenblock, N.K. and Wenger (1990) The Heart, ***7th Edition**, (McGraw Hill Inc., 1990).*

[3] J.S. Stapczynski J.S. Congestive Heart Failure and Pulmonary Edema, *in J.E. Tintinalli, R.L. Krome, and Ruiz E.:* Emergency Medicine *(McGraw-Hill Inc., **4th edition**, 1992) 216-219.*

[4] Diseases of the Heart and Pericardium - Heart Failure (HF), *in* The Merck Manual, *(**15th Edition** 1987), 415-431.*

[5] E.A. Patrick, Fundamentals of Pattern Recognition, *(Prentice Hall, Englewood Cliffs, N.J. 1972), 504 pages.*

[6] J.R. Ullmann J.R., Pattern Recognition, Nature, *1973, **241**, 219-220.*

[7] E.A. Patrick and J.M. Fattu, Artificial Intelligence with Statistical Pattern Recognition, *(Prentice Hall,1986).*

[8] E.A. Patrick, A Theorem of A posteriori of Events Proceedings, MEDINFO'83 *(1983).*

[9] E.A. Patrick and J.C. Hancock, The Nonsupervised Learning of Probability Spaces and Recognition of Patterns, *in* IEEE Intern. Convention Record, Part II *(1965).*

[10] E.A. Patrick and J.C. Hancock J.C., Nonsupervised Sequential Classification and Recognition of Patterns, IEEE Trans. Information Theory, ***IT-12** (3), (1966), 362-372.*

[11] E.A. Patrick, On a Class of Unsupervised Estimation Problems, IEEE Trans. Information Theory, ***IT-14** (3) (1968), 407-415.*

[12] E.A. Patrick and F.P. Fischer III, Cluster Mapping with experimental Computer Graphics, IEEE Trans. Computers, ***C-18** (11), (1969), 987-991.*

[13] E.A. Patrick and F.P. Fischer III, A Generalized k-Nearest Neighbor Rule, Information and Control, ***16** (2), (1970), 128-152.*

[14] E.A. Patrick, Decision Analysis in Medicine, *(CRC Press, 1979), 340 pages.*

[15] E.A. Patrick, The Outcome Advisor, Pattern Recognition, *(Pergamon Press, 1990), **23** (12).*

[16] *B.V. Dasarathy, Editor,* Nearest Neighbor(NN) Norms: NN Pattern Classification Techniques, IEEE Computer Society Press, *(1991).*
[17] *K. Pearson K.,* Contributions to the Mathematical Theory of Evolution, Phil. Trans. Roy Soc. London, *(1894), 185 p71.*
[18] *K Pearson (1902),* On the Systematic Fitting of Curves to Observations and Measurements, Biometricka,***I***, *(1902), p1.*

THE APPLICATION OF BAYESIAN INFERENCE WITH FUZZY EVIDENCES IN MEDICAL REASONING

CHRISTOPH RÖMER
Institut für Statistik und
Wahrscheinlichkeitstheorie
Technische Universität Wien
A-1040 Wien, Austria

ABRAHAM KANDEL
Computer Science Department
University of South Florida
Tampa, FL 33620-5350 USA

1 Introduction

Most approaches in evidential reasoning are mainly based on three theoretical frameworks: *Bayesian probability theory*, *fuzzy set theory* and *Dempster-Shafer theory*. All three theories have been introduced in order to cope with different kinds of uncertainty. Bayesian probability theory is distinguished by its well-developed concepts in decision-making with respect to random experiments, yet it does not provide means for dealing with other uncertainties than those governed by frequential probabilities. Shafer weakens this constraint when introducing his mathematical theory of evidences [30], based on a concept of lower and upper probabilities, first studied by Dempster [6]. Shafer argues [30] that a clear distinction must be made between epistemological and frequential interpretations of probability and proposed a framework for dealing with epistemic probabilities by considering super-additive belief measures, comprising additive Bayesian probability measures as a special case. Hence, it can be viewed as a generalization of Bayesian probability theory by allowing degrees of ignorance due to super-additivity.

Fuzzy set theory was introduced by Zadeh [34] in order to deal with vague information represented by linguistic terms and, though fuzzy set theory and its immediate relative *possibility theory* [9], [16], [36] are still somewhat controversial, they have been used successfully in many real-world applications [14], [22], [23]. Fuzzy set theory is based on the concept of membership functions, introduced as generalizations of characteristic functions, which only can distinguish between either full or non membership to a subsets of a universe. Membership functions ensure a gradual rather than an abrupt transition between full and non membership and are also called possibility densities, in a more general setting. Hence, the basic concepts in Bayesian probability theory can be easily extended to fuzzy events by replacing characteristic functions with membership functions [35]. A problem occurs, when trying to find a consistent extension of conditional probability to fuzzy sets, that is, to define the conditional degree of probability in a fuzzy event B, knowing that fuzzy event A is true. The reason why there is much interest for finding such an extension lies in its potential for evidential reasoning: in classical Bayesian probability theory, the concept of partial belief leads to the so-called *Bayes' Theorem*, a formula used for statistical inference by updating prior knowledge about the unknown parameters of a chance density on the basis of statistical evidences. The problems surrounding partial beliefs conditioned on fuzzy sets, as pointed out in Section 3, renders a corresponding Bayes' theorem for fuzzy evidences in a somewhat controversial manner.

Shafer obtains the Bayes' Theorem as a partial result of a more general concept without employing conditional belief functions [30]. His line of reasoning is based on an idea, known in the statistical literature as the "principle of likelihood". We demonstrate that a similar line of reasoning applies when confronted with fuzzy evidences and therefore, we can derive a generalization of Bayes' Theorem for fuzzy evidences without extending the concept of conditional probability to fuzzy sets. In doing so, we obtain a framework for statistical inference on the basis of fuzzy observations, which allows us to take advantage of all classical Bayesian reasoning methods based on the posterior distributions of the parameter governing the experiment.

One may apply this technique very successfully in medical diagnosis. In analyzing certain disorders and in predicting a variety of outcomes, this tool may end up as the test predictive mechanism. For example, diastolic heart failure, defined as increased resistance to filling of one or both cardiac ventricles, is seen in a variety of disorders as illustrated in [12]. Although there is some degree of diastolic dysfunction in most patients with "heart failure" or "congestive heart failure", as many as 40% of patients with congestive heart failure have normal systolic function and thus have primary diastolic heart failure [4]-[5], [10]-[13], [15]. The extensive medical evidence of diastolic heart failure [17]-[21], [25]-[29], [31]-[33] may be therefore dealt with in an interesting way once it is linked to the Bayesian reasoning with fuzzy evidences.

2 Basics Of Dempster-Shafer Theory

The Dempster-Shafer theory originated from the concept of lower and upper probabilities, first studied by Dempster [6] and extended by Shafer to a mathematical theory of evidences [30]. In Dempster-Shafer theory, probability masses are allocated to subsets of a *frame of discernment* in contrast to Bayesian probability theory, where probability masses are assessed only to singletons. Such subsets with positive mass are called *focal elements* and the family of focal elements is said to be the *basic probability assignment.* Each basic probability assignment $m : 2^\Theta \to [0, 1]$ induces constraints of belief and plausibility over the frame of discernment Θ, given through the lower and upper probabilities

$$\mathrm{Bel}(B) = \sum_{A \subset B} m(A), \qquad \mathrm{Plb}(B) = \sum_{A \cap B \neq \emptyset} m(A),$$

respectively, for all $B \subset \Theta$. Both functions represent the same probabilistic constraint, for they can be obtained from each other by $\mathrm{Plb}(A) = 1 - \mathrm{Bel}(\overline{A})$. One advantage of Dempster-Shafer theory is its ability to express degrees of ignorance, that is the belief in an event and the belief in its complement do not necessarily add up to one like in probability theory, i.e. $\text{Bel}(B) + \text{Bel}(\overline{B}) \leq 1$.

If m_1 and m_2 are two basic probability assignments on the sane frame of discernment Θ, but pertaining to two different evidential sources, the combined basic probability assignment is obtained via Dempster's rule of combination:

$$m_1 \oplus m_2(C) = \frac{\sum_{A \cap B = C} m_1(A) \times m_2(B)}{1 - \sum_{A \cap B = \emptyset} m_1(A) \times m_2(B)} \tag{1}$$

for all non empty subsets C of Θ.

Since only the very basics of Dempster-Shafer theory are presented here, we refer the reader to Dempster [6] and Shafer [30] as well as to reference [7] for further details.

3 Bayesian Posteriori With Respect To Fuzzy Evidences

In this Section we first discuss the issues surrounding Bayesian probabilities conditioned on fuzzy events in the extended probability framework introduced by Zadeh [35]. We demonstrate how a generalized Bayes' theorem for fuzzy events can be obtained by means of Dempster-Shafer theory, by extending Shafer's convention for assessing statistical evidences to fuzzy evidences [30], and without employing conditional beliefs. Subsequently, we give an example of how a such generalized Bayes' theorem can be used for fuzzy evidential reasoning and decision-making. We conclude this section with an remark on non Bayesian priors.

3.1 Partial Beliefs Conditioned On Fuzzy Events

Zadeh has provided a framework for dealing with fuzzy events within the confines of an extension of probability theory [35]. Zadeh defines the (nonfuzzy) probability of a fuzzy event A as the expectation of its membership function μ_A, what reads in the case of the n-dimensional Euclidean space $\mathbb{R}^n$, equipped with a Borel field $\mathcal{B}$ and a probability measure $\mathcal{P}$ on $\mathcal{B}$,

$$\mathcal{P}(A) = \int_{\mathbb{R}^n} \mu_A(x)\, d\mathcal{P}, \tag{2}$$

provided μ_A is $\mathcal{B}$-measurable. It is easy to see that in the case of A nonfuzzy, we obtain the common notion of probability. In accordance with classical probability theory, $\mathcal{P}(A)$ evaluates the degree of probability to which the corresponding experiment belongs to fuzzy event A.

Equipped with this notion, the idea of independent events may be extended in the following way: two fuzzy sets are said to *independent* if $\mathcal{P}(A * B) = \mathcal{P}(A) \cdot \mathcal{P}(B)$, where "$*$" denotes an extension of the intersection operator on $\mathcal{B}$ to fuzzy sets. Hence, the conditional probability of a fuzzy event A given fuzzy event B may be defined as

$$\mathcal{P}(A|B) = \frac{\mathcal{P}(A * B)}{\mathcal{P}(B)}, \quad \text{if} \quad \mathcal{P}(B) > 0, \tag{3}$$

which maintains that $\mathcal{P}(A|B) = \mathcal{P}(A)$ whenever A and B are independent. The question now arises, which operator "$*$" qualifies as an extension of the intersection operator "$\cap$" on $\mathcal{B}$ to fuzzy sets. The common definition of intersection in fuzzy set theory is by means of the the minimum operator "$\wedge$", such that $\mu_{A\cap B} = \mu_A \wedge \mu_B$. But $A \cap B$ does not qualify for conditioning probabilities, since the cylindric extensions of two fuzzy events in two different spaces, respectively, would not be identified as independent with respect to the product measure [35], what is a severe violation of our understanding of the product measure. To retain this property, Zadeh proposed the fuzzy product $A \cdot B$, given by $\mu_{A \cdot B} = \mu_A \cdot \mu_B$, for defining independence and in the sequel partial beliefs conditioned on fuzzy events. However, with such defined conditional probability, the belief in a fuzzy event A, knowing that A is true, does not equal 1 in general, since

$$\mathcal{P}(A|A) = \frac{\mathcal{P}(A \cdot A)}{\mathcal{P}(A)} \leq 1.$$

This inconsistency, which, by the way, does not arise when using the the fuzzy intersection operator, makes the use of the fuzzy product as conditioning operator as least as awkward as the use of the fuzzy intersection. As to our knowledge, no other operators have been considered so far and with the discussed two operators, we either contradict the common sense of independence or the common sense of full dependency of two events. Hence, the Bayes' Theorem used for statistical inference cannot be immediately adapted to fuzzy sets without remaining somewhat controversial.

3.2 A Different Approach

We now give a different approach to a Bayes' theorem for fuzzy evidences by means of Dempster-Shafer theory and without involving conditional probabilities.

Suppose that a certain experiment is governed by one of a class $\{p_\theta\}_{\theta\in\Theta}$ of chance densities on $\mathbb{R}^n$ and that we have observed a fuzzy evidence A pertaining to this experiment. Let, in the continuous case, $\{P_\theta\}_{\theta\in\Theta}$ denote the corresponding family of probability measures on $\mathbb{R}^n$, such that $p_\theta(h) = P_\theta(h)dh$, $\forall\ \theta \in \Theta$. In the discrete case we identify the chance densities with the probabilities.

We further assume that the fuzziness of the observed evidence is relevant in ratio to at least one possible stochastical variation of the experiment. Namely,

$$\exists\ \theta \in \Theta : \quad P_\theta(A) > 0. \tag{4}$$

In other words, there is at least one chance density which might governs the experiment and which renders A a positive probability. Hereafter, we call such fuzzy evidences *genuine fuzzy* evidences with respect to the statistical specification $\{p_\theta\}_{\theta\in\Theta}$.

We are now able to order Θ on the basis of such genuine fuzzy evidence. It is our intuitive feeling that the more probability p_θ, $\theta \in \Theta$ attributes to evidence A the more plausible does such evidence render θ. In other words, A renders $\theta \in \Theta$ more plausible than $\theta' \in \Theta$ whenever

$$P_\theta(A) > P_{\theta'}(A).$$

For discrete statistical specifications $\{p_\theta\}_{\theta\in\Theta}$ and crisp singletons $A = x \in \mathbb{R}^n$, this convention immediately translates into the well known principle of "likelihood" or "relative plausibility", an idea which many classical statistical reasoning methods are based on. For continuous statistical specifications we first may rewrite above inequality as

$$P_\theta(A) \times \lambda(\text{supp}(A)) > P_{\theta'}(A) \times \lambda(\text{supp}(A)),$$

assuming A is having finite support with respect to the Lebegue measure λ, before associating our convention with the principle of likelihood using the likelihood function $l(\theta) = p_\theta(x) = P_\theta(x)dx$.

We now apply the same line of arguing as Shafer did for assessing classical (crisp) statistical evidences ([30], pp. 238) when saying that it is but a short step form this intuition to the idea that A should lend plausibility to a singleton $\{\theta\} \subset \Theta$ in strict proportion to the probability that θ assigns to A. That is, A should determine the plausibility functions Plb_A over Θ obeying

$$\text{Plb}_A(\{\theta\}) = c \times P_\theta(A), \quad \forall\, \theta \in \Theta, \tag{5}$$

where c is a constant not depending on θ. Obviously Eq. (5) does not uniquely define a plausibility function on Θ since plausibility functions are subadditive and thus in general not completely determined by the plausibility indices of the singletons. But Eq. (5) together with the assumption of *consonance*, that is Plb_A also obeys

$$\text{Plb}_A(B) = \max_{\theta\in B} \text{Plb}_A(\{\theta\}), \quad \forall\, B \subset \Theta,$$

completely determines the plausibility function Plb_A, given by

$$\text{Plb}_A(B) = \frac{\max\limits_{\theta\in B} P_\theta(A)}{\max\limits_{\theta\in\Theta} P_\theta(A)}, \tag{6}$$

for all non-empty subsets $B \subset \Theta$. Hence, the corresponding belief function Bel_A reads

$$\text{Bel}_A(B) = 1 - \text{Plb}(\overline{B}) = 1 - \frac{\max\limits_{\theta\in \overline{B}} P_\theta(A)}{\max\limits_{\theta\in\Theta} P_\theta(A)}, \tag{7}$$

for all non-empty subsets $B \subset \Theta$. Note that Plb_A and Bel_A are well defined since A is a genuine fuzzy evidence with respect to the statistical specification $\{p_\theta\}_{\theta\in\Theta}$.

The idea of the proof is due to Shafer ([30], p. 264) and is based on the relation

$$1 = \text{Plb}(\Theta) = \max_{\theta\in\Theta} \text{Plb}(\{\theta\}) = c \times \max_{\theta\in\Theta} P_\theta(A),$$

which holds for all consonant plausibility functions satisfying Eq. (5).

The restriction to consonant plausibility, respectively belief functions has also its intuitive appeal. Since we want to determine a support function based on a single observation, and we do assume that a single observation is homogeneous in the sense that it does not carry any conflicting information, yet it is fuzzy, we also want the sought support function to be free of conflicting information. This is best achieved by consonant support functions, since they are distinguished by their "failure to betray even a hint of conflict in the evidence" because their focal elements are nested and therefore are "pointing in a single direction" only varying in the precision of its focus (Shafer [30], p. 220). Dubois and Prade point out striking relations between consonant belief structures, respectively nested random sets, and fuzzy sets [7], [8].

We are now in the situation to update a Bayesian prior π on Θ with respect to genuine fuzzy evidence A by means of Dempster's rule of combination, yielding the posterior support function

$$\pi(\,\cdot\,|A) = \pi \oplus \mathrm{Bel}_A \tag{8}$$

conditioned on A. Since the combination of a Bayesian belief function with an arbitrary belief function Bel with relative plausibilities $l(\theta) = c \times \mathrm{Plb}(\{\theta\})$ results in a Bayesian belief function $\pi' = \pi \oplus \mathrm{Bel}$ (Shafer [30], p. 205), completely determined by

$$\pi'(\theta) = \frac{\pi(\theta) \times l(\theta)}{\sum\limits_{\theta \in \Theta} \pi(\theta) \times l(\theta)}, \tag{9}$$

the Bayesian posterior $\pi(\,\cdot\,|A)$ conditioned on fuzzy evidence A is given by

$$\pi(\theta|A) = \frac{\pi(\theta) \times P_\theta(A)}{\sum\limits_{\theta \in \Theta} \pi(\theta) \times P_\theta(A)}. \tag{10}$$

It is quite obvious that when confronted with m physical independent trials yielding m genuine fuzzy observations, the posterior is given by

$$\pi(\theta|A_1, \ldots, A_m) = \frac{\pi(\theta) \times \prod\limits_{i=1}^{m} P_\theta(A_i)}{\sum\limits_{\theta \in \Theta} \pi(\theta) \times \prod\limits_{i=1}^{m} P_\theta(A_i)}. \tag{11}$$

This result can either be obtained by combining the evidences on the aleatory level, that is regarding $D^* = (A_1, \ldots, A_m)$ as a single observation of a compound experiment governed by one of the class $\{p_\theta^m\}_{\theta \in \Theta}$ of chance densities on $\mathbb{R}^{nm}$, or by combining them on the epistemic level via support summation, i.e. $\pi(\,\cdot\,|D^*) = (\cdots((\pi \oplus \mathrm{Bel}_{A_1}) \oplus \mathrm{Bel}_{A_2}) \cdots) \oplus \mathrm{Bel}_{A_m}$.

We thus have obtained, by extending Shafer's proposed convention for assessing statistical evidences, what led him to the classical Bayes' theorem, to fuzzy evidences, a generalized Bayes' theorem for fuzzy evidences. It is indeed a virtual generalization, since for $A = x \in \mathbb{R}^n$ and $\{p_\theta\}_{\theta \in \Theta}$ being a discrete statistical specification,

Eqs. (10)-(11) convert immediately into the classical Bayes-Theorem, while for continuous statistical specifications we first may rewrite Eqs. (10)-(11) using the factors $\lambda(\text{supp}(A_i))$, $i = 1, \ldots, m$, in both numerator and denominator before deducing the classical Bayes' theorem from the generalization as a limit case.

It should be noted that Eqs. (10) and (11) cannot be deduced within the confines of an extension of probability theory to fuzzy sets as proposed by Zadeh [35], without using the controversial concept of partial belief functions conditioned on fuzzy events.

Once we have computed the posterior $\pi(\cdot\,|D^*)$ with respect to the observed genuine fuzzy evidences $D^* = (A_1, \ldots, A_m)$, we have access to all Bayesian reasoning methods relying on the posterior distribution $\pi(\cdot\,|D^*)$, such as

- the *posteriori predictive chance density* $p(\cdot\,|D^*)$, given through
$$p(x|D^*) = \sum_{\theta \in \Theta} p(x|\theta) \times \pi(\theta|D^*),$$

- the *posterior estimator* $\hat{\theta}$ for θ, defined as the posterior expectation of $\tilde{\theta}$ and given by
$$\hat{\theta} = \mathbb{E}[\tilde{\theta}|D^*] = \sum_{\theta \in \Theta} \theta \times \pi(\theta|D^*),$$

- the *Bayes' risk* $r(\pi, \delta^*)$ with respect to some loss function $L(\theta, \delta^*)$, defined as the expected posterior loss and given by
$$r(\pi, \delta^*) = \mathbb{E}[L(\tilde{\theta}, \delta^*)|D^*] = \sum_{\theta \in \Theta} L(\theta, \delta^*(D^*)) \times \pi(\theta|D^*),$$
where $\delta^* : \mathcal{F}^m(\mathbb{R}^n) \to \Theta$, with $\mathcal{F}(\mathbb{R}^n)$ denoting the family of genuine fuzzy sets in $\mathbb{R}^n$, is a decision-rule on the basis of fuzzy evidences,

- and *confidence regions* or *HPD-regions*, which are subsets $\hat{\Theta}$ of Θ with posterior probability
$$P(\tilde{\theta} \in \hat{\Theta}|D^*) = \sum_{\theta \in \hat{\Theta}} \pi(\theta|D^*) = 1 - \alpha,$$
and, in the case of HPD-regions, such that $\pi(\theta|D^*) \geq c$, $\forall\, \theta \in \hat{\Theta}$, with c maximal.

Remark on the use of non Bayesian priors: One of the big advantages of Dempster-Shafer theory is its ability to express degrees of ignorance, and in the sequel other than Bayesian belief structures. This is very beneficial, because, supposing the prior knowledge about Θ is given by a non Bayesian support function Bel_0, which may be the case if we want to express complete ignorance regarding Θ, what is properly modeled by a belief function which vanishes everywhere on Θ, or if we have access to fuzzy prior knowledge rather than to Bayesian prior knowledge, what can be modeled in terms of consonant belief functions [7] [8], we still can evaluate a posterior belief function Bel_1, which in general is non Bayesian either. In this case Eqs. (10) and (11) do not hold in general anymore, since they are evaluated with respect to Bayesian priors only, but the posterior can still be evaluated by means of Dempster's rule of combination: $\text{Bel}_1 = \text{Bel}_0 \oplus \text{Bel}_A$.

4 Application To Medical Reasoning

We now give a rather simple example of how such generalized Bayes' reasoning methods for fuzzy evidences can be applied in the field of medical decision making. The present example has the limited objective of showing how ill-defined, or fuzzy, evidences may occur in a medical diagnosis process and how they can be dealt with. We do not attempt to explore in detail any of the steps of the proposed concept, nor do we claim to give a comprehensive or immediately applicable medical diagnosis system.

Example: Suppose we have a set of symptoms $S = \{S_1, \ldots, S_n\}$, which interfere with a certain deceases D and D can be more particular specified by one of the sub-deceases D_1 and D_2. We define a degree of prevalence $\tilde{d}_i$ for each symptom S_i, $i = 1, \ldots, n$, assuming non-negative values on the real line. Suppose we know that $\tilde{d} = (\tilde{d}_1, \ldots, \tilde{d}_2)$ is p_{θ_1}-distributed among patients suffering from decease D_1, while among people suffering from decease D_2, $\tilde{d}$ is known to be governed by chance density p_{θ_2}. The choice of the statistical specification $\{p_{\theta_i}\}_{i=1,2}$ is a problem itself and will not be discussed here.

Suppose a patient shows symptoms S^*, which are quantified by linguistic terms such as "severe", "very pronounced", "apparent" or "barely pronounced", and which can be modeled by means of fuzzy sets of the real line as depicted in Figure 1.

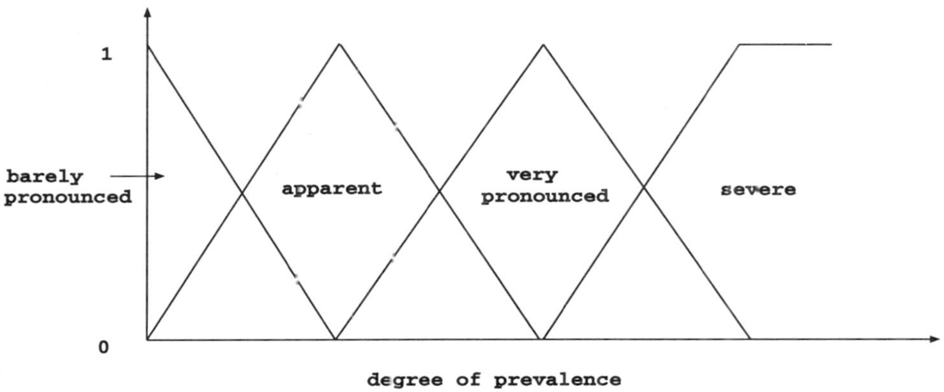

Figure 1: Fuzzy quantifications for the degree of prevalence of a certain symptom.

Due to some other reasons, this patient is more likely to have have decease D_1 rather than decease D_2, a prior knowledge which can be expressed in terms of a Bayesian prior on $\Theta = \{\theta_1, \theta_2\}$, given by $\pi(\theta_1) = p$ and $\pi(\theta_2) = 1 - p$. We now want to decide, with respect to loss function

$$L(\theta, \delta^*) = \begin{cases} L_1, & \text{if } \theta = \theta_1 \text{ and } \delta^* = \theta_2, \\ L_2, & \text{if } \theta = \theta_2 \text{ and } \delta^* = \theta_1, \\ 0, & \text{if } \theta = \delta^*, \end{cases}$$

whether it is more risky to diagnose decease D_1 or decease D_2. We thus have to look at the Bayes' risk

$$\begin{aligned} r(\pi, \delta^*) &= L(\theta_1, \delta^*(S^*))\pi(\theta_1|S^*) + L(\theta_2, \delta^*(S^*))\pi(\theta_2|S^*) \\ &= \begin{cases} L_1\ \pi(\theta_1|S^*), & \text{if } \delta^* = \theta_1, \\ L_2\ \pi(\theta_2|S^*), & \text{if } \delta^* = \theta_2, \end{cases} \end{aligned}$$

and evaluate whether or not $r(\pi, \theta_1)$ is greater than $r(\pi, \theta_2)$.
In the sequel, we may abandon hypothesis D_i in favor of hypothesis D_j, whenever

$$L_i\ P_{\theta_i}(S^*)\pi(\theta_i) > L_j\ P_{\theta_j}(S^*)\pi(\theta_j).$$

It is clear that this procedure can be very useful in dealing with diastolic dysfunction in congestive heart failure, since diastolic dysfunction has a contributory role in most patients with congestive heart failure and a dominant role in some patients [12]. One example of possible use of our technique is the following. Clearly, the rate of myocardial relaxation slows during ischemia and in advanced myocardial hypertrophy [12]. However, in order to achieve a high degree of belief that the assertion whether incomplete relaxation, affecting early, middle, and end-diastolic distensibility occurs or not, one may use the technique described here as a means of applying Bayesian reasoning with fuzzy evidences. To quote Grossman [12]:

> "There is extensive evidence that the relation between left ventricular diastolic pressure and left ventricular diastolic volume commonly shifts upward in patients with angina pectoris induced by exercise [3] or pacing tachycardia [1]-[2], [24], [28] with increases in early, middle, and end-diastolic pressure relative to volume".

It is exactly this kind of an issue, as well as issues related to whether the altered diastolic distensibility results from incomplete relaxation, where our technique can be used in order to achieve results via evidential reasoning using Bayesian technique with fuzzy evidences.

5 Conclusion

In this paper we demonstrate how one can obtain a generalized Bayes' theorem for fuzzy evidences without using the controversial concept of partial belief functions conditioned on fuzzy events. We first discuss the issue of extending the concept of conditional probability to fuzzy events by pointing out that the use of the fuzzy product contradicts the common sense of dependency.

In order to avoid problem, we extended Shafer's convention for assessing statistical evidences to fuzzy evidences by claiming that the principle of likelihood remains plausible and applicable when confronted with fuzzy rather than with crisp statistical evidences. In the sequel, we obtain a generalized Bayes' theorem for fuzzy evidences, which allows us to infer a Bayesian posterior distribution with respect to a classical Bayesian prior and fuzzy observations. Once we have computed the posterior distribution, we have access to all Bayesian reasoning methods relying on the posterior, such as the posteriori predictive chance density, the posterior estimator, the Bayes' risk or HPD-regions.

An example demonstrating how such generalized Bayes' reasoning methods can be applied to medical diagnosis and decision making is given, and a general discussion with regard to the problem of diastolic dysfunction in congestive heart failure is presented.

References

1. Aroesty J. M., R. G. McKay, G. V. Heller, H. D. Royal, A. V. Als, W. Grossman (1985) Simultaneous assessment of left ventricular systolic and diastolic dysfunction during pacing-induced ischemia, *Circulation* **71**, 889-900.
2. Barry W. H., J. F. Brooker, E. L. Alderman, D. C. Harrison (1974), Changes in diastolic stiffness and tone of the left ventricle during angina pectoris *Circulation* **49**, 225-263.
3. Carroll J. D., O. M. Hess, H. O. Hirzel, H. P. Krayenbuchl (1983), Exercise-induced ischemia: the influence of altered relaxation on early diastolic pressure, *Circulation* **67**, 521-528.
4. Carroll J. D., O. M. Hess, H. O. Hirzel, M. Turina, H. P. Krayenbuchl (1985), Left ventricular systolic and diastolic function in coronary artery disease: effects of revascularization on exercise-induced ischemia, *Circulation* **72**, 119-129.
5. Corin W. J., T. Murakami, E. S. Monrad, O. M. Hess, H. P. Krayenbuchl (1991), Left ventricular passive diastolic properties in chronic mitral regurgitation, *Circulation* **83**, 797-807.
6. Dempster A. P. (1967), Upper and lower probabilities induced by a multivalued mapping, *Ann. Mathematical Statistics*, **38**, 325-339.
7. Dubois D., H. Prade (1982), On several representations of an uncertain body of evidences, in *Fuzzy Information and Decision Processes* (M.M. Gupta and E. Sanchez, Eds.), North-Holland, New York, 167-181.
8. Dubois D., H. Prade (1987), The mean value of a fuzzy number, *Fuzzy Sets and Systems* **24**, 279-300.
9. Dubois D., H. Prade (1988), *Possibility Theory*, Plenum, New York.

10. Fragasso G., R. Benti, M. Sciammarella, et. al (1991), Symptom-limited exercise testing causes sustained diastolic dysfunction in patients with coronary disease and low effort tolerance, *J. Am. Coll. Cardiol.* **17**, 1251-1255.
11. Grossman W., L. P. McLaurin, E. L. Rolett (1979), Alterations in left ventricular relaxation and diastolic compliance in congestive cardiomyopathy, *Cardiovasc. Res.* **13**, 514-522.
12. Grossman W. (1991), Diastolic dysfunction in congestive heart failure, *Seminars in Medicine of the Beth Israel Hospital Boston* **325**, No. 22, 1557-1564.
13. Gwathmey J. K., S. E. Warren, G. M. Briggs, et. al. (1991), Diastolic dysfunction in hypertrophic cardiomyopathy: effect on active force generation during systole, *J. Clin. Invest.* **87**, 1023-1031.
14. Hitachi (1987), Fuzzy control ensures a smooth ride, *Hitachi 1987*, 1-23.
15. Humphrey L. S., E. J. Topol, G. I. Rosenfeld, et. al. (1988), Immediate enhancement of left ventricular relaxation by coronary artery bypass grafting: intraoperative assessment, *Circulation* **77**, 886-896.
16. Kandel A. (1980), *Fuzzy Mathematical Techniques with Application*, Addison Wesley, Reading, MA.
17. Kihara Y., W. Grossman, J. P. Morgan (1989), Direct measurement of changes in intracellularcalcium transients during hypoxia, ischemia, and reperfusion of the intact mammalian heart, *Circ. Res.* **65**, 1029-1044.
18. Kitzman D. W., M. B. Higginbotham, F. R. Cobb, K. H. Sheikh, M. J. Sullivan (1991), Exercise intolerance in patients with heart failure and preserver left ventricular systolic function: failure of the Frank-Starling mechanism, *J. Am. Coll. Cardiol.* **17**, 1065-1072.
19. Koretsune Y., M. C. Corretti, H. Kusuoka, E. Marban (1991), Mechanism of early ischemic contractile failure: inexcitability, metabolite accumulation, or vascular collapse?, *Circ. Res.* **68**, 255-262.
20. Lakatta E. G. (1987), Cardiac muscle changes in senescence, *Ann. Rev. Physiol.* **49**, 519-531.
21. Lamas G. A., M. A. Pfeffer (1991), Left ventricular remodeling after acute myocardial infarction: clinical course and beinficial effect of angiotensin-converting enzyme inhibition, *Am. Heart J.* **121**, 1194-1202.
22. Mamdani E. H. (1974), Applications for fuzzy algorithms for the control of a dynamic plant, *IEEE Proc.* **121**, 1585-1588.
23. Mamdani E. H. and S. Assilian (1975), An experiment in synthesis with a fuzzy logic controller, *International Journal of Man-Machine Studies* **7**, 1-13.
24. Mann T., B. R. Brodie, W. Grossman, L. P. McLaurin (1977), Effect of angina on the left ventricular diastolic pressure-volume relationship, *Circulation* **55**, 761-766.
25. McLaurin L. P., E. L. Rolett, W. Grossman (1973), Impaired left ventricular relaxation durin pacing-induced ischemia, *Am. J. Card.* **32**, 751-757.

26. Miyazaki S., B. D. Guth, T. Miura, C. Indolfi, R. Schulz, J. Ross Jr. (1990), Changes of left ventricular diastolic function in exercising dogs without and with ischemia, *Circulation* **81**, 1058-1070.
27. Momomura S. I., A. B. Bradley, W. Grossman (1984), Left ventricular diastolic pressure-segment length relations and end-diastolic distensibility in dogs with coronary stenoses: an angina physiology model, *Circ. Res.* **55**, 203-214.
28. Sasayama S., H. Nonogi, S. Miyazaki, et. al. (1985), Changes in diastolic properties of the regional myocardium during pacing induced ischemia in human subjects, *J. Am. Coll. Cardiol.* **5**, 599-606.
29. Serizawa T., B. A. Carabello, W. Grossman (1980), Effect of pacing-induced ischemia on left ventricular diastolic pressure-volume relations in dogs with coronary stenoses, *Circ. Res.* **46**, 430-439.
30. Shafer G. (1976), *A Mathematical Theory of Evidences*, Princeton University Press.
31. Soufer R., D. Wohlgelernter, N. A. Vita, et. al. (1985), Intact systolic left ventricular function in clinical congestive heart failure, *Am. J. Cardiol.* **55**, 1032-1036.
32. Watanabe J., M. J. Levine, F. Bellotto, R. G. Johnson, W. Grossman (1990), Effects of coronary venous pressure on left ventricular diastolic distensibility, *Circ. Res.* **67**, 923-932.
33. Weber K. T., C. G. Brilla (1991), Pathological hypertrophy and cardiac interstitium: fibrosis and renin-angiotensis-aldosterone system, *Circulation* **83**, 1849-1865.
34. Zadeh L. A. (1965), Fuzzy Sets, *Information and Control* **8**, 338-353.
35. Zadeh L. A. (1968), Probability measures of fuzzy events, *Journal of Mathenatical Analysis and Applications* **23**, 421-427.
36. Zadeh L. A. (1978), Fuzzy sets as a basis for a theory of possibility, *Fuzzy Sets and Systems* **1**, 3-28.

Acknowledgement: This research was done while the first athor was visiting the University of South Florida; the second author was partially supported by the University of South Florida research grant DSR 2108-934-RO.

24 HOUR ANALYSIS OF HEART RATE FLUCTUATIONS BEFORE AND AFTER CAROTID SURGERY USING WAVELET TRANSFORM

METIN AKAY[1], YASEMIN M. AKAY[1], WALTER WELKOWITZ[1], GIORA LANDESBERG[2], DAN SAPOZNIKOV[2]

[1]*Department of Biomedical Engineering*
Rutgers University
Piscataway, New Jersey 08855

[2]*Department of Anesthesiology and Cardiology*
Hadassah University Hospital
Jerusalem, Israel

1. Introduction

Coronary artery disease (CAD) is one of the major causes of mortality in patients undergoing major vascular operations including aortic reconstruction, cardiac endarectomy and lower extremity arterial bypass grafting [1,2]. These are two main reasons for this high mortality during and after operations on the vascular bed [3,4]. The first one is the high prevalence of ischemic heart disease in the population of vascular disease patients [3,4]. The second reason is the operative burden including the volume shifts and hemodynamic derangements, as well as baroreflex disturbances that occur in the carotid operations [5].

The autonomic nervous system (ANS) modulates the cardiovascular control during the traumatic preoperative procedure. Actually, the ANS represents the electrical activity and provides beat-by-beat regulation of the cardiovascular system. In patients with coronary artery disease, myocardial oxygen demand is increased and coronary blood flow is reduced[6].

The application of spectral analysis techniques to beat-to-beat heart rate and blood pressure variations has provided an important tool for noninvasively understanding tonic cardiovascular regulation[7,8]. Results using spectral analysis techniques showed that there are three major spectral regions. The high frequency region (HF, above 0.25 Hz) represents shifts in respiratory rate. The mid-frequency region (approximately 0.15 Hz) is linked to the response of the baroreceptor reflex, and the low frequency region (approximately 0.08 Hz) is related to thermoregulation fluctuation and vasomotor tone (renin-angiotensin system)[7,8].

These spectral components of the heart rate variability data (HRV) and blood pressure can be used clinically to assess the ANS, with separate measures of the sympathetic and parasympathetic systems. The high frequency component in HR variability appears to be mediated solely by the vagal tone since it disappears completely with vagal or muscarinic blockade. The mid-band frequency component is an indicator of the sympathetic tone but is also modulated by vagal activity.

Analysis of HRV data from patients with congestive heart failure shows a large energy decrease at all frequency ranges which show diminished vagal but relatively preserved sympathetic, modulation of HR [9,10]. This provides very important evidence that cardiac parasympathetic function is depressed in patients prone to sudden cardiac death [9-11].

The power spectrum analysis of heart rate has been estimated by using the FFT with short epochs while performing long term monitoring. This traditional method called Short Time Fourier Transform (STFT) may eliminate the effects of the nonstationarity which occur at the expense of low frequency and time localization[13-22].

Little is known about the characteristics of heart rate fluctuations during cardiovascular surgery both in the time and frequency domains. The purpose of this study is to characterize the heart rate fluctuations before and after surgery by determining how the signal changes in the frequency domain during the surgery. Here we introduce the wavelet transform method to analyze the heart rate fluctuations. The wavelet transform method based on multiresolution signal decompositions is free of assumptions regarding the characteristics of the signal and is able to localize the non-stationary signal more accurately (both in the time and frequency domains) than the traditional methods such as the short term Fourier transform[13-22]. This time and frequency localization can be achieved by the wavelet transform since it uses short windows at higher frequencies and long windows at low frequencies. However, the classical methods such as the short time Fourier transform method uses a single size analysis window. This method smears the energy of the signal across the time-frequency plane and fails to adequately represent the signal[13,22]. The spectral resolution of the STFT method can improve with the use of a longer data window. However, using the long window to improve the spectral resolution risks compromising the assumption of stationarity in the chosen window. Choosing the short window produces low spectral resolution. As a result, the wavelet transform (WT) shows better time and frequency resolution than other time-frequency methods, especially for the analysis of **non-stationary** signals, as in the case of the analysis of HRV for a long period.

The WT has been successfully used in analyzing speech processing. The sound produced by turbulence caused by occluded arteries in dogs was measured and analyzed by using the WT. The accurate and reliable time and frequency localization were obtained. A direct correlation between blood flow and sounds due to turbulence was observed in the time and frequency domains[23]. The WT was used in magnetic resonance imaging (MRI)[24]. The use of the WT in MRI was found to be more reliable and accurate than the traditional Fourier transform[24]. The advantages and the proven better performance of the wavelet transform over the traditional methods such as the short time Fourier transform have been very well established in the literature although this method was only recently introduced into signal processing, communication research, image processing, geophysics and biomedical signal processing[13-24].

The wavelet transform may also be preferred in signal processing over the parametric modelling techniques such as the autoregressive (AR) and autoregressive moving average (ARMA) techniques since the wavelet transform is free of any assumptions about the stationarity of the biological signals. The wavelet transform does not require the estimation or assumption of the filter parameters which is the case in the AR and ARMA methods. In practice, the optimal filter order selection is currently a essential and difficult task to get accurate the power spectral density functions.

In our previous studies[29,30,31], we utilized the wavelet transform to characterize autonomic nervous system regulation of cardiovascular activity in order to better understand short-term cardiovascular regulation. The wavelet transform was chosen since it has the ability to localize the change in the characteristics of the non-stationary heart fluctuations during surgery without loosing the time and frequency information[13-24,29,30,31].

The analysis of the heart rate fluctuations using the same data base showed that the power in all the frequency bands were increased only 2 h after declamping. The power in the fourth and third frequency bands were higher 2 h before the declamping.

Although the results obtained using the STFT method vaguely supported the hypothesis that the power in all the frequency bands were increased after declamping, it failed to show the details of the change in the characteristics of the non-stationary heart fluctuations during surgery[29,30,31]. This was not surprising since the STFT method uses a single size analysis window, which could smear the power of the signal across the time-frequency plane and fails to adequately represent the signal[13-22]. The spectral resolution of the STFT method can be improved with the use of a longer data window. However, using the long window to improve the spectral resolution risks compromising the assumption of stationarity in the chosen window. Choosing the short window produces low spectral resolution[13-22]. The other disadvantage of the classical Fourier transform is the leakage of the main lobe in the power spectrum into the sidelobes due to the finite segments of the data in the analysis window[23]. On the other hand the better time and frequency localization was achieved by the wavelet transform since it uses short windows at higher frequencies and long windows at low frequencies. As a result, the wavelet transform (WT) showed better time and frequency resolution than other time-frequency methods in the analysis of Heart rate fluctuations in those studies[29,30,31].

A strong relationship between all four wavelet bands before and after declamping was established using the statistical analysis technique known as as the Kolmogorov-Smirnov (K-S) test, which does not make any assumption regarding the statistical distribution of the data[29,30,31]. Results showed a highly significant relationship between all the wavelet bands and the declamping time. Results also showed that 1 h segments of each wavelet band immediately following declamping is statistically unique, that is, distinguishable from all other segments considered[29,30].

In this study, we would like to explore the use of wavelet transform to characterize 24 h heart rate fluctuations before and after carotid surgery by determining how the signal changes in the frequency domain. Here the wavelet transform was chosen since it shows better time and frequency resolution than any other time-frequency methods, especially for the analysis of the **non-stationary** signals[13-24], which is the case in the analysis of the HRV signal for a long period.

2. Method

2.1 *Wavelet Transform*

The wavelet orthonormal bases provide an important new tool in signal analysis[13-22]. The difference information between the approximation of heart rate fluctuations at resolutions 2^{j+1} and 2^j can be extracted by decomposing the signal on a wavelet orthonormal basis of $L^2(R)$ [27-36]. $L^2(R)$ denotes the vector space of measurable, square-integrable one-dimensional functions f(x). In $L^2(R)$, a wavelet orthonormal basis in the vector space V_{2_j} can be given as a family of functions $[(2^j)^{\frac{1}{2}}\phi(2^j x - n)]_{j,n\epsilon Z}$ which can be built by dilating the unique function $\phi(x)$ called a scaling function. The scaling function $\phi(x)$ can characterize the multiresolution approximation of the vector space V_{2_j}. The projection of the signal f(x) onto the orthonormal bases of $L^2(R)$ can be estimated as follows[13-14]:

$$A_{2^j} = 2^{-j} \sum_{n=-\infty}^{\infty} < f(u), \phi_{2^{-j}}(u - 2^j n) > \phi_{2^j}(x - 2^{-j} n) \tag{1}$$

$n, j \epsilon Z$.

The discrete approximation of f(x) can be estimated by using the inner products at the resolution 2^j, which can be estimated as follows[29]:

$$A^d_{2^j} f =< f(u), \phi_{2^j}(u - 2^{-j} n) > \tag{2}$$

The consecutive $A^d_{2^j} f$ can be explained as a low-pass filtering of f(x) followed by a uniform sampling at a rate 2^j. For each scale change, the higher frequencies of the signal will be eliminated. $A^d_{2^{j-1}} f$ can be calculated by using a recurrence algorithm as follows(15):

$$< f(u), \phi_{2^j}(u - 2^{-j} n) >= \sum_{k=-\infty}^{\infty} \bar{h}(2n - k) < f(u), \phi_{2^{j+1}}(u - 2^{-j-1} n) > \tag{3}$$

where $\bar{h} = h(-n)$ represents the mirror filter of h(n)

$$h(n) = < \phi_{2^{-1}}(u), \phi(u-n) > \tag{4}$$

where h(n) represents the low-pass filter. $A^d_{2^j} f$ can be estimated by convolving $A^d_{2^{j+1}}$ with $\bar{h}(n)$ and storing every other sample of the output[13,14].

The wavelet function, $\psi(x)$, called the orthogonal wavelet can be estimated at resolution 2^j as follows[13,14]:

$$\psi_{2^j} = 2^j \psi(2^j x) \tag{5}$$

The functions of $\psi(x)$, $\psi_{2^j}(x - 2^{-j}n)$, which are an orthonormal bases of the vector space O_{2^j} have good localization properties in the time and frequency domains[13-14].

The orthogonal projection of a signal f(x) on the vector space O_{2^j} can be estimated as follows[13,14]:

$$D^d_{2^j} f = < f(u), \psi_{2^j}(u - 2^{-j}n) > \tag{6}$$

where $D_{2^j} f$ represents the discrete detailed signal. The inner product can be estimated from the higher resolution discrete approximation as follows[13,14]:

$$< f(u), \psi_{2^j}(u - 2^{-j}n) > = \sum_{k=-\infty}^{\infty} \bar{g}(2n-k) A^d_{2^{j+1}}(k) \tag{7}$$

where $\bar{g}(n) = g(-n)$ represents the mirror filter of g(n)[13-16].

$$g(n) = < \psi_{2^{-1}}(u), \phi(u-n) > \tag{8}$$

where g(n) represents the high-pass filter. Since filters g(n) and h(n) are quadrature filters, the high-pass filter g(n) can be estimated as follows [13-15]:

$$g(n) = (-1)^{1-n} h(1-n) \tag{9}$$

The vector space O_{2^j} is orthonormal to the vector space V_{2^j}. As a summary, A_{2^j} and D_{2^j} can be estimated from $A_{2^{j+1}}$ by convolving with the filters h(n) and g(n), respectively. The details of the wavelet transforms have been described elsewhere[13-24].

2.2 Kolmogorov-Smirnov (K-S) Test

The K-S test was successfully applied to the detection of stimulus-related (evoked response) activity in the electroencephalogram[25] and to the distributions of the transition states of the ion channel activity[26]. The value of the K-S test has also been demonstrated in acoustical signal detection associated with coronary artery disease[27].

The K-S test compares the cumulative distribution of sample data sets with that of a known or reference data set. Since the K-S test makes no assumption regarding the type of data distribution, it is applicable to any distribution of data. In our case, the K-S test was an attractive method for statistical analysis of the detailed signal, $|D_j f|^2|$, of the heart rate fluctuations at different frequency bandwidths. Different distribution functions (or data sets) yielded different cumulative distribution function estimates using the K-S test.

The behavior of the distribution functions between the largest and smallest values characterizes the distributions. The K-S distance, D, represents the maximum absolute difference between two cumulative distribution function as follows [25-27]:

$$D = max_{0<x<\infty}|\widehat{F_N(x)} - R(x)| \tag{10}$$

where $F_N(x)$ and $R(x)$ represent the cumulative distribution functions of the sample (unknown) and the reference functions, respectively.

In our case of two unknown cumulative distribution functions, the maximum distance D_i can be calculated as follows(25-27):

$$D_i = max_{0<x<\infty}|\widehat{F_a} - \widehat{F_b}| \tag{11}$$

where F_a represents the cumulative distribution function of the 24 h segment for the RR and the detailed signals after declamping, and F_b represents the cumulative distribution function of the 24 h segment for the RR and the detailed signals before declamping.

3. Results and Discussion

Files of 24-hour R-R intervals before and after surgery were recorded from a Holter Marquette series 8000 analysis system. Files of R-R intervals with their annotations (normal beats, premature ventricular beats, ectopic beats) were transferred to an IBM-386 compatible computer disk. The R-R intervals between two consecutive normal QRS complexes were calculated by noting any irregular beats. Then, the irregular beats were replaced by the values obtained by linear interpolation from the normal beats. The irregular beats were determined by using a threshold obtained by updated averages and standard deviations of the R-R intervals. The details of the recording and interpolation procedures have been described elsewhere[12,28]. Then, the 48 -hour R-R intervals were transferred as a function of time after the interpolation procedure to a Sun 4.0 System for wavelet analysis. We performed multiresolution decomposition for four sets of parameters D_{2^j} where $-1 < j < -3$. The wavelet transform method was applied to the heart rate fluctuations obtained from five patients for 24 h before and 24 h after declamping in patients undergoing carotid endarterectomy. The three wavelet transforms represent the following signal bandwidths: 1. 0.250-0.500 Hz, 2. 0.125-0.250 Hz, 3. 0.062-0.125 Hz.

All the patients ended the surgery with no cardiac or neurological damage. Figures 1a and 1b show the averaged R-R in msec for 24 h before and 24 h after the declamping in five patients undergoing carotid endarterectomy. Figures 1b and 2b show the corresponding power of the three wavelet decompositions which define the power at each time sample, respectively. The patients underwent either right or left carotid endarterectomy with cervical block anesthesia without the need of any additional systemic drug. The average blood pressure of these patients fell from 188/74 to 157/66 within 30 minutes after declamping.

These results show that the power of the heart rate fluctuations in all three wavelet bands was low before surgery and increased after carotid declamping. For this reason, we statistically analyzed the 24 h segment of RR intervals in msec and all three wavelet bands before declamping as well as for the 24 hours after declamping to establish the significance of the 24 h segment after declamping. For each patient, the cumulative distribution function (CDF) values of 24 h segments before and after carotid surgery were estimated for these three wavelet bands.

The standard for comparison is the K-S distance D which can have a maximum of one for extremely contrasting functions and a minimum of zero for functions that are essentially the same. The K-S distances between the cumulative distribution functions of the 24 h segment before declamping and the 24 h segment after declamping following the declamping are shown in

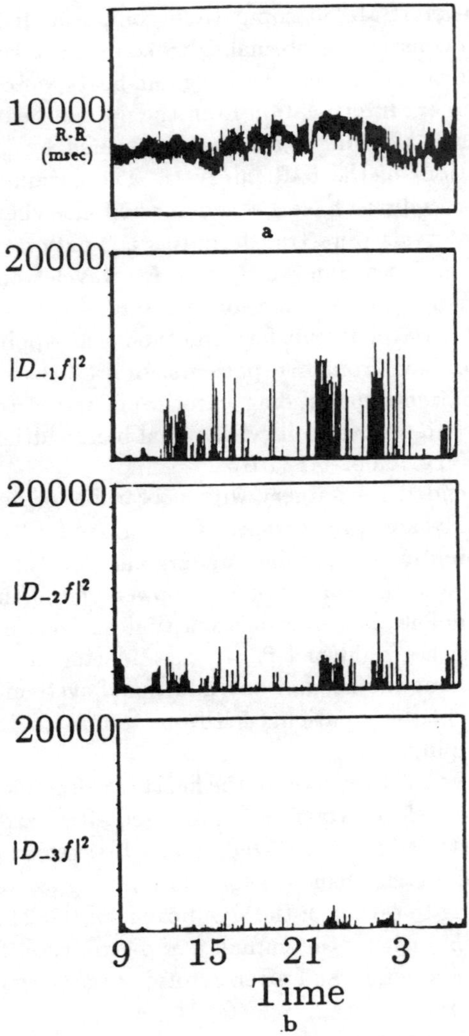

Figure 1: The resolution decomposition of the 24 h averaged R-R intervals obtained from 25 patients who underwent carotid surgery before declamping. a. Averaged R-R intervals. b. The corresponding averaged three frequency bandwidths(discrete detail signals, D_{2^j}) as a function time. From top to bottom the resolution decreases by a power of 2.

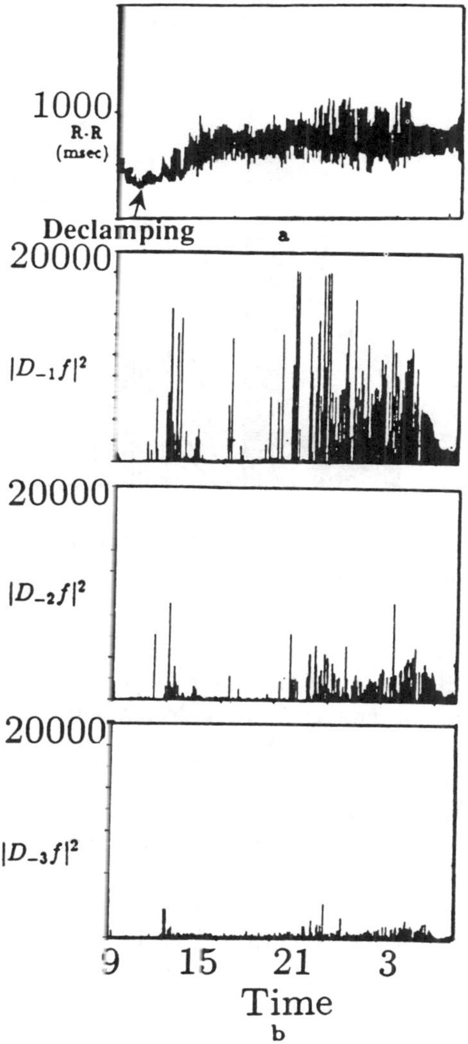

Figure 2: The resolution decomposition of the 24 h averaged R-R intervals obtained from 25 patients who underwent carotid surgery after declamping. a. Averaged R-R intervals. b. The corresponding averaged three frequency bandwidths(discrete detail signals, D_{2^j}) as a function time. From top to bottom the resolution decreases by a power of 2.

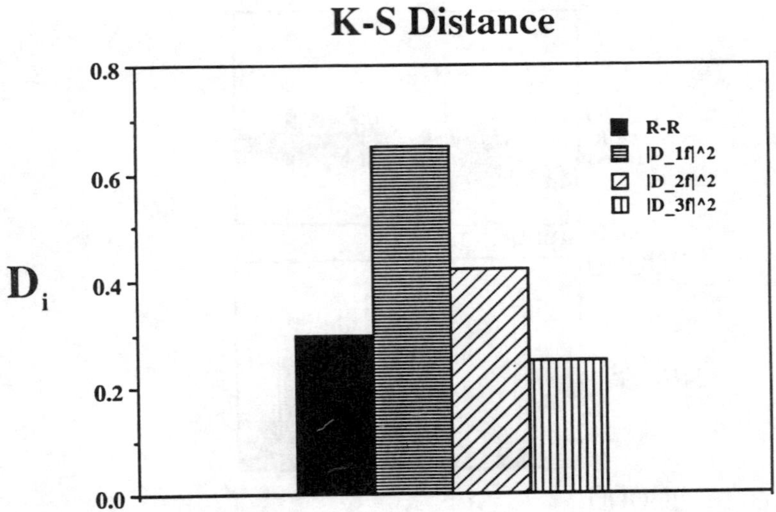

Figure 3: The K-S distance between 24 h segments for the RR and the three wavelet bands before and after declamping.

Figure 3 for the R-R intervals and each of the three wavelet bands. This figure shows that the R-R interval the different statistical patterns before 24 h before the declamping and 24 h after declamping, showing that the heart rate fluctuations were very low 24 hours before declamping compared to the 24 h segment after declamping. The first and second wavelet bands followed the same statistical patterns, which implies that the probabilistic distributions of the 24 h before and 24 h after declamping were significantly different. In other words, the power in the first, second, and third wavelet bands gradually decreased before declamping and drastically increased after declamping. Since the value of S, the K-S test significance, in each case is smaller than 0.001, the results are statistically significant[25-27]. All patients ended the surgery with no cardiac or neurological damage.

4. Conclusion

In this study, the wavelet transform method was utilized to characterize autonomic nervous system regulation of cardiovascular activity in order to better understand the cardiovascular regulation before and after carotid surgery. The wavelet transform was chosen since it has the ability to localize the change in the characteristics of the non-stationary heart fluctuations during surgery without loosing the time and frequency information[13-24].

A strong relationship between all three wavelet bands 24 h before and after declamping has been established using the statistical analysis technique known as as the Kolmogorov-Smirnov (K-S) test, which does not make any assumption regarding the statistical distribution of the data. Results showed a highly significant relationship between all the wavelet bands and the declamping time. Results also showed that the 24 h segment of each wavelet band after declamping is statistically unique, that is, distinguishable from the other segment 24 h before declamping. This implies that the increased power in each wavelet band after surgery is caused by the declamping. Reinstitution of brain blood flow after cleaning the atheroma from inside the artery at the area of the baroreceptors could be responsible for the increase of the power in all frequency ranges. However, the mechanisms responsible for the hemodynamic alterations and even for myocardial ischemic events occurring during carotid clamping and declamping[28] in carotid endarterectomy are not completely understood. Since the behavior of the ANS during major surgery and cardiac ischemic events can be tracked carefully and accurately using wavelet transforms, we believe that this technique will further improve our understanding of the interactions of the control systems with the cardiovascular system.

Acknowledgement

Address correspondence should be made to Dr. Metin Akay, Dept. of Biomedical Engineering, Rutgers University, Piscataway, NJ 08855.

References

1. Blombery PA, Ferguson IA, Rosengarten DS, Stuchbery KE, Miles CR, Black AJ, Pitt A, Anderson ST, Harper RW, Federman J (1987) *The role of coronary artery disease in complications of abdominal aortic aneurysm surgery.* Surgery 101:150-5.

2. Gouny P, Bertrand M, Coriat P, Kieffer E(1989) *Perioperative cardiac complications of surgical repair of infrarenal aortic aneurysms.* Ann Vasc Surg 3:328-34.

3. Herzer NR, Lees CD, *Fatal myocardial infarction following carotid endarterectomy. 335 patients followed 6-11 years after operation*, Ann surg 1981;194:212-218.

4. Tarlov E, Schmidek H, Scott RM, et al.,*Reflex hypotension following carotid endarterectomy: mechanism and management*, J. Neurosurg. 1973;39:323-327.

5. Schomig A, *Catecholamines in myocardial ischemia, systemic and cardiac release*, Circulation 1990;82:13-22.

6. Akselrod S, Gordon D, Ubel FA, Shannon DC, Barger AC, Cohen RJ, *Power spectrum analysis of heart rate fluctuations: a quantitative probe of beat to beat cardiovascular control*, Science 1981;213:220-222.

7. Akselrod S, Gordon D, Madwed JB, Snidman NC, Shannon DC, Cohen RJ, *Hemodynamic regulation investigation by spectral analysis*, Am J Physiol 1985;249;H867-75.

8. Pagani M, Lombardi F, Guzzetti S, Rimoldi O, Furlan R, Pizzinelli P, Sandrome G, Malfatto G, Dell'Orto S, Piccaluga E, et al.,*Power spectral analysis of heart rate and arterial pressure variabilities as a marker of sympatho-vagal interaction in man and conscious dog*, Circ Res 1986;59:178-93.

9. Singer DH, Martin GJ, Magid N, Weiss JS, Schaad JW, Kehoe R, Zheutlin T, Fintel DG, Hsieh AM, Lesch M,*Low heart rate variability and sudden cardiac death*, J Electrocardiol 1988;21:S46-55.

10. Hayano J, Sakakibara Y, Yamada M, Ohte N, Fujinami T, Yokoyama K, Watanabe Y, Takata K,*Decreased magnitude of heart rate spectral components in coronary artery disease. Its relation to angiographic severity*, Circulation 1990;81:1217-24.

11. Hayano J, Yamada M, Sakakibara Y, et al.,*Short and long term effects of cigarette smoking on heart rate variability*, Am J Cardiol 1990;65:84-88.

12. Sapoznikov D, Luria MH, Mahler Y, Gotsman M, *Effects of the lower frequency limit on dtermining high frequency power of heart rate fluctuations*, IEEE EMBS, Paris,1992.

13. Grossman A and Morlet J, *Decomposition of Haar Functions into Square Integrable Wavelets of Constant Shape*, SIAM.J. Math., 15, 723-736.

14. Daubechies I, *Orthonormal bases of compactly supported wavelets*, Commun Pure Appl Math,909-996,1988.

15. Mallat SG, *A theory for multiresolution signal decomposition: the wavelet representation*, IEEE Transactions on PAMI, vol.11, no.7, July 1989.

16. Chui CK, *An Introduction to Wavelets*, Academic Press, NY, 1992.

17. Hlawatsch F and Boudreaux-Barlets GF, *Linear and Quadratic Time-Frequency Representations*, IEEE SP Magazine, pp.21-67, April 1992.

18. Daubechies I, *Time-Frequency Localization Operators: A Geometric Phase Space Approach*, IEEE Trans on Information Theory, vol.34, pp.605-612, July 1988.

19. Daubechies I, The Wavelet Transform, Time-Frequency Localization and Signal Analysis, IEEE Trans on Information Theory, vol.36, pp.961-1005, Sept. 1990.

20. Kronland- Martinet R, Morlet J, Grossmann A, *Analysis of Sounds Patterns Through Wavelet Transforms*, Int. J. Pattern Recognition and Artificial Intelligence, vol.1, pp.273-301, 1987.

21. Yang X, Wang K, and Shamma SA, *Auditory Representation of Acoustic Signals*, IEEE Trans on Information Theory, March 1992.

22. Rioul O and Vetterli M, *Wavelets and Signal Processing*, IEEE SP Magazine, pp.14-38, Oct. 1991.

23. Akay YM, Akay M, Welkowitz W, Lefkowicz S, Palti Y, *Time-frequency analysis of the turbulent sounds produced by femoral artery stenosis in dogs using wavelet transform*, IEEE EMBS, Paris, 1992.

24. Healy DM, Jr. and Weaver JB, *Two applications of wavelet transforms in magnetic resonance imaging*, IEEE Transactions on Information Theory, vol.38, no.2, 840-860, 1992.

25. Bachen NI, *Detection of Stimulus-Related (Evoked Response) Activity in the Electroencephalogram (EEG)*. IEEE BME 6:245-251, 1986.

26. Akay M, Welkowitz W, Semmlow JL, Kostis J, *Application of the ARMA method to Acoustical Detection of Coronary Artery Disease*. Med. Biol. Eng. Comput 29:365-372, 1991

27. Akay M and Craelius W. *Mechanoelectric Feedback in Cardiac Myocytes from Stretch-Activated Ion Channels*, IEEE Trans on BME **in press**

28. Landesberg G, Erel J, Anner H, Eidelman LA, Weinmann E, Luria MH, Sapoznikov D,Berlatzky Y and Cotev S, *Perioperative myocardial ischemia in carotid endarterectomy under cervical block anesthesia and prophylactic nitroglycerin infusion*, J. Cardiothoracic and Vascular Anesthesia (in press).

29. Akay M, Landesberg G, Welkowitz W, Akay YM, Sapoznikov D, *Multiresolution Decomposition of of Heart Rate Fluctuations during Carotid Surgery using Wavelet Transform*, Proc.IEEE EMBS, Paris,1993.

30. Akay M, Landesberg G, Welkowitz W, Akay YM, Sapoznikov D, *Analysis of HRV before, during, and after Carotid Sugery* Interaction Phenomena is the Cardiac System. Sideman and Beyar(Eds), Plenum Publishing

Corporation, NY, 1993.

31. Akay M, Landesberg G, Welkowitz W, Akay YM, Sapoznikov D, *Time-Frequency Analysis of Heart Rate Fluctuations during Carotid Surgery using Wavelet Transform*, IEEE Trans on Biomedical Engineering, (Submitted for publication).

REASONING FOR INTRODUCING A NEW PARAMETER FOR ASSESSMENT OF MYOCARDIAL STATUS - THE SPECIFIC POTENTIAL OF MYOCARDIUM

LJUBA BACHÁROVÁ
National Center for Health Promotion, Limbová 11
833 08 Bratislava, Slovakia

1. Introduction

The development of myocardial hypertrophy is a fundamental adaptive mechanism of the heart in response to increased work load. Initially, the hypertrophied myocardium is capable to meet the increased work demand. However, it has the seeds of deterioration incorporated into its structure. If the stress persists, the hypertrophied heart muscle progresses to the state of irreversible failure. Thus, myocardial hypertrophy may be considered the interface between the normal and failing condition [1]. From this point of view, the recognition and evaluation of left ventricular hypertrophy (LVH) in clinical practice represent important diagnostic and prognostic information.

In noninvasive clinical assessment of LVH two methods are preferred: electrocardiography or vectorcardiography (ECG/VCG) and echocardiography (EchoCG). The diagnostic importance of ECG/VCG in the diagnostics of left ventricular hypertrophy seems to be decreased since echocardiography was introduced into clinical practice.

Reasons for decreasing interest in ECG/VGC are:

* low sensitivity of ECG/VCG criteria for LVH,
* low or even non-significant correlations to left ventricular mass.

Reasons in favor of echocardiographic diagnostics:

* visualization and measurement of cardiac dimensions,
* highly significant correlation between echocardiographically estimated left ventricular mass (LVM) and post mortem findings,
* noninvasive estimation of hemodynamic parameters.

In general, echocardiography is considered to be a clinical electrocardiogram - independent standard ("golden standard") for left ventricular hypertrophy, mainly for its convenient estimation of LVM.

The difference in information content of ECG and other methods of LVM assessment is obvious and generally accepted. But paradoxically, the disagreements between these two approaches in diagnostics have led to stressing the priority of either of the particular methods. Discrepancies between ECG and EchoCG are named "false negative" or "false positive". This is a biased approach to the ECG since the ECG results are considered implicitely to be "false" - e.g. wrong. In the extremes, this approach led to refusal of electrocardiography as an obsolete method of LVH diagnostics.

The aim of this contribution is to describe the reasoning for introducing a new noninvasive parameter - the specific potential (SP) - in the assessment of myocardial status in left ventricular hypertrophy, based on the analysis of the conceptual model used for LVH diagnosis in clinical practice, and its parameters.

2. Recent conceptual model for ecg/vcg diagnosis of LVH

The ECG diagnosis of left ventricular hypertrophy is based on the theoretical assumption that the excitation of the larger and thicker muscle mass results in larger and longer living activation boundaries, which in turn, results in more than usual preponderance of leftward and posteriorly oriented electrical forces.

This theoretical assumption has been supported by results of correlative clinical and postmortem studies, where increased QRS voltage was recorded in a subset of patients with left ventricular enlargement. It is expected that increased voltage magnitude detected in LVH decreased monotonously toward normal values, and the upper limits of normal population are used for ECG criteria for LVH.

The conceptual model for ECG diagnostics of left ventricular hypertrophy is rather simple and can be defined as follows:

1. Input and output of the model:
   input is the measure of hypertrophy, which is represented by left venticular size, or its correlates,
   output is the QRS voltage.

2. QRS voltage is the function of left ventricular size:
   $$QRS = f\ (LVS)$$
   Simple mathematical model is expressed by linear equation:
   $$QRS = a + b\ (LVS)$$

3. Parameters a, b were not defined in the sense of pathophysiological or clinical data.

4. Indirect methods based on the determination of the arbitrary upper normal limits are used for testing the model, i.e. sensitivity, specificity, false negativity, false positivity.

2.1. Input of the model

Before echocardiography was introduced into clinical practice, the assessment of left ventricular hypertrophy was based on the anterio-posterior chest X-ray examination [2], [3], [4], [5], ventriculography [6] and post mortem measurements [7], [8], [9], [10]. Among these methods the autopsy is taken as a basic reference method which allows the direct measurement of heart size and its anatomical parts.

Echocardiographic imaging replaced these methods in LVH diagnostics [11], [12], [13], [14], [15], [16], [17]. M-mode echocardiography allows to measure dimensions of interventricular septum, internal diameter of left ventricle and posterior wall thickness along the ultrasound beam, and these values are used for calculation of left ventricular mass. The most recommended formulas use the cube model of left ventricle [18], [19]. Their accuracy was proved in symmetric left ventricles. Two-dimensional echocardiography, using sophisticated models of left ventricle, provides more accurate estimates of LVM in abnormal hearts [20], [21], [22], [23], [24]. With the aim to reduce the influence of anthropometric differences, the indexing of LVM to body surface area or height were recommended in LVH diagnostics [25], [26].

Main features of echocardiography in diagnostics of LVH are reproducibility in serial studies, and the close correlation with autopsy measurements of left ventricular mass. Clinical diagnostics of LVH is in this way simplified to determination of left ventricular dimensions and/or mass.

2.2. Output of the model - QRS voltage parameters

The development of ECG parameters followed the development of electrocardiologic methods - beginning with standard 12-lead electrocardiography, through orthogonal electrocardiography and vectorcardiography, to the evaluation of the total body surface information on the cardiac electric field - the body surface potential mapping.

2.2.1. The standard 12-lead electrocardiogram

In the standard 12-lead electrocardiography the dominant leftward and posteriorly oriented electrical forces are represented by increased amplitudes of QRS waves in corresponding leads. The **limb leads** (I., II., III., aVR, aVL, aVF) are the leads of frontal plane [27], [28]. Lead axes projected onto the frontal plane reflect leftward and vertical orientation of resultant electrical forces of depolarization. Table 1 gives the list of several recommended limb lead voltage

TABLE 1. List of recommended diagnostic criteria for left ventricular hypertrophy using limb leads of standard 12-lead electrocardiogram.

lead	criterion	author
$(R_I - S_I) + (S_{III} - R_{III})$	17 mm	Lewis 1914 [29]
S_{III}, S_I	$S_{III} > S_I$	Hattori 1966 [30]
Q_{aVR}	14 mm 12 mm	Schack et al. 1950 [31] Murphy et al. 1983 [32]
R_I	13 mm 13 mm 13 mm 15 mm	Manning a Smiley 1964 [33] Gubbner and Ungerleider 1943 [34] Murphy et al.1983 [32] Rodstein and Gubner 1964 [35]
$R_I + S_{III}$	16 mm 16- 25 yrs 17 mm 31- 50 yrs 19 mm 25 mm	Manning and Smiley 1964 [33] Manning and Smileay 1964 [33] Murphy et al. 1983 [32] Rodstein a Gubner 1964 [35]
R_{aVF}	12 mm 14 mm 15 mm 31- 50 yrs 19 mm 20 mm 23 mm 16- 25 yrs	Schack et al. 1950 [31] Murphy et al. 1983 [32] Manning and Smiley 1964 [33] Schack et al. 1950 [31] Goldberger 1947 [36] Manning and Smiley 1964 [33]
R_{aVL}	7 mm 16- 25 yrs 7.5 mm 8 mm 9 mm 31- 50 yrs 11 mm 12 mm 13 mm	Manning and Smiley 1964 [33] Mazzoleni et al. 1964 [37] Murphy et al. 1983 [32] Manning et al. 1964 [33] Sokolow and Lyon 1949 [38] Schack et al. 1950 [31] Goldberger 1947 [36]

parameters of standard 12-lead ECG for LVH diagnostics. The possible sources of false negativity or false positivity are demonstrated using the criterion R_{aVL} as an example (Figure 1).

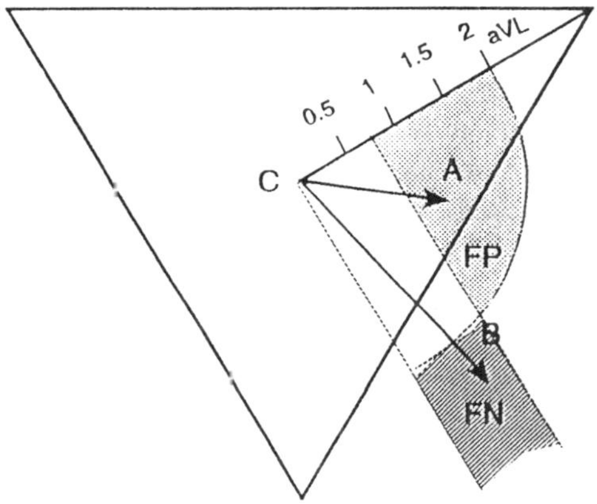

FIGURE 1: Graphic presentation of sources of false positivity and false negativity of diagnostic criterion R_{aVL} in relation to maximum QRS vector magnitude prejected onto the frontal plane.

aVL lead axis is projected onto the Einthowen triangle frame. The scale of aVL axis indicates several recommended upper normal limits. Value of 7.5 mV is used as an example. Area of normal occurrence of QRS vector end-points projected onto the frontal plane according to this criterion is limited by perpendicular line erected from the value of 7.5 mV. The circle defines the area of normal occurrence of maximum QRS vector end-points projected onto the frontal plane.

The vector A represents the vertical position of the electric axis. The magnitude of the maximum QRS vector exceeds the upper normal limit, while according to the aVL criterion it si situated inside the normal area - false negative result.

The vector B represents the horizontal position of the electric axis. The magnitude of the maximum QRS vector is within normal limits, however it surpasses the upper normal limit of aVL - false positive result.

Introducing the set of **chest leads** V1, V2, V3, V4, V5, V6 into standard electrocardiography [39], the important anterio - posterior information was added. The classical criterion for LVH, using chest leads, is the Sokolow-Lyon index [38], which summarizes the leftward oriented maximum deflection in leads V5 or V6 and the posterior deflection represented by the amplitude of S in lead V1 (Figure 2). This index is still widely used in clinical ECG diagnostic of LVH, also several other single or combined voltage parameters using chest leads were recommended (Table 2).

To overcome the limited information of particular leads, or particular planes represented by the set of limb or chest leads, combined parameters were recommended (Table 3). And finally, summing the QRS amplitudes of all 12 leads, increased QRS amplitude in any lead can be included and so no information is missing , as well as disperse borderline voltage increase in any leads can be manifested.

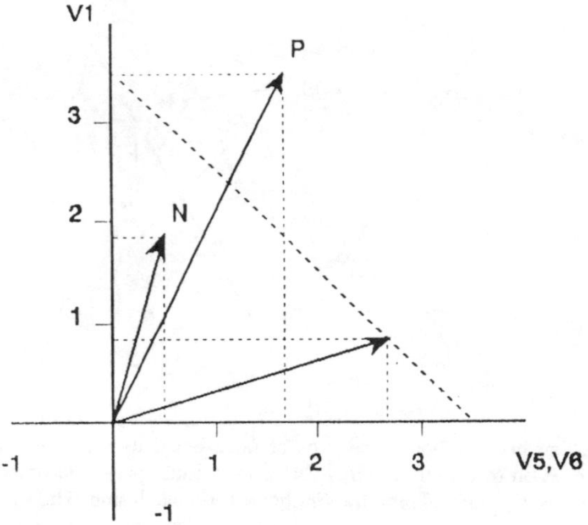

FIGURE 2: Graphic presentation of the positivity of the Sokolow - Lyon index. Lead axes V_1 and $V_{5,6}$ are projected onto the horizontal plane. The area of negative results (N) is defined by a triange: center of coordinate system, value of SV_1 = 35 mm and value of $R_{V5,6}$ = 35 mm. Maximum QRS vector end-points localized leftward and posteriorly with respect to this area exceed the upper normal limit SLI = 35 mm (P).

2.2.2. Orthogonal Electrocardiography and Vectorcardiography

Orthogonal electrocardiography describes the orientation and magnitude of the resultant spatial vector by means of three perpendicular axes of the Cartesian coordinate system. In clinical practice the Frank [52] and McFee-Parungao [53] lead systems are mostly used. The expected posterior and leftward predominace of left venctricle in left ventricular hypertrophy is reflected mainly in leads of the horizontal plane: X (right-to-left) and Z (anterio-posterior). Vectorcardiography visualizes and describes the temporo-spatial relations of these three perpendicular components X, Y, Z in the form of vectorcardiographic loops projected onto the three perpendicular planes - horizontal, frontal and sagittal. Characteristic

TABLE 2. List of recommended diagnostic criteria for left ventricular hypertrophy using chest leads of standard 12-lead electrocardiogram.

lead	criterion	author
$S_{V1} + R_{V5,6}$	30 mm	Wolf 1962 [40]
	33 mm	Murphy et al. 1983 [32]
	35mm	Sokolow and Lyon 1949 [38]
	37	Manning and Smiley 1964 [33]
	31 - 50 yrs	
	40 (45)	Hattori 1966 [30]
	53	Manning and Smiley 1964 [33]
	16 - 25 yrs	
max. $R_{V5,V6}$	26 mm	McPhie 1958 [41]
	33 mm	Manning and Smiley 1964 [33]
	16 - 25 yrs	
	24 mm	Manning and Smiley 1964 [33]
	31 - 50 yrs	
$S_{V1} + R_{V5}$	30 mm	Lepeshkin 1951 [42]
	33 mm	Murphy et al. 1983 [32]
	36 mm	Simonson 1961 [43]
	40 mm	Kimura et al. 1987 [44]
$S_{V1,V2} + R_{V5,V5}$	38 mm	Murphy et al. 1983 [32]
	40 mm	Grant 1957 [45]
S_{V1}	16 mm	Murphy et al. 1983 [32]
	24 mm	Wilson et al. 1944 [39]
$S_{V2} + R_{V5}$	35 mm	Cooksey et al. 1977 [46]
	44 mm	Murphy et al. 1983 [32]
max.R + max.S	40 mm	McPhie 1958 [41]
	49 mm	Murphy et al. 1983 [32]
	45, 35 mm	Grant 1957 [45]
R_{V6}	20 mm	Simonson 1961 [43]
	15 mm	Murphy et al. 1983 [32]
$R_{V6} > R_{V5}$		Holt a Spodick 1962 [47]
		Murphy et al. 1983 [32]
R_{V5}	20 mm	Romhilt et al. 1969 [48]
	20 mm	Murphy et al. 1983 [32]
	26 mm	Sokolow and Lyon [38]
$S_{V2} + R_{V4,V5}$	35 mm	Wolf 1962 [40]

vectorcardiographic features of LVH are the leftward and posterior displacement of the main body of QRS loop and the increased magnitude of maximum QRS vector [54], [55], [56], [57], [58], [59]. Quantitative orthogonal ECG and vectorcardiographic criteria are listed in table 4.

TABLE 3. List of recommended diagnostic criteria for left ventricular hypertrophy combining limb and chest leads.

lead	criterion	author
$R_{aVL} + S_{V3}$	2.8 mV (men) 2.0 mV (women)	Casale et al. 1985 [49]
$QRS_{aVF+V2+V6}$	175 mm	Roberts and Day 1985 [50] Odom at al. 1986 [51]
summa QRS (12 leads)	50 mm 93 mm 16 - 25 yrs 59 mm 31 - 50 yrs	Manning and Smiley 1964 [33] Manning and Smiley 1964 [33] Manning and Smiley 1964 [33]

2.2.3. Body Surface Potential Mapping

Body surface potential mapping provides the total information about the cardiac electric field recorded on the torso surface. Advanced mathematical and statistical methods have been used to achieve improvement of LVH diagnostic classification, anyway, increased voltage is evaluated mainly in individual leads. Sohi et al. [66] constructed departure maps produced by substracting from each patient's voltage patterns the normal range, and described the peak of positivity with a higher amplitude, delayed in onset and longer persisting, on the left anterolateral and upper chest. For identification of the best lead position for optimal separation of normal subjects from patients with LVH, Kornreich et al. [67] constructed discriminant maps. They were obtained by subtracting the normal group mean voltages from the LV hypertrophy group-mean voltages and by dividing the resulting differences by the corresponding pooled standard deviations computed from the population in the training LVH set. Time varying values and discriminant indexes were strictly proportional to Student's t test statistics and reflected the capability of each measurement in each lead to separate LV hypertrophy patients from normal subjects.

TABLE 4: List of recommended criteria for left ventricular hypertrophy used in orthogonal electrocardiography and vectorcardiography

parameter	criterion	author
R_X	18 mm** 1.7 mV* 3.35 mV** 1.84 mV*	Gadzayeva and Alekperov 1984 [60] Yano and Pipberger 1964 [3] Ruttkay - Nedecký 1975 [61] Pipberger et al. 1967 [62]
$R_X + S_Z$	27 mm**	Gadzayeva and Alekperov 1984 [60]
$R_X + R_Z$	3.2 mV* (men) 2.5 mV* (women)	Yano and Pipberger 1964 [3]
$QRS_{max.}$ H plane	1.59 mV* (men) 2.19 mV*	Dower and Horn 1967 [63] Winsor 1973 [56]
$QRS_{max.}$ spatial	2 mV* (<40 yrs) 1.9 mV* (> 40 yrs) 2.47 mV* (men, 22-34 yrs) 2.18 mV* (men, 35-60 yrs) 2.41 mV* (women,22-34yrs) 2.08 mV* (women,35-59yrs) 1.9 mV* (men) 1.82 mV* (women) 2.12 mV*	Chou et al. 1974 [54] Edenbrandt et al. 1987 [64] Dower a Horn 1967 [63] Murata et al. 1964 [65]
$R_{XYZ}:S_{XYZ}$ ratio	1.5**	Gadzayeva and Alekperov 1984 [60]
R_{XYZ}	37 mm**	Gadzayeva and Alekperov 1984 [60]
$QRS_{max.}$ F plane	1.74 mV*	Murata et al. 1964 [65]

The listed electrocardiologic methods and parameters for LVH diagnostics are far from beeing complete and final, but they reflect the generally accepted implication - the hypertrophied left venctricle appears to be the more remote, though more powerful and compact generator. Big variety of recommended leads and the broad scale of the values recommended as criteria for LVH are evident.

2.3. Linear relation

The aims of correlative studies are the elucidation of relation between ECG and signs of anatomical hypertrophy with practical impact - to select the best electrocardiologic parameter and criterion in prediction of LVH and in assessing the severity of LVH. All correlative studies have been using only the linear regression model. Taking into accout the considerable variety of electrocardiologic parameters, as well as of reference non-electrocardiologic methods (as listed above) and their possible combinations, only a limited number of illustrative results could be presented. Table 5 illustrates the scale of correlation coefficients from non-significant to highly significant values. While correlation coefficients are presented in every correlative study as a measure of the fittnes of the linear model, the linear regression equations are not often published. But as well they showed considerable variability (Table 6).

It must be stressed that parameters of the linear model - *a* and *b* - have been presented, but never described or evaluated from the physiological, pathophysiological or clinical point of view.

2.4. Testing the model

The classic and most basic way to evaluate reliability of electrocardiographic criteria for LVH is to investigate the sensitivity and specificity. The main problem of ECG criteria of LVH - considerable overlapping of normal and LVH population - was seen in the classical Sokolow and Lyon work [38]. According to their original results, 32 % of patients with left ventricular hypertrophy had the sum of these two potentials exceeded 35 mm, whereas in no normal person did this sum exceed 35 mm. This of course means that 68 % (!) of LVH population has the voltage parameter within normal limits. As shown in Table 7, this considerable overlapping is reflected monotonously in high specificity and low sensitivity of ECV criteria for LVH. Even the most sofisticated ECG criteria used for computer ECG analysis, which combine all known factors (age, sex, constituional variables, additional ECG criteria including P wave, T wave, QRS duration, QRS axis, e.g.) have nearly the same discriminant power - sensitivity 69 % and 32 %, respectively, specificity 83 % and 89 %, respectively [77], [78].

TABLE 5. Correlation coefficients for selected ECG parameters used for evaluation of left ventricular hypertrophy.

ECG/VCG parameter	r	reference method	author
SLI	0.30 0.39 0.56 0.85	necropsy echocg	Reichek and Devereux 1981 [13] George et al. 1972 [68] Toshima et al. 1975 [69]
R_{aVL}	0.63	echocg	Reichek and Devereux 1981 [13]
S_{V1}	0.63		Reichek and Devereux 1981 [13]
R_{V6}	0.18 0.40		Reichek and Devereux 1981 [13] Gamboa et al. 1965 [70]
$S_{V2} + R_{V5}$	0.48	LVPSP	Gamboa et al. 1965 [70]
summa QRS	0.11	necropsy	Dollar and Roberts 1989 [71]
$QRS_{max.}$ spatial	0.67 0.44 0.88 0.48 0.48	echocg echocg (dilat.) necropsy LVPSP	Toshima et al. 1977 [63] Gamboa et al. 1965 [70] Dower and Horn 1967 [63] Reeve and Kawamoto 1966 [72]
summa 3 MSV	0.51	LVPSP	Reeve and Kawamoto 1966 [72]
summa 4 MSV	0.51	LVPSP	Reeve and Kawamoto 1966 [72]

SLI: Sokolow-Lyon index
LVPSP: left ventricular peak systolic pressure
summa 3 MSV: maximal spatial vector + vectors 0.01 sec before and after the MSV
summa 4 MSV: summa 3 MSV − the vector 0.02 sec after the MSV

2.5. Reasons for the weakness of linear relationship

Low correlations, high number of false negative results and the resulting low sensitivity are attributed mainly to extracardiac factors - sources of interindividual variability within the normal population. In population studies or in the samples of healthy (normal) population, significant differences were found between males and females [43], [62], [79], [80], between different age categories [81], [82], [83], [84],

TABLE 6. Linear equations for selected ECG criteria used for diagnostics of left ventricular hypertrophy.

equation	x, y	author
y = 0.1835x - 7.4415 y = 0.2613x - 17. 0246	SBP, SLI SBP, SLI	George et al. 1972 [68]
y = 1.38x - 1.59 y = 1.47x + 0.01	LVPW, $QRS_{max.}$	Toshima et al. 1977 [69]
y = 40.50x + 75.65	LVPW, $QRS_{max.}$	Gamboa et al. 1965 [70]
y = 0.112x - 2.8 y = 22.7x - 8.7 y = 0.189x - 1.1 y = 37.4x - 10.2	LVT, R_X LVM, R_X LVT, $R_X + S_Z$ LVM, $R_X + S_Z$	Gadzayeva and Alekperov 1984 [60]
y = 303.95 + 88.51x y = 311.68 + 89.14x	$QRS_{max.}$, HW $QRS_{max.}$, HW	Dower and Horn 1967 [63]

[85], [86], [87], [64] and races [88], [86]. Various upper normal limits for QRS voltage, depending on sex, age and race, respectively, are recommended in order to make the diagnotics of LVH more precise. As to the problem of relationship between hypetrophied left ventricle and QRS voltage two main objections arise:

* the above mentioned factors are not parameters of the linear model,
* factors, which influence the normal variability and are used to precise the upper normal limits cannot solve the problem, since they influence both normal and pathologic LVH distributions.

The Brody effect [89] is also often used to explain the weakness of the linear relationship between left ventricular size and ECG voltage magnitude. Originally, Brody concluded, that the relatively large conductivity of the intracavitary blood mass tends to short-circuit the tangential components, but augments the radial components of myocardial doublets, reflected in the decrease of tangentially oriented dipole moment and in the increase of radially oriented dipole moment. However, the citation analysis of the Brody effect shows that its real meaning is not always understood and applied, and changes of intracardiac blood volume instead of changes of intracavitary blood conductivity are often considered. The confusion around the Brody effect is underlined by controversial results of experimental as well as clinical studies under rest and excercise. Results of experimental and clinical studiel support the findings of increased voltage by increasing blood volume [42], [90], [91], [92], [93], [94], [95], as well as decreasing voltage amplitude [96], [97], [98], [99], [100], [101], [102], [103], [104], [105], [106].

TABLE 7. Sensitivity and specificity for selected ECG criteria used for diagnostics of left ventricular hypertrophy.

parameter	sensitivity (%)	specificity (%)	author
SLI	51.9	96.6	Geva et al. 1979 [73]
	21	95 necropsy	Reichek and Devereux 1981 [13]
	53	86 echocg	
	2	100	Vandenberg et al. 1989 [74]
	29	89	Miasuls et al. 1987 [75]
	20 men	100	
	50 women	83	
$S_{V1} + R_{V5}$			
> 30 mm	5	98	Vanderberg et al. 1989 [74]
> 33 mm	50	94	
> 35 mm	56.6	76	Kimura et al. 1987 [44]
> 36 mm	52	97	Warner and Hill 1987 [76]
> 45 mm	24	100	
R_{aVL}			
> 11 mm	25	100	Geva et al. 1979 [73]
	47	99	Reichek and Devereux 1981 [13]
> 13 mm	23	84	Vanderberg et al. 1989 [74]
> 7.5 mm	48	77	
> 11 mm	29	86	
> 12 mm	27	96	
R_{V6}			
> 16	56	97	Warner and Hill 1987 [76]
> 20	7	100	Vanderberg et al. 1989 [74]

Following basic facts in the current ECG/VCG diagnostics of LVH can be summarized:

* in clinical practice the anatomical nature of the LVH is stressed and so the diagnosis of LVH is oriented to increased dimension of the left ventricle or of its parts,
* ECG voltage does not follow proportionally the increase of left ventricular size, and this is considered to be "false" (negative or positive).

3. New approach

We tried to look at this problem from the opposite side:

* a subset of hypertrophied left ventricles really shows increased votlage corresponding to left ventricular mass increase - so called "true possitive" findings,
* but a unneglectable number of hypertrophied left ventricles (already above mentioned 68 % (!) even in classical Sokolow -Lyon work [38]) does not fulfill the expectation of the increased voltage proportionally to increased mass. These findings could be also interpreted that they appear like to have a "voltage deficit" (instead of refusing them as "false negative" results). It could be assumed that they could be less effective generators of cardiac electric field in relation to their mass.

To test the hypothesis of the "voltage deficit" of hypertrophied left ventricle we tried:

* to find a parameter for quantification of the "voltage deficit" using available methods,
* to find possible explanation for this deficit.

Basic issues:

* definition of hypertrophy,
* the information obtained by echocardiography in relation to LVH,
* the information obtained by electro/vectorcardiography in relation to LVH.

3.1. Hypertrophy

Ventricular hypertrophy is an adaptive response of the heart to the hemodynamic overload. According to the results of experimental left ventricular hypertrophy three stages were described [107], [108]:

1. **Stage of damage (stage of developing hypertrophy)**, when the work load exceeds the normal work output of the mass of the heart. During this stage myocardial mass increases 1.5 to 2 times. Increased activity of subcellular structures was described (e.g. activation of energy production and protein synthesis, increase in oxygen comsumption per unit myocardial mass).
2. **Stable state of hyperfunction (compensatory hypertrophy)**, when the work-induced growth of the heart compensates for the increased workload. There is a normal level of activity of myocardial subcellular structures and a corresponding normal level of energy production and protein synthesis. The oxygen consumption per unit myocardial mass is normal, and thus, total oxygen consumption is increased to the same extend as myocardial mass.
3. **Stage of progressing cardiosclerosis and gradual exhaustion (developing heart failure)**, when the workload per unit cardiac mass increases again due to the progressively decreasing force-generation ability of the heart. This

stage is characterized by a decrease in the intensity of protein synthesis, which is responsible for a failure to renew contractile structures and energy-producing components.

LVH is a complex process, which cannot be characterized only by an increase of left ventricular mass, but it is accompanied and conditioned by functional changes (e.g. protein synthesis, energy supply, oxygen consumption, intracellular morphology, structural rearrangement of myocardial tissue, contractility, etc.) These complex functional changes have not (!) linear relationship to the growth of left ventricle during the development of left ventricular hypertrophy. The functional parameters under study (e.g. energy production, oxygen consumtion) are often related to myocardial mass unit with the aim to describe the functional status of hypertrophied myocardium. Analogically it can be assumed, that electrogenesis, as a functional property of myocardium, will not follow proportionally the growth of the left ventricle. It may be expected that the potential contribution of a myocardial unit to the total electric field of the heart could also provide the additional information.

3.2. Information obtained by echocardiography

Echocardiography provides information about the dimensions of the parts of left ventricle. These primary data are used for calculation and estimation of left ventricular mass. The hypothesis for correlative studies EchoCG - necropsy is very simple: the bigger left ventricle at necropsy is reflected in bigger size of left ventricle assertained by echocardiography. Both methods evaluate the same featute - the size (weight). It is natural, that the correlations are tight, significant. These two parameters are not independent and therefore the value of correlation coefficient refelcts the inpreciseness of measuring method. In this context the finding of the correlation coefficient 0.89 is not as methodologically significant, as it is formally statistically significant.

3.3. Information obtained by electro/vectorcardiography

Electrocardiologic methods provide information about the distribution and voltage values of the electric field of the heart on the surface of the body. They characterize the generator of cardiac electric field and not (!) the size of the heart. From endless results of correlative studies it is clear, that the increased voltage is recorded only in a subset of patients with LVH. The most of patients with LVH has voltage "deficit" - reflected as low sensitivity, or high number of false negative results.

With the aim to describe and quantify the discrepancies between ECG and EchoCG findings as well as to preserve both results we tried to introduce another approach and to give another view to so-called "false negative" results. We wanted to turn the attention to the fact, that a large heart needs not to be necesarilly a strong generator of the electric field, and on the other hand, a small-sized heart can generate a stronger electric field.

The following equation, based on distributed dipole and solid angle analysis [109], represents the potential detected at an extracellular recording site:

$$E=\frac{\Omega}{4}(V_{m2}-V_{m1})\,[1+\frac{\sigma_o}{\sigma_i}(\frac{S}{A}-1)]^{-1} \tag{1}$$

where: Ω = solid angle, V_{m2} - V_{m1} = transmembrane voltage difference, σ_i = intracellular conductivity, σ_o = extracellular conductivity, A = area of excitable tissue and S = total cross-sectional area in the conductivity terms.

The solid angle, , represents the spatial determinant of the recorded voltage. It is determined by the actual geometry of the boundary and the electrode distance from the boundary.

Non-spatial determinants of the extracardial voltage magnitude are difficult to assess with clinical diagnostic means. Nevertheless, we tried to approximate them by introducing the concept of the specific potential [110].

4. The specific potential of myocardium

SP was calculated from available clinical data, using equation (1). The part of the equation (1) labeled A (spatial factors) is in direct relation to the left ventricular dimension. In our study the model cross-sectional area of the left ventricle (left ventricular activation area - LVAA) was used, computed from echocardiographic parameters (Figure 3). The part of the equation labeled B (non-spatial factors) can be approximated after some modification and using known parameters:

$$E \approx Vmax. \tag{2}$$

$$A \approx LVAA \tag{3}$$

$$B=\frac{E}{A} \tag{4}$$

$$B \approx \frac{Vmax}{LVAA} \tag{5}$$

$$SP = \frac{Vmax}{LVAA} \tag{6}$$

Using the ratio of spatial factors (A $\approx$ LVAA) the influence of left ventricular size on the resultant spatial vector magnitude is diminished (normalised). The SP value can be considered to be the potential contribution of left ventricular unit area, e.g. the summary parameter of non-spatial factors.

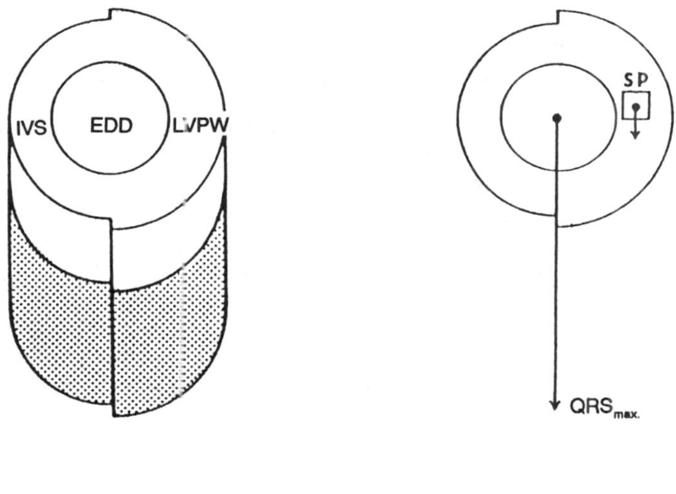

FIGURE 3: The hollow cylinder model of the left ventricle. Left ventricular activation area (LVAA) represents the cross-section of the model left ventricle. Echocardiographic dimensions of interventricular septum thickness (IVS), end-diastolic diameter of left ventricle (EDD) and left ventricular posterior wall (LVPW) were used for calculation of LVAA. Specific potential (SP) is expressed as a potential contribution of a unit area of left ventricular activation area LVAA (= 1 cm2) to the spatial magnitude of the maximum QRS vector (QRSmax.)

4.1. Preliminary results

We used this method in two clinical studies for the evaluation of LVH in patients with hypertension [110,111], as well as in a retrospective analysis of changes of cardioelectric field during the development of experimental LVH [112].

4.1.1. Clinical studies

Frank orthogonal electrocardiograms were recorded in 18 healthy subjects as well as in 47 hypertensive patients. The cross-sectional area of left ventricle (LVAA) was calculated from the M-mode echocardiographic dimensions of interventricular septum, end-diastolic diameter and left ventricular posterior wall thickness. Specific potential was calculated as the ratio of $QRS_{max.}$ and LVAA. Main results of the study [110]:

* no significant correlations were found between $QRS_{max.}$ and left ventricular mass (LVM) or cross-sectional area of left ventricle, respectively,
* $QRS_{max.}$ values above 2.0 mV (considered as the upper normal limit) were recorded in the neighbourhood of 20 cm^2, which represents approximately 200 g LVM, and further in marked left ventricular enlargement with values of LVAA over 30 cm^2. A transient decrease of potential values was observed between these two stages. Such behaviour indicates the possibility of non-linear relationship between $QRS_{max.}$ and left ventricular size (Figure 4),
* SP values decreased with increasing values of LVM (Figure 5). Although it is not a correct correlation (the relationship of basic and derived parameter), gradual decrease of SP can be seen with increased mass of left ventricle.
* SP values were lower in hypertensive patients as compared to healthy persons, while higher values of $QRS_{max.}$ were recorded in hypertensive patients.

Similar results - low correlations between $QRS_{max.}$ and echocardiographical parameters, decreased values of SP with increasing LVM - were obtained in an other study [111], where orthogonal McFee-Parungao electrocardiograms, as well as a different formula for LMV calculation from M-mode echocardiograms were used in a group of 65 hypertensive patients.

4.1.2. Experimental studies

Data of an experimental model of volume overload in rabbits were used to study the changes of SP in defined stages of experimental LVH [113]. Frank orthogonal ECGs were recorded and related to left ventricular mass and area. The specific potential was calculated as a ratio of $QRS_{max.}$ to LVM [112]. After a transient decrease of $QRS_{max.}$ in the early postoperative period, its increase was observed in the stage of compensatory hypertrophy. SP values were decreased during the whole follow-up period. They did not reach the initial values not even

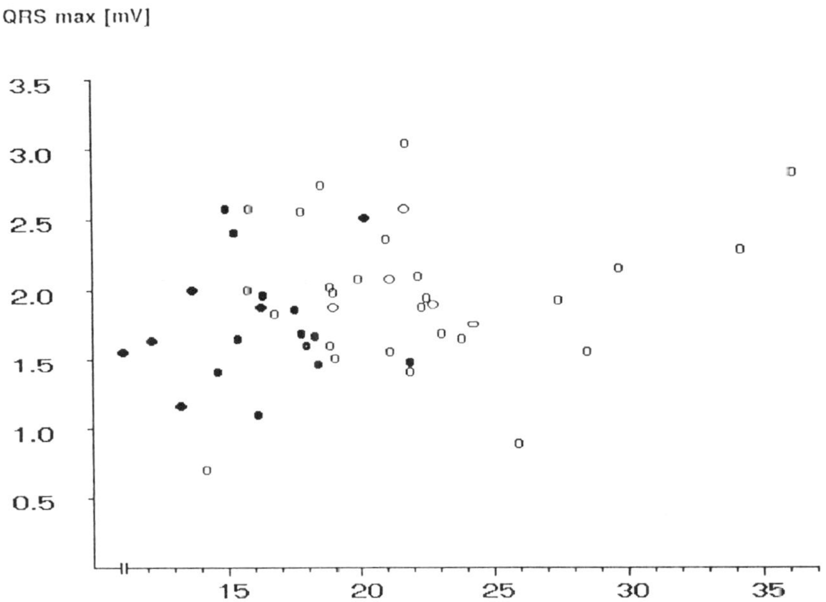

FIGURE 4: Relationship between left ventricular activation area (LVAA) and maximum spatial QRS vector magnitude (QRSmax.) in the mixed group of healthy subjects (solid circles) and hypertensive patients (open circles). Note the transient decrease of QRSmax. values as a function of increased LVAA around the value 25 cm2 of LVAA.

at the stage of developed hypertrophy, when the maximal increase of $QRS_{max.}$ was observed (Figure 6).

Main results of the study:

* Changes of cardioelectric field during the development of left ventricular hypertrophy were not proportional to the increase of left ventricular mass.
* Maximum discrepancies between $QRS_{max.}$ and LVM in experimental LVH were observed during the stages of developing hypertrophy and developing heart failure. These discrepancies could not be explained by a simple interpretation of the Brody efect.
* The suggested new parameter - specific potential - enables the quantification of this relationship.

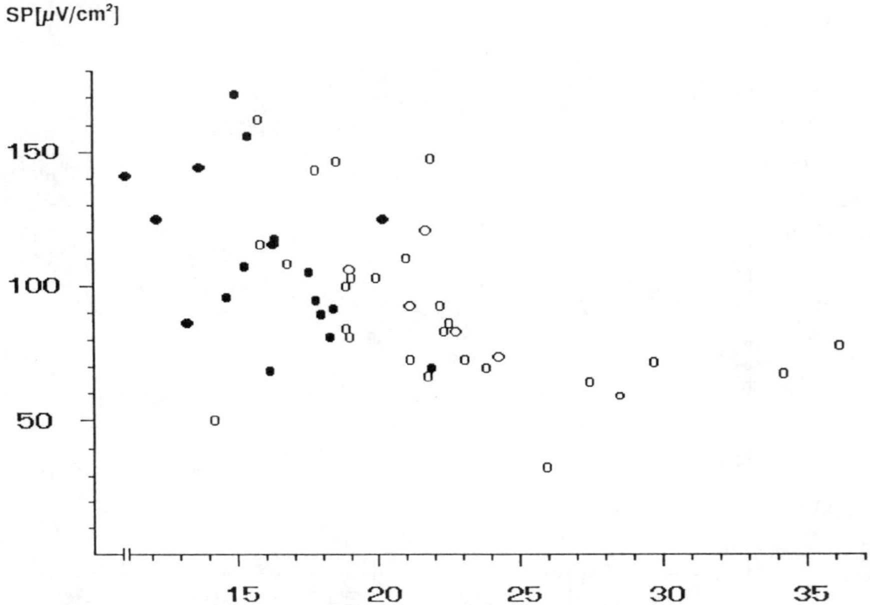

FIGURE 5: Relationship of specific potential (SP) and left ventricular activation area (LVAA) in a mixed group of healthy subjects (solid circles) and hypertensive patients (open circles).

4.2. Relation to the stages of hypertrophy

The concept of the specific potential is based on the assumption that the electrical properties of hypertrofied myocardium are changed in the course of LVH development. Experimental studies give more detailed description of left ventricular hypertrophy under defined model conditions in terms of structure, biochemistry and function [107], [108]. Experimental LVH is described as a dynamic process with continuous changes of anatomical and functional properties of the myocardium. These changes do not show monotonous behaviour in the course of LVH development. The above mentioned autors defined 3 distinct functional stages of cardiac adaptation to overload, instead of using changes of myocardial mass for characterising the stages of myocardial hypertrophy.

The assumption of linear relationship between left ventricular size and ECG potential magnitude, inherent to voltage criteria of LVH, would suggest implicitly that the unit mass of hypertrophic myocardium and the unit mass of healthy myocardium have the same properties, when evaluated as the source of the

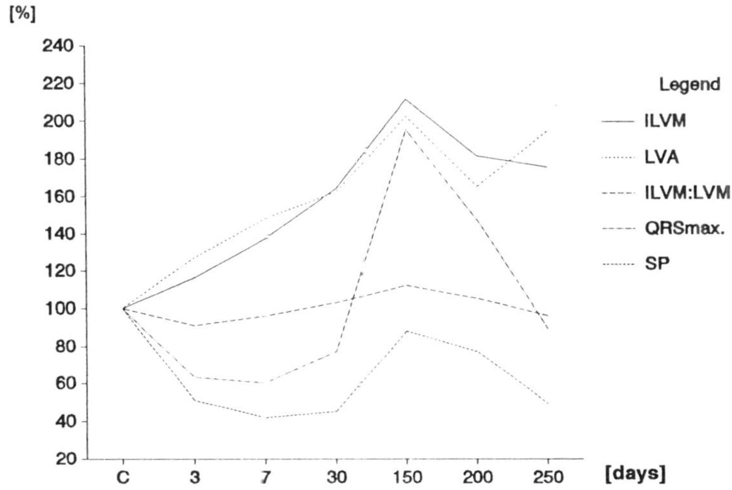

FIGURE 6: Changes of left ventricular mass indexed to body weight (ILVM), left ventricular area (LVA), ILVM:LVA ratio, maximum spatial QRS vector magnitude (QRSmax.) and specific potential (SP) during the course of experimental left ventricular hypertrophy, expressed as per cent of control values.

cardioelectric field. If, on the other hand, the contribution of unit mass of hypertrophic myocardium to the cardioelectric field should be increased, then we would expect an exponential or logarithimic relationship between left ventricular size and the measured potential. This has not been found. On the contrary, the low sensitivity of ECG in evaluation of LVH is notoriously known. It may be supposed that the hypertrophic myocardial unit mass contributes less to the total potential, at least in certain stages of left ventricular hypertrophy.

5. Conclusion

Functional properties of hypertrophied myocardium are influenced by disturbances of metabolism, energy supply, and structure of myocardial cells, ionic composition of extracellular fluid and structure of non-muscle cells of myocardial tissue, as well as by changes in regulatory mechanism. All the above mentioned factors are involved in non-spatial determinants of extracardial potential magnitude and can counterbalance the influence of increased left ventricular size. We are aware of rough estimation of "non-spatial factors" expressed as SP, but we would like to give a new point of view to the analysis of so-called false negative and false positive results in clinical ECG diagnostics of LVH in terms of summary functional properties of myocardium as a generator of the cardioelectric field.

6. References

1. N.R. Alpert (ed.), *Cardiac hypertrophy* (Academic Press, New York, London, 1971)
2. S. Jonsell, *Acta Radiol.* **20** (1939) 352
3. K. Yano and H.V. Pipberger, *A. Heart J.* **67** (1964) 44
4. P.M. Chikos, M.M. Figley, L. Fisher, *Am. J. Roentgenol.* **128** (1977) 367
5. C.P. Rose, and H.O. Stohlberg, *Invest. Radiol.* **11** (982) 139
6. W.A. Baxley, H.T. Dodge, H. Sander, *Circulation*, **37** (1968) 509
7. P.M. Zeek, *Arch. of Path.* **33** (1942) 820
8. B.J. Allenstein and H. Mori, *Circulation* **21** (1960) 401
9. L. Wolf, R. Wolf, M.D. Samartzis, et al., *Circulation* **23** (1961) 880
10. E.D.Geiser and K.E. Bove, *Arch. Pathol.* **97** (1974) 13
11. H.H. Kaye, M. Tyman, S. Hunter, *Br. Heart J.* **37** (1975) 371
12. T.M. Mc Farland, M. Alam, S. Goldstein, et al., *Circulation* **57** (1978) 1140
13. N. Reichek and R.B. Devereux, *Circulation* **63** (1981) 1391
14. A.E. Weyman, *Cross - sectional echocardiography* (Lea and Febiger, Philadelphia, 1982)
15. R.B. Devereux, P.M. Casale, R.R. Eisenberg, et al., *J. Am. Coll. Cardiol.* **3** (1983) 82
16. J.N. Woythaler, S.L. Singer, O.L. Kwan, et al., *J. Am. Coll. Cardiol.* **2** (1983) 305
17. D. Levy, D.D. Savage, R.J. Garrison, et al., *Am. J. Cardiol.* **59** (1987) 956
18. R.B. Devereux and N. Reichek, *Circulation* **55** (1976) 613
19. D.J. Sahn, A. De Maria, J. Kisslo, et al., *Circulation* **58** (1978) 1072
20. B.J. Maron, J.S. Gottdiener, R.O. Bonow, et al., *Circulation* **63** (1981) 409
21. N. Reichek, J. Helak, T. Plappert, et al., *Circulation* **67** (1983) 348
22. N.B. Schiller, C.G. Skioldebrand, E.J. Schiller, et al., *Circulation* **68** (1983) 210
23. B.F. Byrd, D. Wahr, Y.S. Wang, et al., *J. Am. Coll. Cardiol.* **6** (1985) 1021
24. H.W. Collins, M.W. Kronenberg, B.F. Byrd III, *J. Am. Coll. Cardiol.* **14** 1989) 672
25. R.B. Devereux, E.M. Lutas, P.N. Casole, et al., *J. Am. Coll. Cardiol.* **4** (1984) 1222

26. S.R. Daniels, R.A. Meyer, Y. Liang, et al., *J. Am. Coll. Cardiol.* **12** (1988) 703
27. W. Einthowen, G. Fahr, A. De Waart, *Pfugers Arch. ges. Physiol.* **150** (1913) 275
28. E. Goldberger, *Am. Heart J.* **23** (1942) 483
29. T. Lewis, *Heart* **5** (1914) 367
30. M. Hattori, *Jap. Circulation J.* **30** (1966) 655
31. J.A. Schack, R.H. Rosenman, L.N. Kate, *Am. Heart J.* **40** (1950) 696
32. M.L. Murphy, P.H. Thenabadu, L.R. Blue, et al., *Am. J. Cardiol.* **52** (1983) 1275
33. G.W. Manning and J.R. Smiley, *Circulation* **29** (1964) 224
34. R.S. Gubner and H.E. Ungerleider, *Arch. Int. Med.* **72** (1943) 196
35. M. Rodstein and R.S. Gubner, *Am. J. Cardiol.* **13** (1964) 619
36. E. Goldberger, *Unipolar lead electrocardiography 2nd ed.*(Lea and Febiger, Philadelphia, 1947)
37. A. Mazzoleni, R. Wolff, L. Wolff, et al., *Circulation* **30** (1964) 808
38. M. Sokolow and T.P. Lyon. *Amer. Heart J.* **37** (1949) 161
39. F.N. Wilson, F.D. Johnston, F.F. Rosenbaum, et al., *Am. Heart J.* **27** (1944) 19
40. L. Wolff, *Electrocardiography. 3rd ed.* (WB Saunders, Philadelphia, 1962)
41. J. McPhie, *Aust. Ann. Med.* **7** (1958) 317
42. E. Lepeshkin, *Modern electrocardiography* (Williams and Wilkins Company, Baltimore, 1951)
43. E. Simonson, *Differentiation between normal and abnormal in electrocardiography.* (CV Mosby, St. Louis, 1961)
44. M. Kimura, S. Matsushita, K-I. Nakahar, et al., *J. Electrocardiology* **20** (1987) 369
45. R.P. Grant, *Clinical electrocardiography* (Mc Graw - Hill Book Company, New York, 1957)
46. J.D. Cooksey, M. Dunn, E. Massle, *Clinical vectorcardiography and electrocardiography (2nd ed.)* (Year Book Medical Publishers, Chicago, 1977)
47. D.H. Holt., D.H. Spodick, *Am. Heart J.* **63** (1962) 65
48. D.W. Romhilt, K.E. Bowe, R.J. Norris, et al. *Circulation* **40** (1969) 185
49. P.N. Casale, R.B. Devereux, P. Klingfield, et al. *J. Amer. Coll. Cardiol.* **6** (1985) 572
50. W.C. Roberts and P.J. Day, *Am. J. Cardiol.* **55** (1985) 431
51. H. Odom II, J.L. Davis, H.A. Dinh, et al., *Am. J. Cardiol.* **58** (1986) 801
52. E. Frank, *Circulation* **13** (1956) 737
53.R. McFee and A. Parungao, *Amer. Heart J.* **62** (1961) 93
54. T-Ch. Chou, R.A. Helm, S. Kaplan, *Clinical vectorcardiography (2nd ed.)* (Grune and Straton, New York, 1974)

55. J. Wartak, *Simplified vectorcardiography* (J.B. Lippincott Company, Philadelphia, 1970)
56. T. Winsor, *Primer of vectorcardiography* (Lea and Febiger, Philadelphia, 1972)
57. I. Ruttkay-Nedecký and E. Vanžurová, *Bratisl.lek.Listy* **64** (1975) 516, in Slovak, Summary in English
58. I. Ruttkay-Nedecký, *Electric field of the heart* (Veda, Bratislava, 1983) in Slovak, summary in English
59. L. Bachárová, *Atlas of clinical vectorcardiography* (Kabel Publishers, Rockville, 1993)
60. F.U. Gadzayeva and I. Alekperov, in: *Electrocardiology 83* ed. I. Ruttkay - Nedecký, P. MacFarlane, (Excerpta Medica, Amsterdam, 1984)
61. I. Ruttkay-Nedecký, *Bratisl. lek. Listy* **59** (1973) 682, in Slovak, summary in English
62. H.V. Pipberger, M.J. Goldman, D. Littmann, et al., *Circulation* **35** (1967) 536
63. G.E. Dower and H.E. Horn, *Am. Heart J.* **74** (1967) 368
64. L. Edenbrandt, B. Jonson, B. Lundh, et al., *Clinical Physiology* **7** (1987) 525
65. K. Murata, H. Kurihara, S. Hosoda, et al., *Jap. Heart J.* **5** (1964) 543
66. G.S. Sohi, E.W. Green, N.C. Flowers, et al., *Circulation* **59** (1979) 1277
67. F. Kornreich, T.J. Montague, P. Rautaharju, et al. *Amer J Cardiol.* **62** (1988) 1285
68. F.C. George, A.M. Brecken, C.T. Dollery, *British Heart J.* **34** (1972) 618
69. H. Toshima, Y. Koga, N. Kimura, *Am. Hear J.* **94** (1977) 547
70. R. Gamboa, P.G. Hugenholtz, A.S. Nadas, *Brit. Heart J* **27** (1965) 344
71. A.L. Dollar and W.C. Roberts, *Am. J. Medicine* **87** (1989) 377
72. R. Reeve and K. Kawamata, *Circulation* **34** (1966)
73. B. Geva, U. Elkayam, W. Frishman, *Chest* **76** (1979) 557
74. B. Vandenberg, K. Sagar, W. Paulsen, et al., *Am. J. Cardiol.* **63** (1989) 1080
75. E. Maisuls, A. Lorber, T. Margulis, et al., *Int. J. Cardiol.* **17** (1987) 137
76. R.A. Warner and N.E. Hill, *J. Electrocardiology (suppl.)* **89** (1987)
77. M.L. Murphy, P.M. Thenabadu, N. De Soyza, et al. *Am. J. Cardiol.* **53** (1984) 1140
78. G.C. Timmis, D.M. Bakalyar, S. Gordon, *J. Am. Coll. Cardiol.* **8** (1986) 301
79. I. Sotobata, H. Richman, E. Simonson, *Circulation* **37** (1968) 438
80. M. Nemati, J.T. Doyle, D. Mc Cauhan, et al.: *Am. Heart J.* **95** (1978) 12
81. J. Liebman, T.D. Downs, A. Friede, in: *Vectorcardiography II*, ed. I. Hoffman (North - Holland Publishing Co., Amsterdam, 1971)
82. W. Schonberger, J. Michaelis, E. Scheidt, et al.: *Adv. Cardiol.* **16** (1976) 102
83. K. Ishikawa, *Am. Heart J.* **92** (1976) 152
84. M. Tuna, C. Liedtke, *Adv. Cardiol.* **21** (1978) 286
85. L.W. Perry, H.V. Pipberger, H. Pipberger, et al.: *Am. Heart J.* **111** (1986) 721

86. P.M. Rautaharju, A.Z. LaCroix, D.D. Savage, et al. *Amer. J. Cardiol.* **62** (1988) 59
87. P.W. McFarlane and T.D.V. Lawrie, in: *Comprehensive electrocardiology* ed. P.W. McFarlane, T.D.V. Lawrie, (Pergamon Press, New York, 1989)
88. P.S. Rao, M.K. Thapar, R.J. Harp, *J. Electrocardiol.* **17** (1984) 239
89. D.A. Brody, *Circulation Research* **4** (1956) 731
90. W.A. Baxley, H.T. Dodge, H. Sandler, *Circulation* **37** (1968) 509
91. M. Manoach, S. Gitter, E. Grosman, et al. *Am. Heart J.* **84** (1972) 72
92. R.W. Millard, B.C. Hodgkin, C.V. Nelson, *Am. J. Physiol.* **H182** (1978)
93. J.A. Paroskoa, H. Gratema, W.S. Walker, et al., *J. Electrocardiol.* **16** (1983) 161
94. S. Daniels, A.S. Iskandrian, A.H. Hakki, et al., *Am. Heart J.* **107** (1984) 711
95. T. Feldman, K.M. Borow, A. Neumann, et al., *Am. J. Cardiol.* **55** (1985) 1168
96. C.V. Nelson, M. Chatterjee, E.T. Angelakos, *Am. Heart J.* **62** (1961) 83
97. C.V. Nelson, P.W. Rand, P.G.Hugenholty, et al., *Circulation* **36 (suppl.II)** (1967) 198
98. C.V. Nelson, P.G. Hugenholtz, E.T. Angelakos, et al., *Circulation* **39 (suppl. III)** (1969) 154
99. K. Ishikawa, M. Kini, H.V. Pipberger, *Circulation* **48** (1971) 565
100. M. Manoach, S. Gitter, E. Grossman, et al., *Amer. Heart J.* **82** (1971) 55
101. A. Battler, V. Froelicher, R. Slutsky, et al., *Circulation* **60** (1979) 1004
102. J. Lekven, K. Chatterjee, J.V. Tyberg, et al., *Am. Heart J.* **98** (1979) 200
103. G. Tommasini, C. Poluzzi, A. Masa, et al., in: Computers in Cardiology, I.E.E.E. (1981)
104. H. Ohlmeier, H. Mannebach, U. Gleichmann, *Clin. Cardiol.* **6** (1983) 29
105. D. David, M. Naito, Ch.C. Chen, et al., *Circulartion* **63** (1981) 1364
106. J. Myers, S. Ahnve, V. Froelicher, et al., *J. Am. Coll. Cardiol.* **6** (1985) 603
107. F.Z. Meerson, *Circulation Research* **24 - 25 (suppl.)** (1969)
108. R. Zak, in: ed. L. Opie, *The heart* Grune and Straton, London, 1984)
109. M.F. Arnsdorf, *Electrophysiology of the heart, 1110 Electrocardiography, Applied Theory I.* (American Physiological Society, 1978)
110. L. Bachárová, J. Melotová, K. Sedláková, et al., in: *Electrocardiology 1988* ed. H. Abel, (Elsevier Science Publisher, Excerpta Medica, Amsterdam, 1989)
111. L. Bachárová, F.U. Gadzayeva, J. Melotová, in: *Teorija i praktika avtomatizacii kardiologičeskich issledovanij*, ed. J. Blužas, (Kaunas 1990), in Russian, summary in English
112. L. Bachárová, M. Bernadič, A. Fízeľová, in: *Electrocardiology 91*, ed. J. Jagielski and M. Górnicki, (World Scientific, Singapore, 1992)
113. M. Bernadič, A. Fízeľ, A. Fízeľová, et al., *Bratisl. lek. Listy* **84** (1985) 683

CORRECT DIAGNOSIS OF CHEST PAIN BY AN INTEGRATED EXPERT SYSTEM

Deodato Assanelli, Massimo Strambini, Giuseppe Maifredi, Livio Cazzamalli, Maria L. Poeta, Maurizio Marconi, Odoardo Visioli.

Department of Cardiology, University of Brescia ,Brescia, 25100 Italy

1. Introduction

Coronary artery disease (CAD) is still the leading cause of mortality and morbidity in Western countries. Acute myocardial infarction and other forms of acute coronary ischemia are still difficult to recognize correctly and to stratify prognostically in many patients. Therefore, much effort has been devoted during the last decade to improving treatment of acute and chronic phases of myocardial ischemia and to preventing complications and recurrences. To this end, many new diagnostic, monitoring and treatment strategies have been developed, such as the coronary care unit, coronary angiography, coronary by-pass surgery, percutaneous coronary angioplasty, hemodynamic monitoring and treatment with intraaortic balloon counterpulsation. In addition, many new drugs have been introduced and widely used in recent years. All these new strategies have reduced short-term prognosis after acute coronary ischemia, while long-term prognosis improvement after hospital discharge has not been demonstrated since 1960 [1]. All but one internally controlled study [2] showed no improvement in long-term prognosis. The progression of underlying CAD or the failure to influence variables that affect discharge survival could be the main explanation as postulated [3]. Early thrombolytic therapy could improve long term prognosis of many CAD patients by reducing post-infarction congestive heart failure (CHF) [4]. The clinical value of thrombolytic therapy in acute myocardial infarction has been clearly established but nowadays only about 20% of eligible patients are still treated [5]. Primary care internists or family practitioners are faced with the majority of patients with impending or evolving myocardial infarction. There is still a wide gap between the diagnostic and therapeutic opportunities for CAD patients in specialized cardiology departments and the poor diagnostic possibilities at home, during ambulance transfer to the hospital and sometimes even in emergency departments inside the hospital. This gap is mainly cultural and it also concerns the delay of correct input and transfer of main clinical and instrumental information from inside and outside the cardiology department.

The electrocardiogram (ECG) has been used for many years as a key non-invasive method in the diagnosis and early detection of CAD [6].

2. ECG

It has been clearly demonstrated that correct interpretation of ECG abnormalities can give very important diagnostic information. Several studies have already reported the association between ST-T segment abnormalities during typical chest pain or during treadmill test and the increased risk of mortality in patients with previous acute myocardial infarction (AMI) or with chronic ischemic heart disease , and also in high risk asymptomatic patients. Correct analysis of ECG abnormalities when the patient comes to the emergency room has been found to be a useful prognostic means, particularly in patients with rest angina and non-Q myocardial infarction. All these patients are a high risk group for the development of recurrent angina (needing revascularization with either angioplasty or coronary artery by-pass graft), precocious acute myocardial infarction or sudden death. Some papers have pointed out that, in these patients, the presence on the entrance ECG of significant ST or T abnormalities suggesting ischemia (underdevelopment of ST segment greater than or equal to 1 mm and T wave abnormalities) in 2 leads at least, has good sensitivity and good specificity, and is also a good predictor of undesiderable clinical events. All these parameters become even more predictive if, during clinical evaluation, the patient complains of typical chest pain. These studies show that an easy test like the ECG can be reliable in predicting the risk of unfavourable events and can help guide the patient through the best clinical and instrumental triage. The main limitation is that the ECG's predictive value has only been demonstrated in patients treated with thrombolytic therapy, while there are some limitations to the use of the same criteria in the general population. Thus, since pre-existing left ventricular hypertrophy can reduce the ECG's predictive value, since the lack of chest pain reduces its sensitivity, and also because of the presence of minimal ECG abnormalities, in the presence of chest pain, the risky situation of multivessel coronary disease cannot be excluded [7].

In patients with angiographically documented CAD, ischemic ECG abnormalities of ST-T segment that appear during cycle-ergometer effort, both with and without chest pain, have a discrete prognostic value. It has been demonstrated that patients with symptomatic underdevelopment of ST segment during effort have a more rapid course of the disease and a worse prognosis in comparison to patients with silent ischemia, and thus independent of other risk factors. No difference has been found in the prevalence of diabetes, hypertension or smoking. Lastly, the presence of angina during effort test is associated with a significantly higher prevalence of 3-vessel coronary artery disease [8].

Ambulatory monitoring of ST segment, with a 24/48-hour Holter, can be used to show and quantify the episodes of ischemic ST underdevelopment in patients with known CAD. In patients with stable angina who have been medically treated, a significantly higher probability of undesired events has been shown when Holter ST abnormalities appear. In the same cohort of subjects with known stable angina and positive effort test, the extension (number of leads) of ST down-sloping appears to be useful in predicting unfavourable clinical events. Several papers have already proved that there is a a correlation between the effort test severity and the frequence of ischemic episodes during Holter monitoring.

Nevertheless, if models of risk prediction, such as Cox's method, are added to the evaluation of the presence, frequency and time of ischemia, together with ischemia parameters of effort test, or ambulatory ECG evaluation of ischemia, it is possible to have more information on the prognosis of such a patient than without these models (of risk prediction), while effort test alone cannot have such prognostic power. These rules are true for all the subgroups of coronary artery diseased patients at different stage of the disease.

In subgroups of CAD patients with positive effort test (which in these patients has proved useful for the prognosis), Holter monitoring of cardiac ischemia is much more accurate in identifying subgroups at high risk for unfavourable events [9]. From all these data it appears evident that a correct integration of different sources of information can be very helpful from both the diagnostic and the prognostic point of view.

It is estimated that more than 100 million standard electrocardiograms are recorded yearly in the European Community (EC) for routine diagnostic and screening purposes [10]. It is estimated that over 50 percent of the 100 millions ECGs recorded annually in the United States are interpreted by means of a computer [10].

Although many studies have evaluated such computer programs [11,12], systematic quality assessment has only been undertaken in recent years. The results of some recent research [13] demonstrate that computer programs with the best performance are almost as accurate as the best cardiologist in classifying the ECGs of patients in seven common diagnostic groups. However,all the programs studied can still be improved. Most cardiologists performed better than the programs in confirming normality and were more sensitive in diagnosing anterior myocardial infarction. The authors of this paper wish to point out that,in some cases,computer interpretation of ECGs may be correct and cardiologists incorrect when their diagnoses are tested against the clinical evidence, although the opposite is twice as likely (14.7 % vs. 6.3 %) when an average computer program and an average cardiologist are compared. Standard ECG reading computer programs can assist clinicians in achieving more consistent interpretations of ECGs [14]. Unfortunately all the information available with computerized ECG interpretation, which is increasingly reliable, still has to be exploited in clinical practice.The lack of a standard was probably the main obstacle to the correct widespread use of such programs.

Almost all new electrocardiographs nowadays use digital recording, interpretation and communication techniques. These stand-alone, microcomputer or personal computer based machines can be connected to each other, and to larger minicomputers or personal computer based management servers for long-term storage and serial comparison [15]. To this end, various manufacturers have used different techniques.

It is in the general public's interest for users not to be restricted in their options by incompatible technical features and services of different systems. ECG processing is increasingly being integrated with various other data processing techniques in health care. This evolution will have considerable impact on the storage and communication of ECG data. There are many different end users who, for various reasons, (patient care back-up, management,research and education) want to obtain a copy of the signal data, interpretative report and/or measurement results. Being one of the very first systems for medical decision back-up, computerized ECG interpretation ranges from hospital cardiology departments to general practitioners in primary and health care centers. In life-threatening acute myocardial infarction, ECGs are being used in ambulances by paramedical personnel to assess the need for administering thrombolytic agents, with long-distance monitoring whenever possible.

To enable the interconnectivity of various systems it was of utmost importance for a standard communications protocol for computer-aided electrocardiography (SCP-ECG) to be established [16]. The primary aim of this standard is to ensure that ECG reports and data from any make of computerized ECG recorder can be transmitted on a direct connection serial line to a central ECG management system of another make. The same standard should also allow standardized transmission of digitized ECG data and results between various computer systems. For all these reasons it was important that a standard communication protocol (SCP) for computerized electrocardiography should be established.

ECG computer processing can be reduced to 3 main stages:

1) data acquisition, encoding, transmission and storage
2) pattern recognition and feature extraction, i.e. ECG measurement
3) diagnostic classification.

In each of these stages there are important needs for standardization and quality assurance testing. Such a standardization task is difficult, especially when commercial factors are at stake, and can only be obtained by means of international collaboration between clinicians, engineers and computer specialists. The different solutions developed by individual manufacturers can only be merged by a wide consensus approach. This has to include contributions and expertise from different university research centres with an international reputation, industry and user cardiologists from all over the world. The basic aim of the SCP-ECG project was to arrive at a standard communication protocol to enable the interconnection and exchange of ECG data between different computerized ECG analysis and other information sytems. This pre-standard was worked out and submitted to European Community. When this pre-standard becomes a real standard, many programs using it will be produced by several manufacturers at an affordable cost and this will allow a correct and more widespread use of computerized ECG.

3. Chest pain symptoms

The symptoms described by the patient are very important for diagnostic and prognostic purposes in cases with certain or suspected coronary ischemia, as has already been pointed out by various authors. Chest pain analysis, in particular, seems to be more helpful if all the information given by the patient himself is recorded correctly since cardiologists in the past did much better than modern ones. One of the major limitations of chest pain is that the description is frequently interpreted subjectively and the pain threshold can change in different patients and in the same patient at different times .

The questionnaire was proposed in the past [17] to avoid, as far as possible, the subjective aspect of the information and to standardize it, in an attempt to compare different patients correctly and to better define discriminant rules to differentiate chest pain arising from the heart from pain of different origin (mainly musculo-skeletal or gastro-oesophageal). It has proved of great value in indicating CAD, with a fairly good sensitivity and specificity. In addition, a positive result to the questionnaire probably suggests a higher risk of developing CAD even in patients with atypical chest pain who are clinically considered as subjects without angina pectoris. This type of questionnaire would be much more useful if the presence of individual risk factors, particularly arterial hypertension and high cholesterol level, was also evaluated.

4. Data integration

All the work that has been done on the ECG will increase its diagnostic accuracy but there are still some daily problems in individual patients that only a correct integration with clinical data and risk profile can improve. Each method used for the detection of myocardial ischemia has its own limitations, which is why new instruments are needed to help doctors correctly estimate individual risk of developing CAD by improving diagnostic accuracy of devices used today. They might also improve the possibility of a correct prognostic stratification for the best diagnostic course and therapeutic treatment.

Many studies have already demonstrated the importance of a correct epidemiological evaluation starting from main risk factors [18,19]: a correct analysis of these factors can indeed contribute to a better clinical and prognostic classification. Even today in clinical practice, particularly in the emergency room, risk profiles are realized with a superficial procedure, while epidemiological procedures, with better methodology, are only used in cohorts of subjects that are presumably healthy. When correctly performed, in fact this evaluation can be very helpful, in particular as exclusion criteria in selected patients.

Alongside epidemiological studies [20], diagnostic aids have been developed with different philosophies based on the use of questionnaires aimed at a correct discrimination of thoracic pain of cardiac origin in patients with similar symptoms. Important information can also be obtained by the correct interpretation and integration of traditional clinical and instrumental data, particularly for EKG abnormalities.

5. To test or not to test

Recently, different techniques such as echocardiography, scintigraphy, spect, coronary angiography, etc. have proved to be more powerful in recognizing cardiac ischemia at an earlier stage than ECG during the ischemic cascade, but, for various reasons, none of them are used in spite of ECG for routine detection of cardiac ischemia: cost-effectiveness is one of the major explanations. The recent technical and cultural development of many techniques has encouraged the use of many non-invasive tests to increase the diagnostic power of more traditional techniques like ECG and chest pain and risk evaluation. Unfortunately, whereas knowledge has increased, the habit of integrating different sources of information correctly has been lost. The tests cost time and money and it is important to know if and when they could be useful in doing a particular patient a real service. Generally speaking, the less selective a diagnostic approach, the less the predictive value of the method to be used. Indeed the predictive power of a test is not an intrinsic property of the test itself, it is exponentially correlated with the prevalence of the disease in this particular population; even a specific test, when applied to a population with a fairly high chance of developing a certain disease, will give many false positives. Similarly, negative results of a highly sensitive test applied to a high risk population would probably be false negatives. The ideal situation is to have techniques with a good predictive value both in extreme conditions and in all these intermediate situations, which are very frequent in clinical practice and sometimes difficult to classify. Several papers have already stressed the diagnostic accuracy and the possibility of prognostic predictions can be improved by correct integration of various sources of information for each patient [8,9,18,19]. Such information is represented by clinical evaluation, plus an estimation of individual risk factors, an analysis of Rose's questionnaire and correct ECG interpretation. In particular, ST-T abnormalities typical of ischemia during chest pain, effort test or Holter monitoring are very important in reaching this goal. This seems to be the best route to follow for improved clinical and prognostic definition in individual patients, whether those with known CAD or high risk asymptomatic subjects.

6. Risk profile

Many epidemiological studies, performed on different populations have found important correlations between the possibility of developing a coronary artery disease and risk factors estimated both individually and in association: the results of studies frequently did not agree, probably because they were performed in populations with different and heterogeneous risk profiles. Some of the more classic factors have a fairly significant correlation with the following appearance of CAD. The major factors are age, total cholesterol, systolic and diastolic hypertension, sex, smoking habit and physical activity. Other factors, such as thickening skin folds (as an obesity index), body mass index, vital capacity, heart rate and other anthropometric indices, have a minor value, frequently negligible, and no independent predictive value [20]. Now we shall analyse individual risk factors so as to understand their role.

Several studies performed on patient groups with ischemic cardiopathy documented by angiography, compared to control groups, showed that the former had a higher frequence of lipid abnormalities, in particular HDL reduction. The prevalence of LDL increasing, on the contrary, was demonstrated as being similar in both groups. The prevalence of others risk factors too, such as hypertension, was clearly higher in the CAD group. It then became evident that both morbidity and mortality from CAD increase with lipid levels: this statement was proved in subjects with a pre-existing CAD and also in subjects without any evidence of CAD .In the latter, the high cholesterol level increases the death risk from CAD to even higher levels than in subjects with known CAD but low cholesterol. This relation would also appear to be true for LDL [18]. There is also evidence that a reduction in lipid level is able to reduce both cardiovascular morbidity and mortality.

Repeated angiographic studies with quantitated angiography have already shown that when total cholesterol is lowered and LDL and HDL are improved, there is a slower progression or even a more important regression of coronary atherosclerotic lesions. It has not been fully ascertained whether and to what extent lipid lowering treatment can prevent the development and progression of CAD [18].

- The role of hypertension, in both systole and diastole as risk factor for the development of CAD has been known for a long time and does not require further discussion. Almost all studies done in the past have shown that hypertension was present, with an increasingly high prevalence, in subjects with CAD as compared to normal controls.

- Familiarity has proven to be a significant and independent factor for the development of CAD; the effect is more pronounced in males and it does not seem to be particularly influenced by the presence of other risk factors. This suggests that increased individual risk, associated with the presence of standard factors, is not significantly different in patients with positive familiarity when compared to those with negative familiarity. In addition, positive familiarity can help to predict the occurence of CAD in subjects with low traditional risk factors. Some studies suggest that familiarity for CAD is not a consequence of other similar major risk factors in the family. The major risk could be interpreted as being due to one of the following: 1) subjects with positive familiarity could be more sensitive to the deleterious effects of traditional risk factors; 2) family history could be associated with events that are not only due to usual risk factors; 3) less known factors like LPa lypoprotein or phybrinogen level can make a difference with patients without cardiovascular familiarity. The possible presence of genetic components in the appearance of CAD still has to be defined [21]. Studies concerning the familial recurrence of CAD that began at early age have shown, in these cases, that familiarity is very important. This same factor decreases in importance with increasing age at the first ischemic episode,and becomes negligible in cases in which the disease appears for the first time at an older age. The same study also proved that the hereditary component certainly plays a major role in the predisposition to the disease of subjects who have CAD at an early age. In older patients the hereditary component plays a minor role, and this suggests a major role of environmental factors in the latter group of subjects [22].

7. Acute coronary ischemia diagnosis

Correct and rapid recognition of acute coronary ischemia is still a difficult problem since, even in emergency rooms, about 40% of patients nowadays are hospitalized in the USA every year due to a false positive diagnosis, while 5-8 % are sent home with a false negative diagnosis and they develop a myocardial infarction after emergency room discharge [23,24]. The number is about 30,000/year in the USA.

Correct integration of clinical, epidemiological and electrocardiographic data could be performed for faster recognition of acute myocardial ischemia in individual patients. This integration would probably allow better treatment, correct prognostic stratification and an improved triage of useful tests to perform at different stages of CAD.

To ensure that patients receive thrombolytic therapy in a timely manner, a public education campaign must be mounted as important authors have already underlined [5]. Another alternative or combined strategy to reach the same goal of quick and correct diagnosis of acute coronary ischemia could be computer integration of different sources of information routinely used to monitor, on-line, coronary ischemia and correctly interpret chest pain in individual patients by correctly coding, compressing and transmitting by phone the main information required to make a quick correct decision in individual patients with cardiac ischemia, whether certain or suspected.

Some authors have developed an algorithm that allows trained paramedics, under the direction of a hospital based physician, to identify in the field patients eligible for thrombolytic therapy. In patients potentially eligible for such therapy, the electrocardiogram can be transmitted to the hospital by portable phone. With recent cultural and technical developments in medical informatics, diagnostic aids have been designed to help doctors make decisions. The former are done with an algorithm that tries to give correct weight to the main symptoms as deduced from the histories of patients with acute myocardial infarction. This weight is obtained by assigning each symptom or clinical sign a numerical coefficient [23,24]. These systems can be helpful but use a formula that is quite rigid and cannot easily be changed as soon as the knowledge of the problem increases. Another limitation is that medicine is part science part art. A classic algorithmic approach is usually not well accepted by the doctor because it sacrifices the creative aspect of medical knowledge.

Another approach which is more similar to the reasoning mechanism of the doctor can be an expert system [25]. Such a system tries to emulate the reasoning procedure of the human brain of an expert in the field, which is the result of:

1) his basic knowledge
2) the frequently unconscious improvement in his decisional capacity obtained by solving many individual patients' problems (the experience)
3) the comparison of clinical and instrumental data for each patient with similar situations already solved in the past.

This allows the expert to give different weight to the same symptoms in different patients in relation to the clinical context. This complex knowledge, which progressively increases with experience, enables the expert to reduce the field of reasoning to problems that are important in guiding the best decision for each patient,at each step of CAD.

8. Uncertainty models and "ad hoc" reasoning software

During both analysis and synthesis the cardiologist can manipulate symbolic information such as symptoms, diseases and instrumental tests [25,26]. Very frequently the decision is made using information that is neither complete nor certain. Experience enables one to arrive at the correct diagnosis, using euristic judgment built up on a few behavioural rules and acquired over the years [27-31]. An expert system uses a process that is very similar to human reasoning [32]. It can also explain at each step of the diagnostic course why it made certain choices and why it asked the patient certain questions; it can simulate the reasoning procedure of the expert cardiologist to trasmit this logical approach to students. It can be improved by changing,, increasing or modifying the rules of reasoning: its decisional ability with the new version can then be tested in all patients in the data-base to validate the new changes. In 1987 a decision was made to build up a prototype expert system for all these reasons, and because the commercial shells of the expert system did not completely satisfy our requirements. This system might use an ad hoc reasoning mechanism aiming to recognize in the emergency room acute coronary ischemia as well as the main differential diagnoses, whether of cardiac musculo-skeletal or gastro-oesophageal origin. The prototypal version was implemented in UNIX AIX. Lisp language and C was used to write the program. A modified Rose's questionnaire was used to input data concerning chest pain peculiarities of each patient with suspected coronary ischemia. The doctor also introduced, with a guided procedure, anamnestic data and main clinical signs and symptoms, ECG abnormalities and the comparison with previous ECG when avaliable.The third main input added to chest pain and the ECG was, in this version of the program as well, individual risk estimation made by calculating the risk of major events in the next five years, applying Cox's method estimated in an Italian population [20,33]. When a very high risk profile was found, the system arbitrarily increased the power of major rules. After the system integrated all these data with the results of new questions it considered important for this working session,the system concluded in 10-15 minutes whether the problem was cardiac, if so whether the patient had an acute myocardial infarction or not,etc.,until the doctor considered the session finished. To reach this goal, a detailed analysis of the expert doctor's knowledge and reasoning mechanism when faced with a patient with chest pain was made. Both the knowledge and the reasoning mechanism are imprecise and uncertain, two opposing dimensions of knowledge. Many mathemathical procedures used in the past to define an uncertainty scale were algorithmic: the doctor usually did not like to codify the uncertainty level on a numerical scale. That is why more recently, in spite of Baye's, Zadeh's, Prade's or Demstershafer's theories [34-37], symbolic approaches have been used, more similar to the doctor's unconscious representation of the uncertain knowledge that is qualitative not quantitative. Among these symbolic approaches is Driankow's theory to the model proposed by Bonissone.

This method used two orthogonal factors to define the incertitude level and, at the end of the reasoning procedure, can distinguish between ignorance and contradiction in all the information input by the system. Driankow's theory represents the credibility of a piece of information with a pair of fuzzy numbers (s,p), where s and p are part of the verbal scale and express the degree of support or the degree of conviction that the statement is true (s), and the degree of plausibility (p): my degree of certainty in excluding the contrary of the same affirmation. Each pair of factors can allow the subjects to conclude how true the conclusions are. This method distinguishes between incertitude, contradiction and ignorance in all the information input by the system. The amplitude of symbolical intervals modulates the discriminant level of the operator: a verbal scale with seven intervals was used at an intermediate level of granularity, because it better fitted the doctor's habits. The architecture of the system is made up of four main modules: the supervisor, the inferential engine, the diagnosis support system and the system managing the knowledge base. The supervisor manages all the procedures of initialization, checking and guiding the whole system. The inferential engine has the goal of reaching a correct diagnosis, modulated by the incertitude level. The inferential engine, like each expert system, is guided by rules, obtained mainly from a modified version of Rose's questionnaire [17]. These rules are the static knowledge of the system. This system being a prototypal version, the number of rules was progressively increased, and some rules were formulated differently to find, together with the expert,the best rule sequence for the purpose of diagnosis.

In addition to static knowledge, the system also uses dynamic or short-term knowledge (fig.1): the system creates dynamic knowledge for each patient and for every working session from the responses of the patient, anamnestic data, guided clinical evaluation and individual risk estimation.

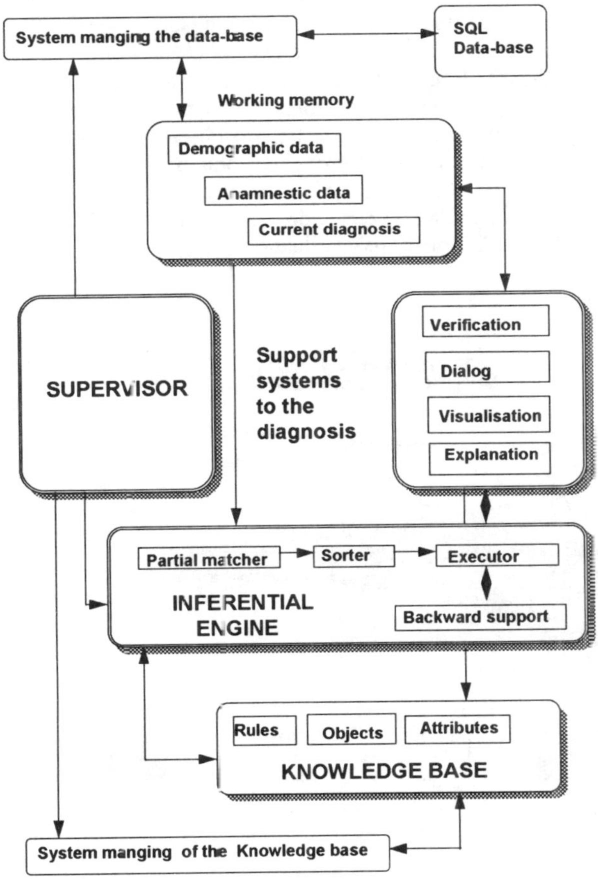

Figure 1: Architecture of the prototypal version of the expert system, running on minicomputer, in UNIX. The inferential engine uses, on line, the knowledge base for the working memory (dynamic memory, different for each patient). There is a direct connection with both the data base of patients studied with this prototypal version and the cardiology department data base. Different supports for the diagnosis can be used and the knowledge base can be changed. The system inputs the patient's demographic and anamnestic data and makes a clinical evaluation to reach the correct diagnosis. Supports for the diagnosis are: explanation system, rules tree, input and output of clinical data, alternative dianostic.

The storage of dynamic knowledge makes it possible to record the questions, the rules activated and the conclusion reached: all this information can be re-utilized in a similar working session. The system utilizes static knowledge to build up dynamic knowledge. When activated, the inferential engine chooses a rule and, by a forward concatenation, decides whether the rule is true in this particular patient by using guided questions. If it is, the system updates the contents of the fact base with the consequence of the activated rule. At the same time there is a reverse check (fig. 2): it evaluates whether the consequence of the rule fitted well with one of the objectives of the fact base.

Both procedures have some limitations, which is why they were used together (mixed procedure), which in our mind is better for differential diagnoses. In the end, all the dynamic knowledge for each patient gives one or more diagnoses with a high credibility level (I am certain), to obtain contradictory conclusions (very rare) or the system does not have enough data to conclude (I do not know). Main inputs of the system are: ECG, Chest Pain and Coronary risk evaluation.

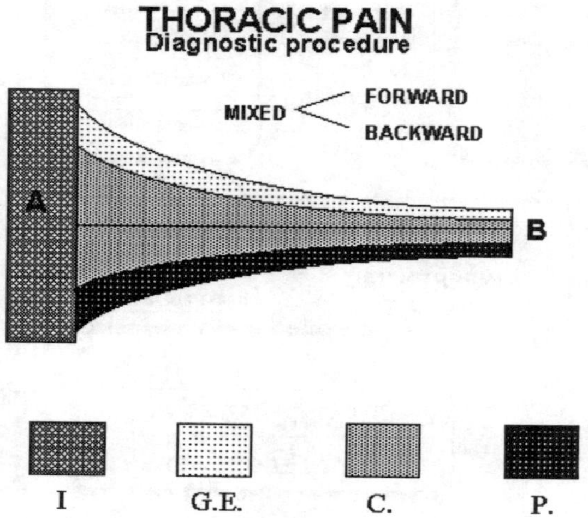

Figure 2: The prototype works with a forward sequence of rules at the beginning (B), when the diagnostic process is at the very first stage, and with a mixed procedure (predominantly backward) when the diagnosis of the patient is more defined as being cardiac, gastro-oesofageal or musculo-skeletal.

9. Chest pain

The term "angina pectoris" was introduced in 1768 to define that cumule of clinical manifestations essentially characterized by painful chest symptomatology excellently described by William Heberden [38]. Therefore angina pectoris is a clinical symptom [39] and this is the definition that strictly belongs to it; however, it is now common practice to identify angina pectoris with transient myocardial ischemia with or without chest pain. Transient myocardial ischemia is defined as a temporary condition of insufficient blood supply with functional compromission deriving from the transient change from an aerobic metabolism to an anaerobic one.

Pain signals the presence of potential or effective tissutal damage caused by lesive factors leading to stimuli which are communicated to higher nerve centres by means of peripheral nerves in the likelihood of bioelectrical signals. There are two kinds of pain:

1) visceral

characteristics:	dull, heavy, widespread
conducting anatomical ways:	C nerve fibres
characteristics:	small diameter
	amyelinic
	slow conduction

2) somatic

characteristics:	sharp and highly localized
conducting anatomical ways:	A nerve fibres
characteristics:	large diameter
	myelinic
	fast conduction

Afferent sensitive cardiac fibres run within superior, median and inferior cardiac nerves to cervical and thoracic ganglions in the sympathetic system; they arrive at the posterior roots of the medulla spinalis, between vertebra T1 and T5 in common with afferent sensitive fibres from the oesophagus, aorta, mediastinum and thoracic wall.

Pain fibres from parietal pleura and the diaphragmatic surface of the pericardium run within phrenic and intercostal nerves.

Anginal pain generally has precise features of quality and anatomical site, starting and ending mode and duration:
it generally refers to the precordial and retrosternal area in the dermatomes corresponding to T1-T2-T3-T4-T5, but it can irradiate to the left arm, particularly to the distribution surface of the ulnar nerve (dermatome corresponding to C8), or even to both arms.

It can also irradiate to dermatomes corresponding to T6 and C3-C4-C5-C6-C7. It rarely extends beyond C3 and T6. In atypical cases it can be present only in the irradiation sites, for example the mandible or arm. It is extremely rare for it to be so localized that it can be indicated with a finger.

It can be constricting
heavy
rarely burning
extremely rarely transfixing

It is perceived as deep and usually accompanied by hyperhydrosis.

It often arises in recurrence of effort and disappears within 10 minutes after rest or assumption of oral TNG.

The duration is short, usually 1-5 minutes. If it persists longer than 15-20 minutes it can be a matter of prolonged myocardial ischemia or myocardial infarction. Continuous pain is never of cardiac origin.

Chest pain screening is closely related to the question of chest pain threshold and the complex, highly-debated question of silent ischemia. The latter has various effects depending on the groups selected from among population: about 2.5 % in subjects without previous manifestations of CAD, 25-34 % in subjects suffering from significant coronary atherosclerosis, 50 % in patients with unstable angina, up to 92 % of all ischemic events.

Up to now, the following mechanisms have been used to eplain silent ischemia:

1) pathological alterations of the neurosensorial system (particularly frequent in diabetes mellitus and the elderly)
2) insufficient coronary ischemia duration for angina to appear: pain often appears as much as 30 minutes after balloon occlusion during coronary angioplasty
3) abnormally high pain threshold: the relevant works are conflicting. Indeed some authors have found high serum Beta endorphin levels in patients with silent ischemia [40] and some refuse to admit the leading role of Beta endorphin serum concentrations in pain threshold changes. However, a high pain threshold seems to have been proved in athletes and in the elderly [41,42].

9.1 Other cardiovascular causes of chest pain

PERICARDIAL: visceral pericardium does not have painful afferences
parietal pericardium has painful afferences only in the diaphragm area

Pericardial pain can run along intercostal nerves (producing a precordial localization of pain) or phrenic nerves (producing a painful irradiation to the left shoulder).

It increases with deep inspiration and decreases in the seated or forward inclined position.

AORTIC: aortic dissection usually gives chest pain; in typical cases pain is frontal, posteriorly irradiating the interscapular zone. Very often chest pain is frontal in the dissecting aneurysm of the ascending aorta and posterior in that of the thoracic descending aorta.

Other cardiovascular causes are represented by myocarditis, mitral valvular prolapse, aortic stenosis and hypertrophic cardiomyopathy (in the latter two, pain can be anginal)

9.2 Thoracic causes

PLEURAL: visceral pleura does not have painful afferences
parietal pleura has painful afferences
Pleural pain is mediated by intercostal nerves when the lesion is localized at the costal parietal pleura or lateral diaphragmatic zone.
It is mediated by phrenic nerves when the lesion is

localized in the central diaphragmatic zone

Characteristics of pain: usually localized on one side only; intense, burning, exacerbated by deep respiration and sometimes by movements of the chest.

PULMONARY: pulmonary embolism can produce a chest pain similar to angina pectoris. The mechanism is discussed and can involve:

- acute dilation of the pulmonary artery
- right ventricular acute ischemia
- pain of the pleural kind when a pulmonary infarction occurs.

MEDIASTINIC: the pain is dull and badly localized when caused by:

- mediastinitis
- mediastinic tumours

In other cases the pain is precordial or sub-sternal with possible irradiation to neck, jaw or arm.

9.2.1 Digestive causes

OESOPHAGEAL: the pain is generally localized at the dermatomes of nervous radicula included between C7 and T12.

Causes of oesophageal pain:

- gastro-oesophageal reflux
- motility disturbances (spasm)
- infections
- tumours
- oesophageal connective diseases
- CREST-Syndrome

In oesophageal spasm the pain is thoracic, heavy and usually occurs after meals or effort. It can be reduced by TNG and /or calcium-antagonists.

In gastro-oesophageal reflux, the pain is usually retrosternal, burning (which defines the so-called "gastric pyrosis"), particularly frequent after meals, in clinostatism and during antiflexion of chest (lowered position); it is reduced by antiacids. It is due to direct irritant action of HCl on nervous terminations of oesophageal mucosa with subsequent oesophageal spasm.

COLICYSTIC: the pain is usually localized at the epigastrium and/or right hypochondrium with typical irradiation to right back or right shoulder; sometimes it is retrosternal.

PANCREATIC: the pain is generally epigastric with irradiation to the back; sometimes it is retrosternal.

It is often reduced by seated position and forward inclination, with flexed chest and knees gathered toward chest.

GASTRO-ENTERIC: peptic ulcer pain can be burning or constricting and simulate an attack of angina.

It generally appears 1-2 hours after meals and responds to antiacids but not to nitrates.

The Splenic flexure Syndrome is characterized by heavy pain localized at the left hypochondrium which can irradiate to the left shoulder. It is due to gaseous hyperdistension of the descending colon and to a subsequent diaphragmatic irritation.

9.2.2. Osteo-arthro-muscular causes

Costal fractures: traumatic or from neoplastic metastasis.
The pain is increased by cough, respiration and chest flexion

Costal chondritis: the pain is often dull and constricting, but it is evoked by manual pressure of the chest.
The 2nd, 3rd and 4th ribs are most frequently involved.

Tietze's Syndrome: painful, non-inflammatory tumefaction of one (more frequently) or more (rarely) chondro-costal synchondrosis

Xiphoiditis and xiphodynia: pain is retrosternal and deep and can irradiate to the epigastrium and precordium. It is evoked by pressure on xiphoid process.

Vertebral osteo-arthritis (cervical or thoracic): the pain is evoked by pressure of nervous radicula of intervertebral foramens.
Sometimes retrosternal pain is present, even heavy (the so-called "cervico-precordial angina), with irradiation to neck, jaw or arms. However, it generally accompanies cervical pains.
Painful symptomatology is usually triggered by movements of neck, arms or chest, but it can be present even after a prolonged seated or supine position.

Other osteo-articular causes:
- primitive costal tumours
- chest-wall infections
- osteoporosis (with costal fractures or crushing of one or more vertebras)

Muscular strains: when affecting accessory muscles of respiration this can produce heavy, continuous and deep chest pain, with possible irradiation to a shoulder or an arm. A restriction in the range of muscular movement is usually present and manual pressure of painful muscular points often evokes pain and even a muscular spasm.

9.2.3. Neurological causes

Intercostal neuralgias: - from viral involvement (Herpes Zoster and post-herpetic neuralgia)

- from metastatic invasion or local invasion of chest tumours
- from a post-thoracotomic process of healing

The pain, usually burning, involves a pathway on one side, with localization at one or more thoracic dermatomes.

In Herpes Zoster, before the typical rush occurs, there is a band of hyperestesia with dermatomeric distribution.

9.2.4 Other causes

Painful heals: they provoke pain, even of the burning kind, which extends outside the anatomical limits of heal.

It can be increased by thermic changes, tactile stimuli, local pressure, emotional matters.

This pain is attributed to imperfect nerve regeneration, with formation of disarranged nerve elements.

Breast removal: painful syndrome subordinate to radical breast removal, generally producing a burning pain in the axillary area and in the upper part of chest with possible homolateral irradiation to the arm.
It is probably due to resection of the intercosto-brachial nerve.
The pain rarely persists for over three months, in which case it represents a chronic painful syndrome indefinitely localized at the front thoracic wall, with extreme sensitivity to tactile stimuli.

After we reviewed all the possible causes of chest pain, it appeared evident that the need to discriminate anginal pain from all other pains becomes inevitable for the heart specialist. Indeed, the predictive value of this symptom is connected with a discriminant ability based up to now on distinctive features of anginal pain.

The definition of chest pain was made by CASS (Coronary Artery Surgery Study) on the basis of evaluation of painful symptoms according to three fundamental characteristics (43):

1) site: is pain retrosternal?
2) causal mode: is pain caused by effort?
3) remission mode: does pain disappear within ten minutes after rest or sublingual TNG?

On the basis of the results obtained in answer to these three questions it is possible to distinguish four class of subjects:

1) typical angina if the answer to all three questions is affirmative
2) atypical angina if the answer to two questions is affirmative
3) non-anginal chest pain if the answer to only one question is affirmative
4) asymptomatic subject if there is no pain above the diaphragm

According to this subdivision[44], quantized the risk of CAD in each subject, according to sex and the different age ranges.

These data led to the conclusion that patients with typical angina have a high probability of CAD, but also patients with atypical angina or with non-anginal chest pain are candidates for further diagnostic check-ups.

Asymptomatic subjects have about a 5 % probability of CAD if considered altogether [45]. This probability can be further defined, in addition to age and sex, by the presence of so-called "risk factors", which are:

- smoking
- hypertension
- hypercholesterolemia
- diabetes mellitus

These data show that asymptomatic subjects with multiple "risk factors" have approximately the same probability of CAD as subjects with atypical angina. The probability is higher in male subjects and with increasing age and risk factors[46]. Nevertheless, other works [47] have demonstrated the usefulness of associating electrocardiographic analysis with the study of symptoms and risk factors. The interpretation of data from these three different and important sources of information produces a far more precise evaluation of disease probability and indeed informatics system is based on just that.

Angina pectoris is a symptom which has always been used to identify and correctly stratify patients with ischemic heart disease. At present angina pectoris is too frequently evaluated with a dichotomic procedure as being typical or atypical: this procedure has determined the loss of much useful anamnestic information. Unfortunately, too often invasive examinations are performed without correctly analysing and evaluating all the characteristics of thoracic pain. New techniques have reduced the role of angina pectoris and of epidemiological estimation for diagnostic purposes, although many papers point out that, in cardiac patients, diagnostic accuracy may be increased and prognostic stratification improved by a correct integration of different sources of information in individual patients. In a large cohort of patients a checklist of typical history and physical examination criteria can help correctly screen possible candidates for thrombolytic therapy, mainly by increasing the specificity of ECG alone [48] . When this information is not enough to identify patients with impending, sustained or constituted intracoronary thrombosis, only early angiography can help because biologic markers are still not sufficiently specific [49]. A systematic integration of ECG and chest pain and individual

history can help correctly recognize candidates for emergency angioplasty or coronary by-pass as well as to judge the efficacy of new anticoagulants and direct antithrombin agents [49]. In symptomatic patients with CAD, it has been demonstrated that the more frequent or progressive the anginal symptoms, the poorer the prognosis [28]. Thus prognostic stratification is improved by considering both subjective and objective markers of ischemia. Some authors have worked in this area in patients with stable angina: they suggest that the ischemic cascade sequence remains unchanged but timing and hemodynamic level at the onset of the ischemic event varies with ischemic threshold. In patients with low level ischemia, chest pain is a precocious and very important marker. Other authors have pointed out that shortness of breath, syncope or stroke can be the main symptoms associated with acute myocardial infarction in elderly patients [42].
A patient who enters hospital with a generic diagnosis of thoracic pain can be affected by several cardiac or non cardiac diseases. This is a sample of 1400 men hospitalized in Brescia for chest pain in 1987 (fig. 3): 9.6 % of them had thoracic pain of musculo-skeletal origin. This percentage of healthy people reaches 20 % in females hospitalized for the same reasons (fig. 4).

We have built up an expert system to tackle correctly all the problems related to chest pain. The prototype works with a forward sequence of rules at the beginning, when the diagnostic process is right in the initial stage, and with a mixed procedure when the diagnosis of the patient is better defined as being cardiac, gastro-enterological or musculo-skeletal (fig. 2).

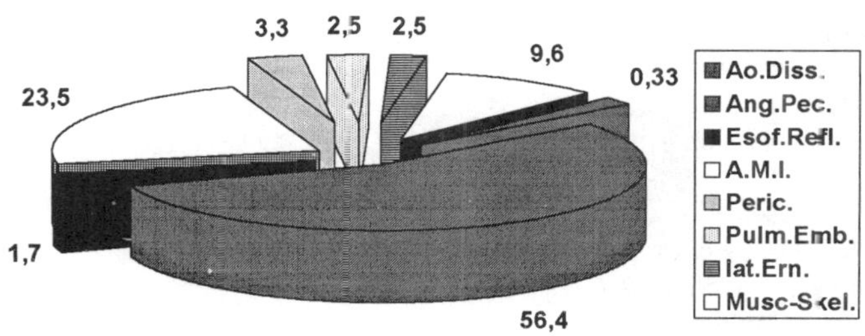

Figure 3: Percentage of main discharge diagnoses in 1480 males hospitalized in 1987 in Brescia Hospital, in different departments, due to problems related to chest pain: aortic dissection (ao. diss.), angina pectoris (ang. pec.), acute myocardial infarction (AMI), pericarditis (Peric.), pulmonic embolisation (Pulm. Emb.), oesofageal reflux (Esofag. Refl.), iatal hernia (Iat. Ern.), musculo-skeletal pain (Musc-Skel).

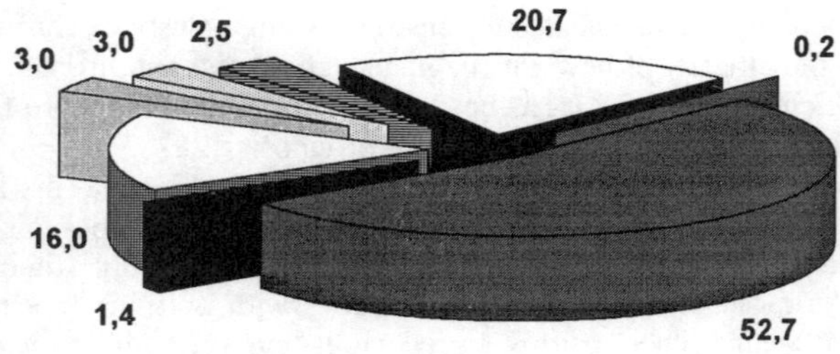

Figure 4: Percentage of main discharge diagnosis in 1380 femakes hospitalised in 1987 in Brescia Hospital, in different departments, due to problems related to chest pain: same legend as for Figure 3.

10. ERIC

Many traditional expert systems have proved useful in solving only limited and very specific problems. This is why in the first diagnostic stage, when there are many possibilities and none excludes the other, many system use an algorithmic method. In the past, some algorithms were elaborated for routine diagnosis of chest pain. In 1988 the Multicenter Chest Pain Study [23] introduced an algorithm for recognizing acute myocardial infarction based on 9 clinical parameters:

1) patient's age
2) interval since occurence of pain
3) pain duration
4) characteristics of pain irradiation
5) kind of pain
6) presence or absence of angina or AMI history
7) pain evokability by chest palpation
8) pain comparison with a previous angina or AMI
9) electrocardiographic data

This is a protocol was developed using the statistical method of "recoursive subdivision" presented as a decision tree wich classifies patients into 14 groups.Those associated with a recurrence of AMI higther than 7% are considered "AMI groups", the other as "non-AMI groups. The expert system only intervenes at a late stage, when the problem is better defined. Such an approach is very interesting but unfortunately it takes a lot of data to decide the right direction because it uses a standardized procedure for every patient and for every disease. We tried to overcome the problem by dividing the diagnostic process into different stages. Our approach to the system is different and aims to recognize the area of patient problems right from the beginning. This reasoning structure is more similar to that of the expert cardiologist and is better accepted. It works by confirming or excluding whether the problem is car c. If the problem is cardiac, the system makes a quick prognostic stratification for the best diagnostic and therapeutic triage. During each stage in this diagnostic process it is possible to move directly from one diagnostic course to another if some requisites expressed by specific rules are satisfied: forward and backward (mixed). The advantage of such a mixed procedure is new in the medical field and allows a separate exploration of all the diagnostic apects of the knowledge that is useful in this particular patient, by using the information that has been progressively stored. The first version was based solely on rules and it needed a lot of hardware resources. The system had some positive aspects: 1) it was able to decide correct diagnosis in a good percentage of patients; 2) it was linked directly to the data-base of all patients hospitalized in our department since 1987, about 12,000 with 31% of patients hospitalized more than once, 3) it evaluated individual risk, 4) it stored all the caractheristics of chest pain in individual patients. The last prototypal version (figg. 1,2) had 33 rules and it worked quite correctly as clinical validation has shown. The performance of this prototypal version was tested in 190 CAD patient hospitalized in our department. Global diagnostic accuracy was 85% in such patient in recognizing that it was a cardiac problem in the emergency room. It was much higher , 95% in normal controls (already hospitalized for suspected chest pain), higher than 3 expert cardiologists. Some rules turned out to be very useful for cardiac patients or normal subjects with suspected chest pain and they were modified several times to get the best solution for diagnostic purposes. A second version of the software was implemented in DOS in 1991 using paradox language and running on personal computer. In both versions the main inputs were the same:

1) ECG trace in 12 leads, interpreted by the doctor interactively with the computer in the old version, directly from an electrocardiograph in the new one through a RS232 port. This system also made an interpretation of the tracing and it reported many measurements concerning the ECG trace in each lead

2) Chest Pain by Rose's questionnaire modified and integrated with guided clinical observations

3) epidemiological estimation of individual risk using Cox's method.

This system was called ERIC from Electrocardiogram, RIsk and Chest pain. The functional scheme of the new ERIC (Fig.5) takes information from the data-base, Rose's questionnaire, other questions and clinical evaluation by an algorithmic procedure and it concludes whether the patient is healthy or cardiac.

If the patient is cardiac it makes a prognostic stratification and it can recommend the best department and the best treatment for each stage of ischemia. In the case of incertitude it starts expert consultation (Fig. 6). This is a complicated procedure that attempts to imitade the cardiologist's method with informatic devices. The program uses a number of experts than can be considered single expert system by themselves and have the task of giving the correct diagnosis.

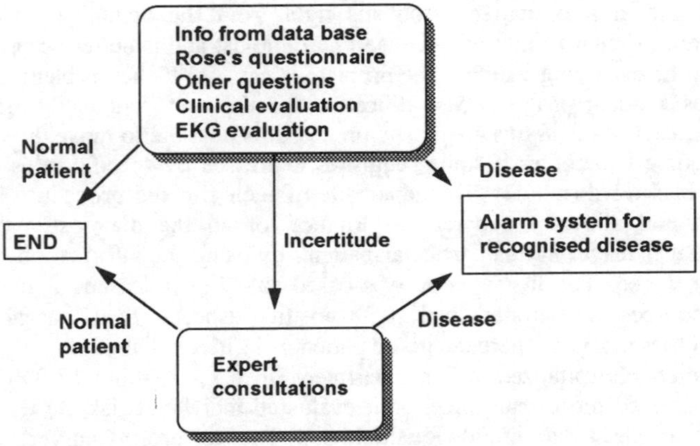

Figure 5: Functional scheme of ERIC (Ecg, RIsk, Chest pain): it takes information from the data base, modified Rose's questionnaire, other questions, clinical evaluation and automatically interpreted ECG, measures, and trace in 12 leads. It works with an algorithmic procedure and concludes whether the patient is healthy or cardiac. If the patient is cardiac, it makes a prognostic stratification and advises the best department and the best treatment for each stage of ischemia. In case of incertitude, it commences the expert consultation.

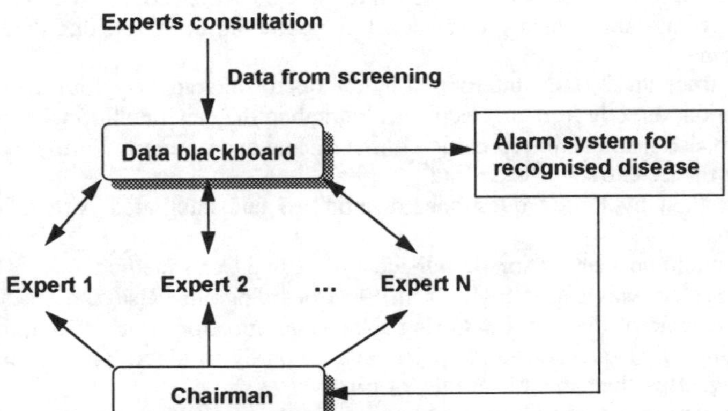

Figure 6: ERIC uses a number of experts that can be considered single expert system by themselves and have the task of providing the correct diagnosis; it is also a chairman that collects all the data and gives the final conclusions. All the data from screening are memorized using so-called blakboard polling. This word is used in engineering and indicates the way the chairman follows to choose the expert. All the experts use data listed on the blackboard, and when they have enough information, they elaborate a new diagnostic hypothesis that will be memorized on the blakboard. At each step the blackboard is controlled by an alarm system, like a traffic light that informs the chairman of the diagnostic situation. At each point the chairman controls the expert's job and decides whether to question them and in which order (polling).

One expert analyses the symptoms, one interprets the signs, etc., all coordinated by a chairman (fig. 6) who asks each expert to solve specific problems, puts all the data together and makes the final conclusion. All the screening data are memorized on a so-called blackboard by a mechanism called blackboard polling. This word is used in engineering and indicates the way in witch the chairman chooses the expert.

All the experts use data listed on the blackboard, and when they have enough information, they elaborate a new diagnostic hypothesis that will be memorized again on the blackboard. At each step the blackboard is controlled by an alarm system, like a traffic light, which keeps the chairman up to date on the diagnostic situation. At each point the chairman checks the experts and decides whether to question them and in which order (polling). The expert can infer by using three types of reasoning: 1) rule based, 2) algorithmic evaluation, 3) costraints propagation. The latter method is based on progressive reduction of the area of interest until certainty of the disease is reached. Thanks to the new development of ERIC, the computer user can follow on-line (fig.7) in 5-10 seconds at each step the evolution of diagnostic procedure until each diagnostic probability is below 10% or over 90% and so he can form his own opinion about the value of the rules used in each single patient.

This is more rapid ans easier to understand than the classic rule tree that was used in the prototypal version. It was helpful at this stage to understand the usefulness of each one, but too slow for routine use. This version of ERIC has proved useful in distinguishing typical chest pain from pains arising from outside the heart (musculo-skeletal or gastro-esophageal) in the first stage (Fig. 8,9,10) and also acute coronary ischemia (unstable angina or acute myocardial infarction) in the second stage (Fig. 11).

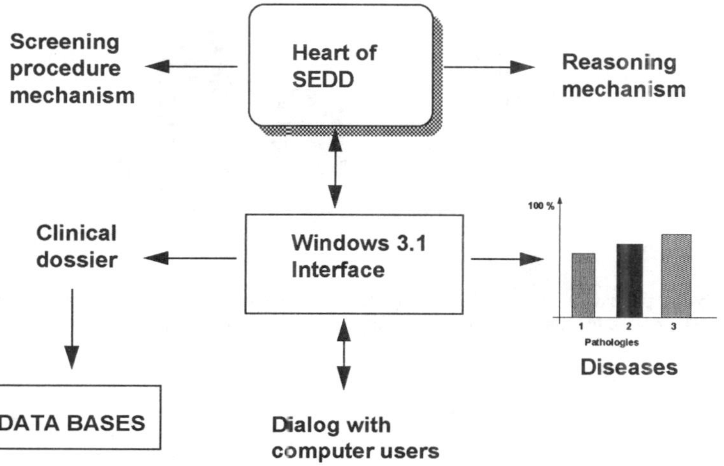

Figure 7: ERIC's heart uses screening procedure mechanisms and reasoning mechanism. It is connected to the data base through the Window's interface, and has on-line graphic display of the main diagnostic conclusions.

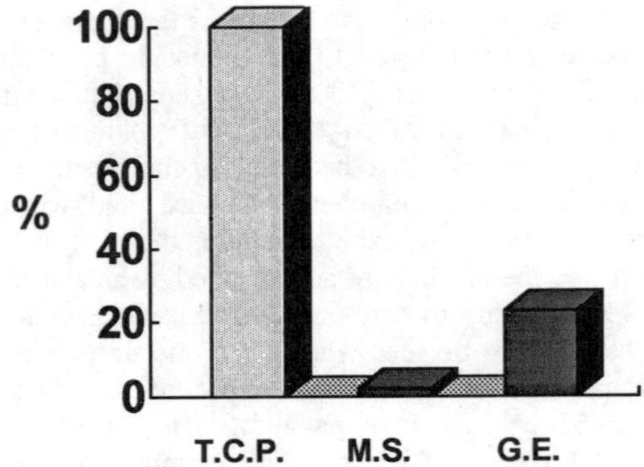

Figure 8: Sample of diagnostic conclusions in 48 years old male with mid left ventricular hypertrophy due to hypertension at the ECG, medium risk profile and typical effort chest pain with stable threshold. The probabilities of alternative causes (Musculo-Skeletal, M.S. and Gastro-Esophageal, G.E.) are low enough to decide whether the problem is cardiac and the chest pain is typical (T.C.P.).

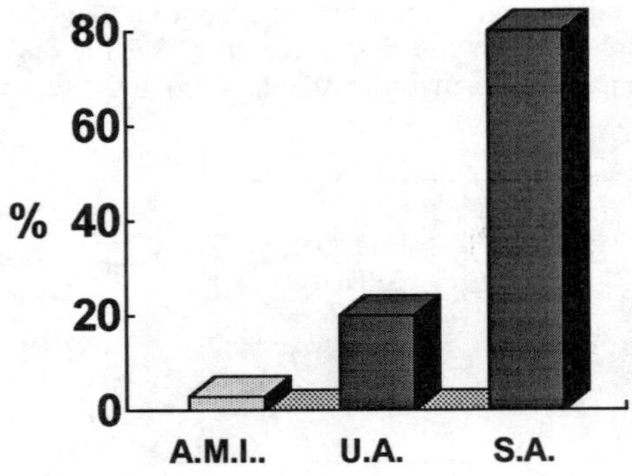

Figure 9: Same patient as in Figure 1: the system decides whether the anginal pain is stable (S.A.), unstable (U.A.) or due to an acute myocardial infarction (A.M.I.) and it is rigt.

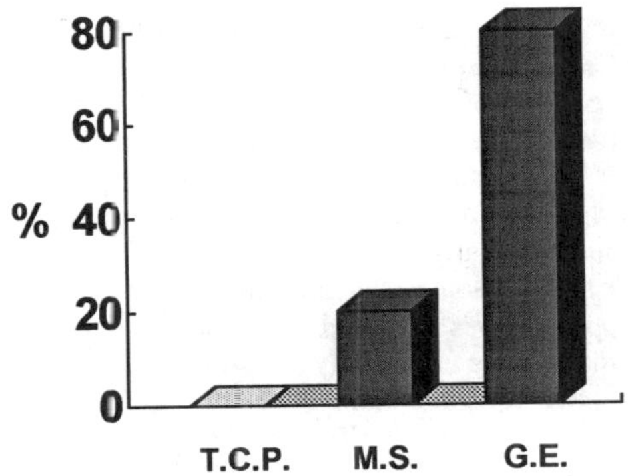

Figure 10: Sample of diagnostic conclusions in 60 years old male with previous inferior A.M.I., hgh risk profile and unchanged ECG during doubtful chest pain. The system concluded that the main problem was gastro-esophageal, as a 24-h manometry and phmetry later confirmed. Two month later ERIC was able to recognised in the same patient with similar ECG abnormalities a post-infarction angina with more typical chest pain.

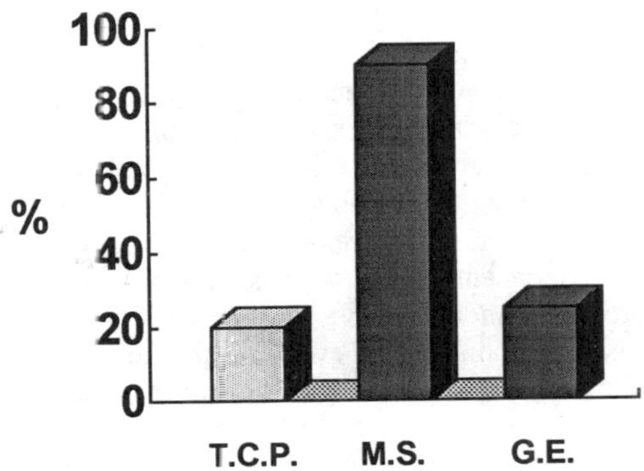

Figure 11: Sample of a female patient 42 years old, with low risk profile, incomplete budle branch block at the ECG and doubtful chest pain, mainly atypical. ERIC concluded that the chest pain was Muscular-Skeletal (M.S.) origin as the holter, treadmill test and MIBI scintigraphy later confirmed.

This second version of the program has proved useful in recognizing cardiac ischemia in patients with typical chest pain, high risk and normal ECG. It can help in patients with abnormal ECG but without cardiac chest pain and in low-risk patients with panic situation and slightly abnormal ECG. It allows a real time graphic evaluation of the diagnostic procedure at each stage in order to understand interactively the best reasoning mechanism in different cohorts of subjects. This program can be useful for a quick and correct diagnosis of acute myocardial infarction in the emergency room or at home so as to recognise candidates for systemic thrombolysis and correctly alert the cardiology department when some specific procedures such as coronary angiography , angioplasty or counter-pulsation can be life or myocardial saving. The chest pain is evaluated using a modified Rose's questionnaire. Some new questions,concerning the gastro-oesophageal origin. This complete approach was also used in the old version because we are convinced that it was very important to solve completely the problem of chest pain in each individual patient. Most patients have at some time in their lives either gastro-oesophageal or musculo-skeletal chest pain: a complete analysis of the symptom can be decisive in making a quick and correct decision.

- The ECG: it is possible to store both the digital trace on 12 leads and the interpreted analysis by Hannover program [13] in a compressed form : it occupies about 5 Kbytes and can be rapidly decompressed and quickly transmitted to the PC or to another ECG in RS232 by modem using an ordinary or portable phone,The systems available today can afford a reliable interpretation both in CAD patients and in normal controls. Many measures made on the ECG are used only partially, for a serial comparison of different traces of the same patient for early detection of cardiac ischemia and to judge the effect of cardiovascular drugs.

The system could utilize for diagnostic purposes the main conclusion of the interpreted analysis but it could also use some quantitative measurements in 12 lead, such as ST down-sloping or up-sloping, R wave amplitude,QRS axis etc.,already expressed both numerically and by a description of major findings in the program we use. In the present version only ECG conclusion and interactive comparison with old EKGs are used but we are working on a serial analysis of ECG, stored digitally.

This system can be interfaced with any automatic EKG that utilises ESC protocol [13].

- The risk of major cardiac events: this input made an individual risk estimation using Cox's method with the coefficients obtained in an Italian population using major risk factors: total cholesterol,age, smoking habit, systolic and diastolic arterial pressure and sex [20]. The output is the probability of events in the next 5 to 25 years: the system increases the power of main rules when the risk is higher than an arbitrary cut-off point in such patient. We chose this solution because to our knowledge there are no data allowing the use of epidemiological coefficients for diagnostic purposes. The graphic interface (figg. 7-11) allows on-line assessment of the correct diagnosis. Now our next step will be to obtain a better definition of the cut-off point between the characteristics of both ECG and chest pain in normal controls and CAD patients with different age, sex and risk profile: we are going to test it in a large population of normals, the intensive care unit, the emergency room and the ambulance. The aim is to take advantage of all the invaluable information in the automatic ECG interpretation and measurements and to better clarify the so-called atypical chest pain particularly in cohorts of high risk subjects. We also plan to improve the educational possibilities of ERIC to interactively build up a correct decisional capacity in students both and general practitioners.

References

1. de Vreede JJM, Gorgels APM, Verstraatem GMP, Vermeer F, Dassen WRM, Vellems Did prognosis after acute myocardial infarction change during the past 30 years? A Meta-Analysis. J Am Coll Cardiol 1991;18,698-706.
2. Gomez-Marin O, Folsom AR, Kcttke TE, Wu SH, Jacobs DR, Gillum RF, Edlavitch SA, Blackburm H Improvement in long-term survival among patients hospitalized with acute myocardial infarction, 1970 to 1980. N Engl J Med 1987;316,1353-1359.
3. Goldberg RJ, Gore JM, Alpert JS, Dalen JE. Incidence and case fatality rates of acute myocardial infarction (1975-1984): the Worcester Heart Attack Study. Am Heart J 1988;115,761-767.
4. Simoons ML, Vos J, Tijssen JGP, Vermeer F, Verheught FWA, Krauss XH, Cats VM Long term benefit of early thrombolitic therapy in patients with acute myocardial infarction: 5 year follow-up of a trial conducted by the University Cardiology Institute of the Netherlands. J Am Coll Cardiol 1989;14,1609-1615.
5. Braunwald E Optimizing Thrombolitic Therapy of acute Myocardial Infarction. Circulation 1990;82,1510-1513.
6. Bruce RA, Yarnall SR. Reliability and normal variations of computer analysis of Frank electrocardiograms by the Smith-Hyde program. 1972 ;Am J Cardiol 29,389-396.
7. Cohen M., Hawkins L , Greenberg S., Fuster V.Usefullness of ST-segment changes in >_ 2 leads on the emergency room electrocardiogram in either unstable angina pectoris or non-Q-wave myocardial infarction in predicting outcome. Am J Card 1991; 67,1368-1372.
8. Mark DB, Hlatky MA, Califf RM, Morris JJ, Sisson SD, McCants CB, Lee KL, Harrel FE, Pryor DB Painless exercize ST deviation on the treadmill: long-term prognosis. J Am Coll Cardiol 1989: 14,885-892
9. Rocco M.B., Nabel E.G., Campbell S., Goldmann L., Barry J., Mead K., Selwyn A.P. Prognostic importance of myocardial ischemia detected by ambulatory monitoring in patients with stable coronary artery disease. Circulation 1988;78,877-884
10. Drazen E, Mann N, Borun R, Laks M, Berson A. Survey of computer assisted electrocardiography in the United States. J Electrocardiol 1988; 21,Suppl S98-S104.
11. Caceres CA, Hocheberg HM. Performance of the computer and physician in the analysis of the electrocardiogram. Am Heart J 1970; 79,439-443.
12. Pipberger HV, Corfield J What ECG-computer program to choose for clinical application: the need for consumer application. Circulation 1973 47,918-920.
13. Willems JL, Abreu-Lima C, Arnaud P, van Bemmel JH,Brohet C, , Degani R,Denis B, Gerhing J,Graham I,van Herpen G, Machado H, Rubel P,Zywietz C. The diagnostic performance of computer programs for the interpretation of electrocardiograms. N Engl J Med 1991;325,1767-1773
14. Milliken JA, Burgraf GW, McCans JL The impact of the computer reported vectocardiogram on the cardiologist interpreter of the scalar electrocardiogram. J Electrocardiol 1977 10,375-378

15. Willems Jl,Ed. SCP-ECG Project. Standard Communication Protocol for Computerized Electrocardiography. Final specifications and recommendations. aď nced Informatics in Medicine (AIM *1015), isbn-90-73402-01-7.Past experience on reaching consensus for the standardization of medical systems,the example of the aim * 1015 scp-ecg project. ACCO Publisher 1991, Leuven
16. Mertins V, Fischer R, Joseph G, Zywietz C, Malossi C, Wack(1992) Implementation of the SCP-ECG Protocol into standard-alone Electrocardiographs, in Murray A and Arzbecher R (Eds) IEEE 1992;Computers Society Publisher, Los Alamitos, pp.83-86
17. Heyden S, Bartel AG, Tabesh E, Cassel JC, Tyroler HA, Cornoni JC, Hames CG Angina pectoris and the Rose questionaire. Arch Intern Med 1971;128,961-964.
18. Pekkanen A.J., Linn S., Heiss G., Suchindram C.M., Leon A., Rifkind B.M., Tyroler H.A. Ten-year mortality from cardiovascular disease in relation to cholesterol level among men with and without preexisting cardiovascular disease. Protocol to predict myiocardial infarction in emergency department patients with chest pain. N Engl J Med 1991;318,797-780
19. Genest J.J., McNamara J.R., Salem D.N., Schaefer E.J. Prevalence of risk factors in men with premature coronary artery disease. Am J Cardiol 1991;67,1185-1189.
20. Menotti A. La stima quantitativa del rischio coronarico. Giorn Ital Cardiol 1972;2,665-668
21. Myers R.H., Kiely D.K., Cupples L.A., Kannel W.B. Parental history is an independent risk factor for coronary artery disease: The Framingham study. Am Heart J 1990;120,963-969.
22. Rissanen A.M. Familial occurrence of coronary heart disease: effect of age at diagnosis. Am J Card 1979;44,60-66
23. Goldman L, Cook E F, Brand DA, Lee TH, Roman GW, Weisberg MC, Acampora D, Stasiulewicz C, Walshon J, Terranova G, Gottlieb L, Kobernick M, Goldstein-Wayne B, Copen D, Daley K, Brandt AA, Jones D, Mellors J, Jakubowski R A computer protocol to predict myocardial infarction in emergency department patients with chest pain. N Engl J Med 1988;318, 797-803
24. Goldman L, Weinberg M, Olshen R, Cook E F, Sargent R K, Lamas G A, Dennis C, Wilson C, Deckelbaum L, Fineberg H, Stiratelli R, and the Medical Staff at Yale-New Haven Hospital and Brigham and Women's Hospital A computer derived protocol to aid in the diagnosis of emergency room patients with acute chest pain. N Engl J Med 1982;307,588-596
25. Pollock BH,Diamond GA Accuracy of heuristic and algorithmic interpretation of cardiac stress test in comparison to expert clinicians. Am J Noninv Cardiol 1988;2:339-346
26. Ransohoff D F, Feinstein A R Problems of spectrum and bias in evaluating the efficacy of diagnostic tests. New Engl J Med 1978;299,926-930
27. Goldstein S, Lakier J(1986) Spasmo Coronarico: puntualizzazione. Medicine illustrated 1986;2,245-252
28. Selker HP Sorting out chest pain. Emergency decision. Circulation 198564(2),8-17

29. Lee KL, Pryor DB, Harrel FE, Califf RM , Behar VS, Floyd W, Whalen RE, Rosati RA Predicting outcome in coronary disease. Statistical models versus expert clinicians. Am J Med 1986;80(4),553-560
30. Fattu J M, Blomberg D J, Patrick E A Consult learning system applied to early diagnosis of chest pain, in Murray A. and Arzbecher R.(Eds): Computers in Cardiology, IEEE 1987;Computers Society Publishers, Los Alamitos, pp. 171-177
31. Hlatky M, Botvinick E, Brundage D Diagnostic accuracy of cardiologist comparated with probability calculating using Bayes' rule. Am J of Cardiol 1982; 6(49),1927-1931
32. Dubois D, Prade H Handling uncertainty in expert systems: pitfalls difficulties remedies. Lab L S I, Univ Sabatier P, Touluse (France)1988;123-137
33. Menotti A, Corradini P, Capocaccia R, Farchi G, Mariotti S, Puddu V(1975) La previsione della cardiopatia coronarica. Applicazione di un modello matematico a materiale epidemiologico italiano. Giorn It Cardiol 843-851
34. Prade H(1983) A computational approch approximate and plausible reasoning with applications to expert systems. Vol.3. IEEE Computers Society Publisher, Los Alamitos.
35. Driankov D Uncertainty calcules with verbally defined belief-intervals. Linkoping Univ 1986(Sweden)
36. Bonissone PP: Summaring and propagating uncertain information with triangular norms. General Electric Corporation Research and Development, Schenectady, 1988 New York
37. Bonissone PP, Decker SK Selecting uncertainty calculi and granularity: an experiment in trading-off precision and complexity. General Electric Corporation Research and Development, Schenectady, 1986 New York
38. Heberden W Some account of a disorder of the breast. Med Trans Coll. London 1772;2,59-67
39. Masoni A Sindromi cliniche e storia naturale dell'ischemia miocardica transitoria, in Fazzini PF, L'Abbate A (Eds): Il punto su la diagnostica dell'ischemia miocardica transitoria. OIC Medical Press, 1987 Firenze p.19
40. Sheps DS, Adams KF, Hinderliter A, Price C, Bissette J Orlando G,Margolis B, Koch G Endorphins are related to pain perception in coronary artery disease. Am J Cardiol 1987; 59,523-527
41. Miller PF, Sheps DS, Bragdon EE, Herbst MC, Dalton BS, Hinderliter AL, Koch GG, Maixner W, Ekelund LG Aging and pain perception in ischemic heart disease. Am Heart J 1990; 120,22-30
42. Bayer AJ, Chanda JS, Farag RR, Pathy MS Changing presentation of myocardial infarction with increasing old age. J Am Geriatr Soc 1986 34,263-266
43. CASS:Principal Investigators and Their Associates: National Heart, Lung and Blood Institute Coronary Artery Surgery Study Circulation 1981;63(PartI Suppl)1-10
44. Diamond GA A clinically relevant classification of chest discomfort. J Am Coll Cardiol 1983;1,574-575
45. Diamond GA, Forrestor JS Analysis of probability as an aid in the clinical diagnosis of coronary artery disease. N Engl J Med 1979; 300,1350-1358

46. Pryor DB, Harrel FE Jr, Lee KL, Califf RM, Rosati RA Estimating the likelihood of significant coronary artery disease. Am J Med 1983; 75,771-780
47. Giagnoni E, Secchi MB, Wu SC, Morabito A, Oltrona L, Mancarella S, Volpin N, Fossa L, Bettazzi L, Arangio G, Sachero A, Folli G Prognostic value of exercise EKG testing in asymptomatic normotensive subject. N Engl J Med 1983;309,1085-1089
48. Kudenchuck PJ, Ho MT, Weaver WD, Litwin P, Martin JS, Eisemberg MS, Hallstrom AP, Cobb LA, Kennedy JW,for the MITI Project Investigators Accuracy of computer-interpreted electrocardiography in selecting patients for thrombolytic therapy. J Am Coll Cardiol 1991;17,1486-1491
49. Brochier M, Raynaud P, Rioux P, Charbonnier B, Desveaux B Thrombosis and thrombolysis in unstable angina. Am J Cardiol 1991; 68,105B-109B

PHONOCARDIOGRAM ANALYSIS OF CONGENITAL AND ACQUIRED HEART DISEASES USING ARTIFICIAL NEURAL NETWORKS

DIETER BARSCHDORFF♦, STEPHAN ESTER♦, ECKHARD MOST♦♦

♦*Electrical Measurement, University of Paderborn*

♦♦*St.-Vincenz-Hospital Paderborn, Paderborn, Germany*

1. Introduction

Particular heart diseases like aortic and mitral stenosis, aortic or mitral incompetences as well as arrhythmia's can be diagnosed in a primary examination using the classical methods of electrocardiography (ECG) and ultrasonic echocardiography but also by auscultation with a stethoscope. Auscultation is certainly one of the oldest and easiest to be applied methods. Its effectiveness, however, is based on the physicians sense of hearing and the subjective evaluation of characteristic sounds. Also, a natural draw back is the fact, that an important part of the sound energy within the heart sound is centered around frequencies below the human audition cut-off frequency. While auscultation yields direct information on myocardial and valvular deterioration or on hemodynamic abnormalities, it should not fall into oblivion, that ECG mainly manifests the electrophysiology of the heart. In any case, the accurate diagnosis of complicated heart diseases requires the diagnostic verification by cardiac catheterization.

Both ECG and stethoscopic auscultation are frequently used in medical education and in the daily practice of physicians. With respect to acquired and congenital heart diseases, the results from ECG, mostly displayed in graphical form, are limited. Many attempts have therefore been undertaken to utilize the diagnostic potential of the phonocardiogram (PCG) for an automatic classification of heart diseases [11], [12], [20]. These concepts need either sophisticated sensor systems like low frequency accelerometers or high computational capacities, both not being easily available in the daily practice of physicians.

Our new phonocardiographic approach is based on two concepts, the noise removal from the auscultation signal by adaptive filtering techniques and the learning capabilities of artificial neural networks. An analytical description and programming is substituted by learning from examples. The filtering procedure yields sound signals with reduced acoustic disturbances and is therefore easy to handle in practice. Utilizing the extraorbitant computational and graphical capacities of modern personal computers, a PC-based diagnostic assistance for fast monitoring and documentation during a primary examination are the goals of our concept [2-7].

2. Methodical approach

2.1. Heart sound recording in noisy environment

Background noise from speech, door closing, air-conditioning etc. is unavoidable in almost every practical auscultation. Disturbances can be removed from the stethoscope signals by using a second microphone and an adaptive filter. This method is known from speech recognition techniques. Figure 1 shows our concept of noise cancelling during a PCG-recording.

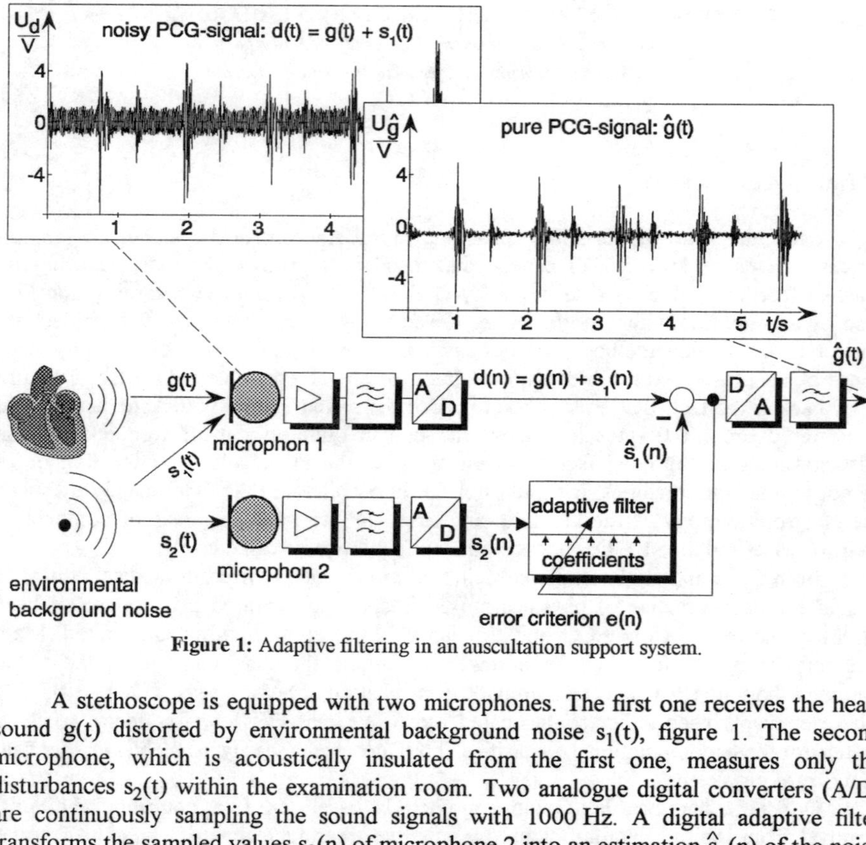

Figure 1: Adaptive filtering in an auscultation support system.

A stethoscope is equipped with two microphones. The first one receives the heart sound g(t) distorted by environmental background noise $s_1(t)$, figure 1. The second microphone, which is acoustically insulated from the first one, measures only the disturbances $s_2(t)$ within the examination room. Two analogue digital converters (A/D) are continuously sampling the sound signals with 1000 Hz. A digital adaptive filter transforms the sampled values $s_2(n)$ of microphone 2 into an estimation $\hat{s}_1(n)$ of the noise in the PCG-signal (microphone 1). The root value of the error criterion e(n) is minimized by modifying the filter coefficients using the LMS rule (least mean square) for each sampling. If the noise estimation $\hat{s}_1(n)$ and the noise component $s_1(n)$ in the PCG-signal d(n) are equal, the subtraction of both components yields a pure PCG-signal $\hat{g}(t)$ at the output of the digital analogue converter (D/A) [5], [6]. Real time computing is achieved via a Digital Signal Processor (DSP, TMS320C30).

2.2 Segmentation of heart sound

It has been shown earlier that the sound signal of nearly every single heart cycle contains quite the same information about the specific heart disease [3-6]. Therefore in a preprocessing phase of the stethoscope signal the segmentation of the continuous heart sound signal into single cycles is performed. For an automatic detection of these single cycles the well known systolic time intervals [1], [10], [16-19] can be used. They are defined by the relationships between the heart sound and two synchronously measured reference signals, the ECG-signal and an infrared plethysmography at the fingertip, figures 2 and 4 (above).

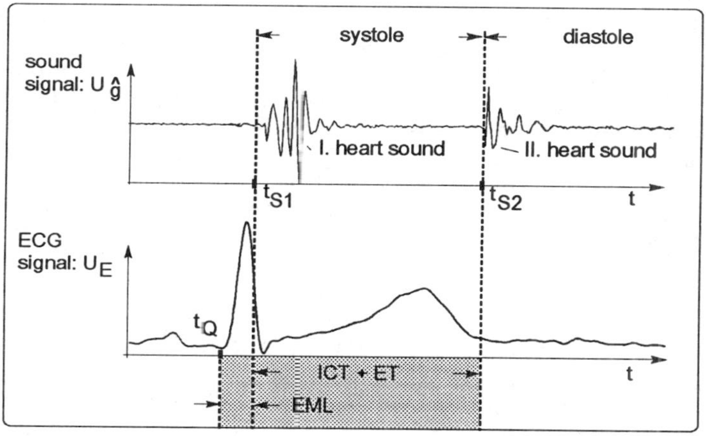

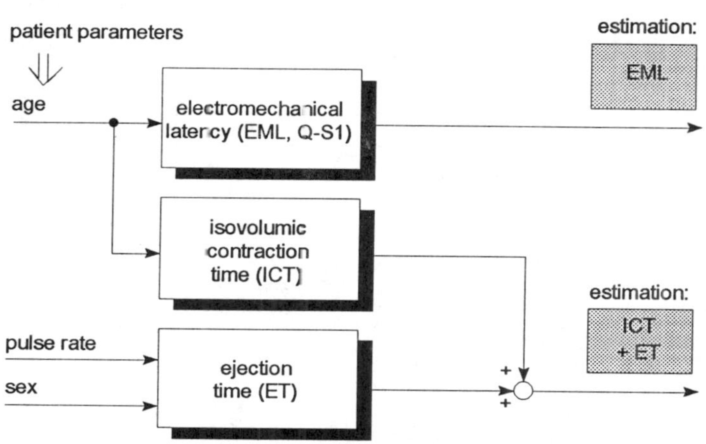

Figure 2: Relationships between PCG- and ECG-signal (above) and the mathematical models (below).

2.2.1 Statistical models

During recent years systolic time intervals have been estimated using statistical models. Several approaches in form of regression functions are known [1], [15-19]. They need parameters like blood pressure, heart rate, patient age, sex etc. as inputs and are well suited for being solved on a computer. Due to these known relationships and an own field study, carried out in the cardiology department of St. Vincenz Hospital (81 patients: 20 normal and 61 heart failures), the methodical approach was divided into two parts, outlined in figures 2 and 4.

Figure 2 shows simultaneously recorded heart sound and ECG-signals. Beginning at the positive slope of the QRS-complex at t_Q in the ECG recording, the duration t_Q-t_{S1} (electromechanical latency, EML) marks the beginning of the first heart sound t_{S1}, the duration t_Q-t_{S2} marks the beginning of the second heart sound at t_{S2}. This way the beginning of the systolic and diastolic phase in the heart sound signal can be determined.

The selection of input parameters of our own models is based on the results of the above mentioned researches of **Weissler** et al., figure 3. He showed the linear dependency of pulse rate (PR) and ejection time (ET) subdivided into two equations for male (Eq. 1), and female (Eq. 3) patients, respectively [17]. Extending this approach we are including persons with heart diseases and obtain the following equations, which are based on the patient set of our own field study.

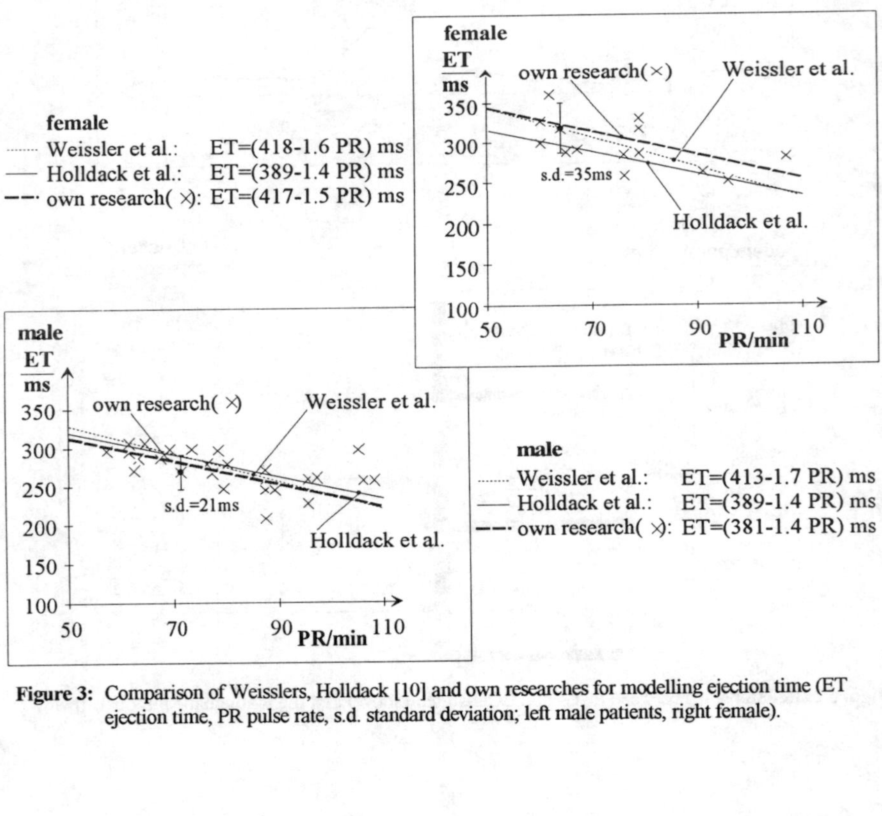

Figure 3: Comparison of Weisslers, Holldack [10] and own researches for modelling ejection time (ET ejection time, PR pulse rate, s.d. standard deviation; left male patients, right female).

Linear dependency of pulse rate (PR) and ejection time (ET):

male:	Weissler:	$ET = (413 - 1.7 \cdot PR)$ ms		(1)
	own:	$ET = (381 - 1.4 \cdot PR)$ ms	(r = -0.65)	(2)
female:	Weissler:	$ET = (418 - 1.6 \cdot PR)$ ms		(3)
	own:	$ET = (417 - 1.5 \cdot PR)$ ms	(r = -0.51)	(4)

(ET ejection time, PR pulse rate, r correlation coefficient)

In accordance with the article "Bedside technics for evaluation of ventricular function in man" from Weissler [19] we found in our analysis of 61 patients with heart diseases nearly the same behaviour of ejection time (ET) and pulse rate (PR). Weissler had used 140 normal (70 male and 70 female) individuals for modelling the Eqs. 1 and 3, figure 3. Holldack [10] mentioned a regression function without distinguishing in patient sex.

Some authors regard the isovolumic contraction time (ICT) as a constant [18]. In our field study we found a low correlation of ICT with the patient age (r = 0.41). Therefore we correct the constant of the ICT by a function proportional to the age (years):

$$ICT = (21.7 + 0.408 \cdot \text{patient age})\ \text{ms} \qquad (r = 0.41) \qquad (5)$$

For modelling the Q-S1 interval (EML) we found a correlation with patient age (r = 0.53) as well:

$$EML = (13.11 + 0.38 \cdot \text{patient age})\ \text{ms} \qquad (r = 0.53) \qquad (6)$$

Altogether we received a standard error for Q-S1 estimation of 18 ms and for Q-S2 of 26 ms.

Figure 4 shows the corresponding procedure for the heart sound and the volume pulse signal (digitalis). We use an infrared transmission signal from a commercial finger clip sensor for tracing the volume pulse. The initial phase of ventricular contraction is followed by a pulse onset t_O in the transmission signal, which is fundamentally delayed by the pulse wave spreading time (PWST).

Subtracting the isovolumic contraction time (ICT) from the pulse onset t_O, which must be corrected by the PWST delay, yields automatically the beginning of the first heart sound at t_{S1}. A corresponding addition of the time interval ET-PWST indicates the beginning of the second heart sound at t_{S2}. Usually the PWST is measured between the aortic component of the second heart sound and the well known incisure (notch) in the pulse signal [10].

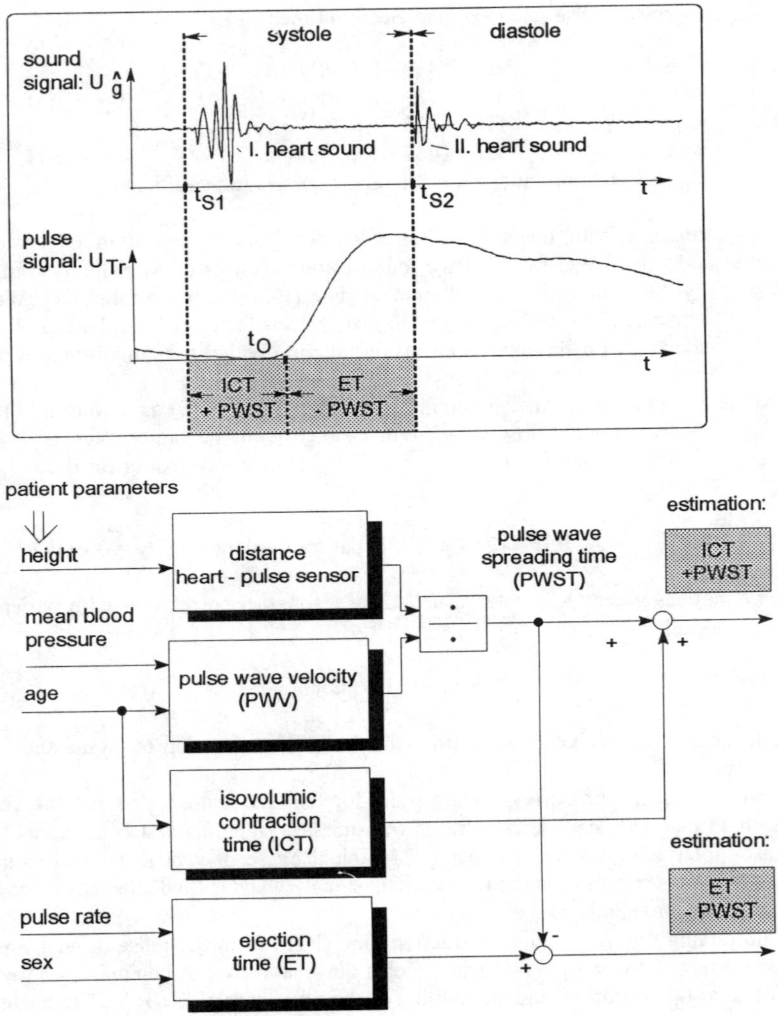

Figure 4: Relationships between PCG- and volume pulse signal (above) and the mathematical models (below).

Due to problems distinguishing among incisure and dicrotic wave (effect of reflection) in general, we substitute the measurement procedure by a model for estimation the PWST. It is derived from the ratio of the distance between heart and pulse sensor location and the pulse wave velocity (PWV), figure 4 and Eq. 8. The heart-sensor distance can be estimated from the patients height.

A non-linear relationship of mean blood pressure ($\overline{p}$ [mmHg]) and patient age, which yields the necessary pulse wave velocity (PWV) was given by Schimmler [15]. We compute the following non-linear regression function from data, published by **Schimmler** (nearly 2500 healthy probands):

$$\mathrm{PWV} = \begin{bmatrix} (3.68\cdot 10^{-12}\cdot \overline{p}^2 - 1.38\cdot 10^{-8}\cdot \overline{p} + 1.58\cdot 10^{-6})\cdot (\text{patient age})^4 + \\ (-8.88\cdot 10^{-11}\cdot \overline{p}^2 + 1.36\cdot 10^{-6}\cdot \overline{p} - 1.62\cdot 10^{-4})\cdot (\text{patient age})^3 + \\ (-5.34\cdot 10^{-8}\cdot \overline{p}^2 - 2.55\cdot 10^{-5}\cdot \overline{p} + 3.82\cdot 10^{-3})\cdot (\text{patient age})^2 + \\ (3.86\cdot 10^{-6}\cdot \overline{p}^2 - 2.57\cdot 10^{-5}\cdot \overline{p} - 3.34\cdot 10^{-3})\cdot (\text{patient age}) + \\ (-6.79\cdot 10^{-5}\cdot \overline{p}^2 + 3.34\cdot 10^{-2}\cdot \overline{p} + 2.83) \end{bmatrix} \cdot \frac{\mathrm{mm}}{\mathrm{ms}} \quad (7)$$

$$\mathrm{PWST} = \frac{\text{heart} - \text{pulse sensor distance}}{\mathrm{PWV}} \quad (8)$$

$\overline{p}$ mean blood pressure [mmHg]
PWV pulse wave velocity [mm/ms]
PWST pulse wave spreading time

The calculations of the isovolumic contraction time (ICT) and the ejection time (ET) are based on the same statistical regression models as the PCG-ECG-modelling in figure 2. Altogether we obtain a standard deviation for the error in the ICT+PWST estimation of 26 ms and in the ET-PWST interval of 32 ms.

The result of this investigation are two independent model concepts for the extraction of single sound cycles using either the ECG signal or the volume pulse signal as reference. For a first examination for example in case of an emergency the time-consuming application of the ECG-electrodes is not necessary. The system estimates the corresponding time intervals from the volume pulse reference signal alone with good accuracy.

2.2.2 Artificial Neural Networks

During recent years, artificial neural networks (ANN) have proven to be powerful tools in signal classification as well as in modelling of numerical data [2-8], [14]. The most important advantage of ANNs consists in their "learning capability", often substituting the requirement of an analytic description and programming of a problem [8], [13]. Naturally, biological (human) systems depend on a great variety of individual parameter variations. Therefore, exact mathematical relations in biomedical systems cannot easily be formulated in a closed form. Instead of applying time consuming methods for an analytical description of the problem, multi-layer ANNs are able to represent even nonlinear relations with good accuracy by learning from examples [9].

Figure 5 depicts a multi-layer perceptron, which can be trained following the back propagation rule [14]. There are three layers, an input, one hidden and an output layer. Each layer contains a number of feed forward connected "neurons". The strength of each connection is described by a weight, w_{kj}.

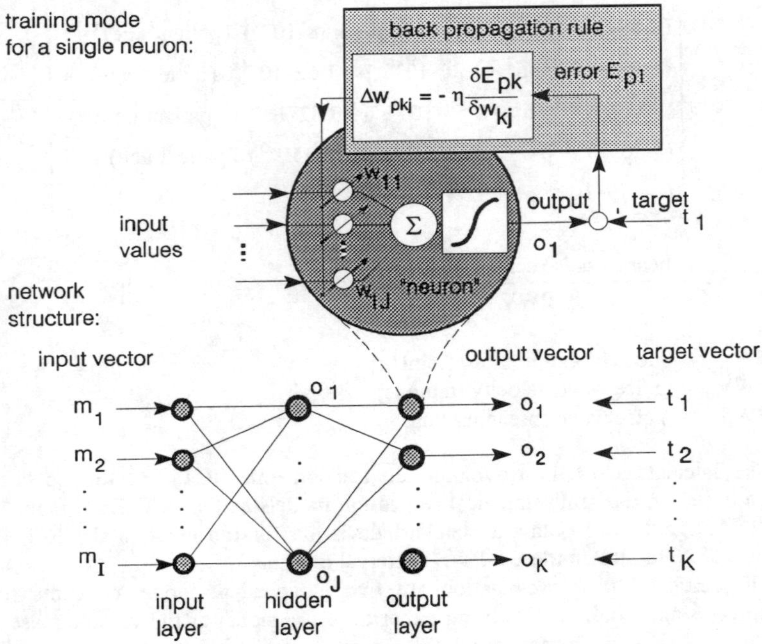

Figure 5: Simplified training mode (above) and structure (below) of an artificial neural network (ANN).

In general we have to distinguish between two network modes, the training and the propagation mode. The **training mode** is shown in the upper part of figure 5 for one single neuron:

The input values are multiplied with the weights w_{1j}. The results are summed up. This value serves as input for an S-shaped transfer function, which has some similarity with the activation function of a biological neuron. The resulting neuron output o_1 is compared with the desired output t_1, called target. During the training mode this difference (error E_{P1}) has to be minimized for all neurons and for all given examples (patterns) P by changing the weights w_{kj}. After the training phase the following condition for the total error E is true:

$$E = \frac{1}{2} \cdot \sum_{p=1}^{P} \sum_{k=1}^{K} \left(t_{pk} - o_{pk} \right)^2 \Rightarrow \text{minimum} \tag{9}$$

Following the described training mode we can store the weights and start the **propagation mode**:

In this mode, the net performs a transformation, which represents the unknown nonlinear regression function between input values and the output. This transformation was learned from examples during the training phase.

This concept was used to increase the accuracy of the time interval estimation. We have added an ANN in parallel to each statistical model, figure 6. The task of the neural model is to reduce the estimation error e due to individual variations of patient parameters. Detailed analytic descriptions of the error relationships are unknown. Figure 6 shows a block diagram of the statistical model and a parallel neural network.

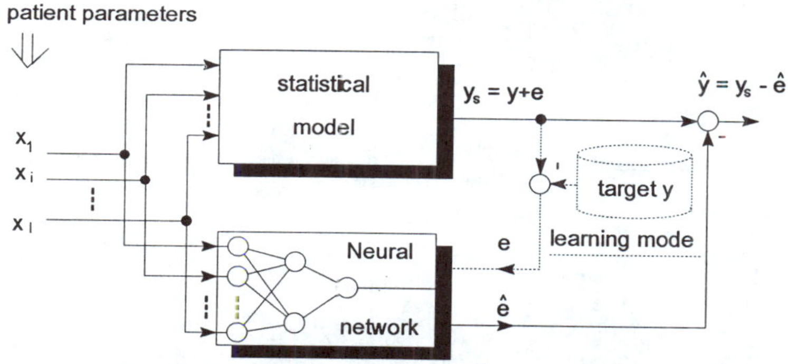

x_i input parameter (such as systolic blood pressure)
y target (true value)
y_s output value of the statistical model (for example ejection time, ET)
$\hat{y}$ estimation of the real value y
e error between y and y_s
$\hat{e}$ error estimation

Figure 6: Concept of statistical model with a parallel neural network (dashed line: learning mode).

The input values of the statistical model and the neural network are identical. In assumption that the error e of the statistical model is an unknown nonlinear function of model input parameters $e(x_1..x_I)$, we trained the network with the statistical error e as the target (dashed line in figure 6). The target values in the training set are measured out manually. After training, the neural net delivers an error estimation $\hat{e}$ of the statistical model which is subtracted from the output y_s. Utilizing this procedure we observed two advantages for estimation of time intervals:

1. The performance of the estimation is increased by a robust model behaviour in spite of parameter variations.
2. If the statistical parameters of the patient set change in time, the user can simply retrain the system with the actual data without a complete new regression analysis to optimize the model performance.

The results of the model based extraction procedure are single heart sound cycles, which now can be classified by a second neural network.

2.3. Feature generation and classification of the heart sound

Every algorithm for pattern recognition needs characteristical input information. During auscultation, a physician as an experienced expert performs the subjective diagnosis of heart murmur by a time and frequency evaluation of the listened sound [10]. Our PC-based system analyses the heart sound in a very similar way.

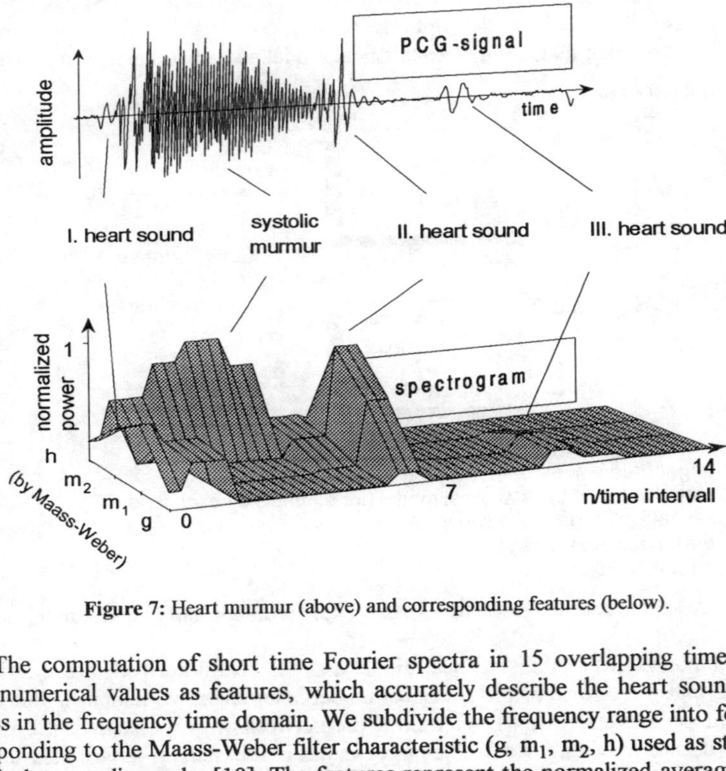

Figure 7: Heart murmur (above) and corresponding features (below).

The computation of short time Fourier spectra in 15 overlapping time intervals yields numerical values as features, which accurately describe the heart sound characteristics in the frequency time domain. We subdivide the frequency range into four bands corresponding to the Maass-Weber filter characteristic (g, m_1, m_2, h) used as standard in clinical phonocardiography [10]. The features represent the normalized average spectral power within each time segment. Figure 7 shows an example of one heart sound cycle of a mitral incompetence. The high frequency systolic murmur directly following the first heart sound together with a third heart sound can clearly be seen. Arranging the calculated numerical values in a so called feature vector with sixty elements yields the input information for a neural classifier.

Heart sound classification and diagnostic proposals are performed using the same network principle as for modelling.

Instead of physiological model parameters the net is fed with the 60 elements of the mentioned sound signal feature vector as input information. The output and the target vector consist instead of analogue values of a so-called "1 out of K" binary code. Each single output neuron represents a certain diagnostic result when active, figure 8. For example the output binary combination 010000 marks an aortic incompetence. For the training of the ANN data from about sixty input patterns of typical heart diseases, which were additionally verified by heart catheterization, are presented to the net combined with corresponding target vectors. After training, the net was tested with 106 patterns of single sound periods, which were not included in the training set.

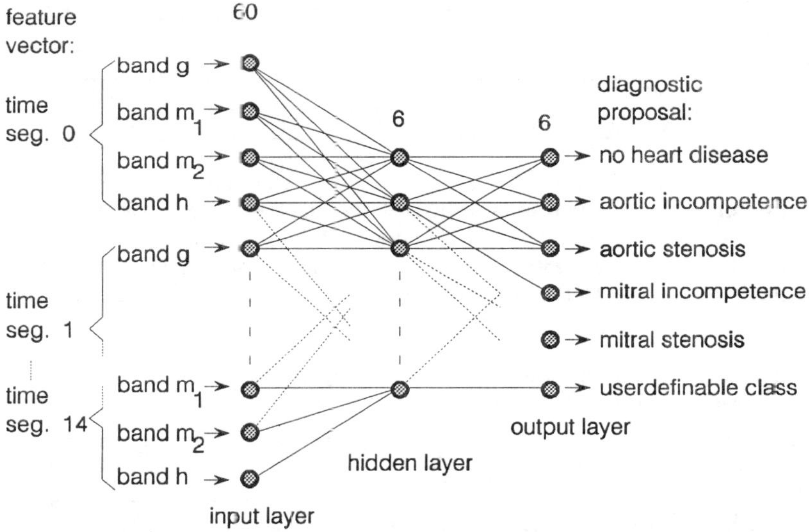

Figure 8: Structure of a second neural network for classification of sound patterns.

3. Results

The field study with our auscultation support system yields three main results to be discussed. The first one stresses the increased accuracy of the systolic time interval estimation using a combination of statistical and neural models. The second one indicates accuracy of the diagnostic proposals given by the system during the auscultation. A possibility to determine the stroke volume index of the heart, using the model-based estimation of systolic time intervals is the third result.

The advantages of the **neural model-based time interval estimation** are shown in table 1, which contains the mean square estimation errors. This result is based on time intervals of 162 single heart cycles from 81 patients in the field study. The third column lists the mean square estimation error of the statistical model alone and the fourth the corresponding error of statistical model in combination with a parallel neural network.

The first 100 cycles with different heart diseases are used for building the statistical model and training the parallel neural network. The remaining 62 cycles represent the test set. Except of the EML interval, all estimation errors of the unknown test set can be reduced significantly using a parallel neural model, figure 6.

Table 1: Errors of the time interval estimation using a combination of a statistical and a neural model (ICT isovolumic contraction time, PWST pulse wave spreading time, ET ejection time, EML electromechanical latency).

reference signal	time interval	mean square estimation error /ms	
		only statistical model	with parallel neural model
volume pulse	ICT+PWST	26	22
	ET-PWST	32	23
ECG	EML	18	18
	EML+ICT+ET	26	24

Next we discuss the second result, i.e. the system capability to support a **physician with automatic diagnostic proposals** by analysing the heart sound. Table 2 emphasizes the high accuracy of the neural classifier, figure 8. The system was tested with 103 single heart sound cycles from patients which were not included in the training set and therefore were a priori unknown to the classifier. Nearly 93% of unknown pattern are correctly classified.

Table 2: Classification results of 103 single heart sound cycles, which were not included in the training set.

diagnosis	pattern	correct	misclassified
normal	23 (22%)	23 (100%)	0 (0%)
aortic incompetence	12 (12%)	10 (83%)	2 (17%)
aortic stenosis	46 (45%)	44 (96%)	2 (4%)
mitral incompetence	14 (14%)	12 (86%)	2 (14%)
mitral stenosis	8 (7%)	7 (88%)	1 (12%)
Σ	103 (100%)	96 (93%)	7 (7%)

Figure 9 shows an example of a certain (above) and an uncertain (below) diagnostic proposal using signals from two patients with an aortic stenosis. The dashed line in the upper part of the figure marks the typical systolic sound behaviour of an aortic stenosis. The signal in the lower part has a systolic decrescendo (dashed line) directly following the first heart sound, which is a characteristic indication for a mitral incompetence too. Therefore, the automatic diagnostic proposal "uncertain" in this case is basically correct. If misclassification occurs, the diagnostic proposal can be modified manually by an editor. After a few minutes of retraining, the system has additionally learned the new pattern and classifies now accurately.

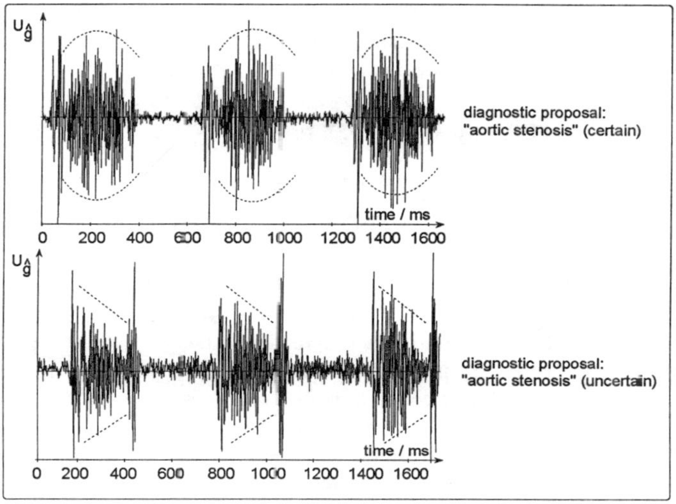

Figure 9: Examples of certain (above) and uncertain (below) automatic diagnostic proposals.

At last we are discussing a possibility, how the **stroke volume index** of the heart can be determined using the above mentioned model-based estimation of systolic time intervals. **Weissler** et al. published in the 60-ties a method for calculating the stroke volume index (SVI, stroke volume/body surface) from the ratio PEP/ET (pre-ejection period / ejection time of the left ventricle) [1], [16-19]. He showed a correlation coefficient of $r = -0.82$ between PEP/ET and SVI of 34 patients with heart diseases. Due to the PWST, we are also able to calculate the PEP/ET ratio, figure 10.

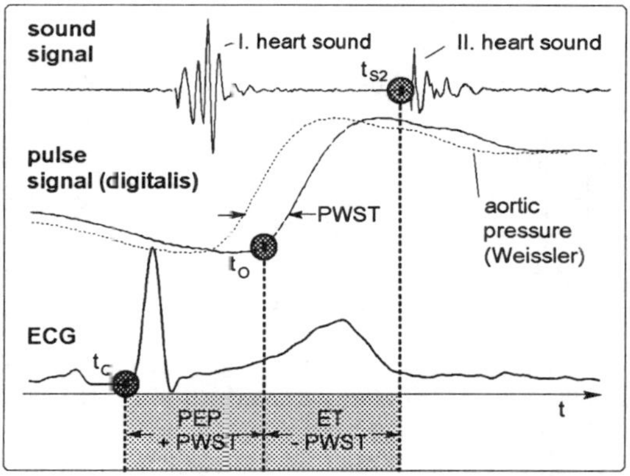

Figure 10: Determination of PEP and ET in consideration of the pulse wave spreading time (PWST).

We are substituting the aortic pressure, which is used in **Weisslers** approach, by the infrared volume pulse signal (digitalis). We obtain the following equations for the calculation of the SVI for a beat to beat analysis.

$$PEP = t_O - t_Q - PWST = EML + ICT \tag{10}$$

$$ET = t_{S2} - t_O + PWST \tag{11}$$

$$SVI = \left[-58.38 \cdot \frac{PEP}{ET} + 62.29 \right] \cdot ml / m^2 \tag{12}$$

t_O	time of onset in the infrared volume pulse signal
t_Q	time of corresponding Q-serration in the ECG signal
PWST	pulse wave spreading time
PEP	pre-ejection period
ET	ejection time (left ventricle)
EML	electromechanical latency
ICT	isovolumic contraction time
SVI	stroke volume index

The time intervals PWST, ET, EML, ICT and the instant of t_Q and t_O in Eqs. 10-12 are detected automatically by a computer program using the above mentioned models for the systolic time intervals [1], [19]. The regression function (Eq. 12) is based on data which was published by Weissler. Table 3 depicts first results between invasive $SVI_{thermod.}$ (thermodilution) and non invasive $SVI_{calcul.}$ (calculation, Eqs. 10-12) measurements of 5 patients with heart disease. The thermodilution was part of the heart catheterization in the clinical cardiology department. The fifths column in table 3 shows the absolute error e of the difference between $SVI_{calcul.}$ - $SVI_{thermod.}$.

Table 3: Comparison of calculated $SVI_{calcul.}$ and invasive by thermodilution $SVI_{thermod.}$ determined relative stroke volumina.

Patient no.	PEP/ET	$SVI_{calcul.}$[ml/m^2]	$SVI_{thermod.}$[ml/m^2]	e [ml/m^2]
1	0.40	39	44	-5
2	0.54	31	37	-6
3	0.62	26	29	-3
4	0.62	26	25	+1
5	0.68	23	25	-2

In this first test of the system we performed our poly-cardiographic measurements (heart sound, volume pulse and ECG) after catheterization for thermodilution, when the psychological stress of the patient and hence the SVI had decreased. This effect may cause the systematic mean error of −2.4 ml/m^2 between the two methods. For a next study, we are planning synchronous registrations. Based on these first results both methods indicate a significant correspondence.

Figures 11 demonstrates the capability of the complete diagnostic system. During a first medical check-up, a patient index card can be printed directly. It contains all the information about the current auscultation, including the automatic diagnostic result and parameters of cardiac performance. Physicians obtain a direct diagnostic and documentation assistance from their primary examination.

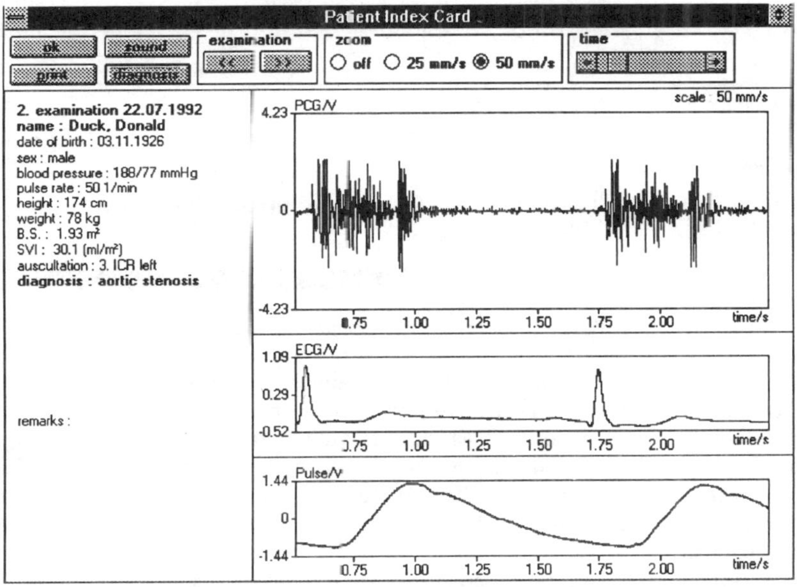

Figure 11: Example of a "patient index card".

4 Summary

Figures 12 and 13 show a scheme of the complete PC-based system The program is written in the programming language "C" and runs under Microsoft® Windows™ using an additional Digital Signal Processor (DSP TMS320C30). Three synchronously recorded time signals as well as six additional patient parameters are the required input information. In the succeeding preprocessing mode single heart cycles are extracted from the sound signal using a combination of a statistical and a neural model. For each cycle characteristical sound features are calculated. A second neural network (neural network II in figure 12) proposes a diagnosis based on the computed sound features. This diagnosis together with a graphic display of the recorded time signals and the calculated SVI is printed on a patient index card, figure 11.

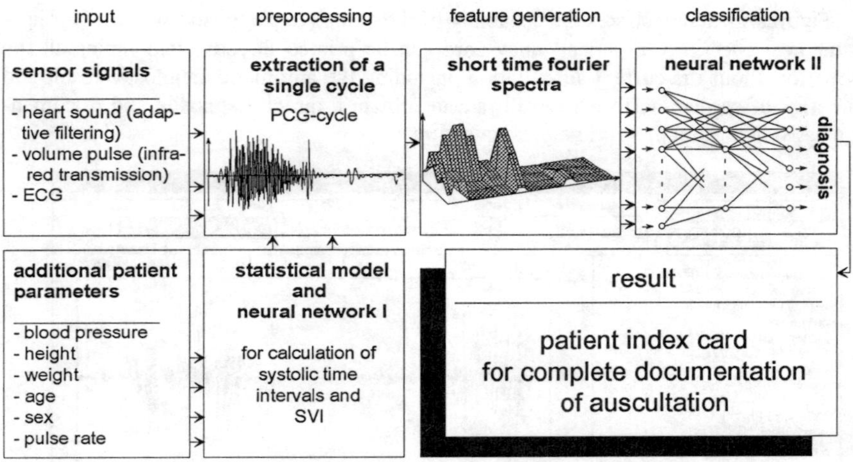

Figure 12: Structure of the complete system.

The advantages and the broad field of applications of artificial neural networks in biomedical instrumentation are evident. In this specific investigation, the systolic time intervals of healthy persons as well as patients with heart diseases, estimated by a combination of statistical and neural models were found to be in significant correspondence with the measured values. In addition, the sound pattern recognition results (table 2) demonstrate the good accuracy though training and test sets originated from different patients.

The system serves in mass screenings as well as in medical education. All measurements can be stored on the harddisk of the PC and replayed at any time. The recorded heart sounds can be played back into a head phone or via an audio amplifier into a speaker for a large auditorium, figure 13. The effect of noise cancelling by the adaptive filter technique emphasises the acoustic impression of the noise cancelled heart sound.

It should be mentioned that this new auscultation concept is designed for the primary examination situation in physicians practice. The diagnostic results are mainly regarded as proposals. It is not our intention to substitute a human expert for auscultation by a computer system, which has learned from examples. Since medical experts have selected the training examples, the accuracy of the diagnostic proposals cannot be higher than the performance of the human experts.

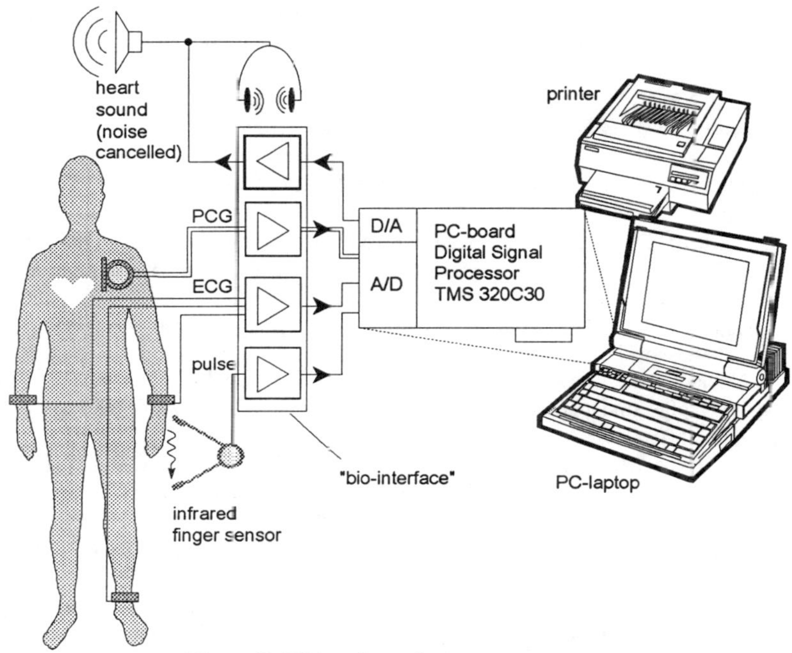

Figure 13: PC-based auscultation support system.

References

[1] Arnoud, K., and Faust, U. (1985) The measurements of systolic time intervals. Medical Progress through Technology, Vol. 10, No. 4, pp. 229-238.

[2] Barschdorff, D., Bothe, A., and Rengshausen, U. (1989) Heart Sound Analysis using Neural and Statistical Classifiers: A Comparison. Computers in Cardiology, 19.-22. Sept. 1989, Jerusalem, Israel, Proc., pp. 415-418.

[3] Barschdorff, D., Ester, S., Dorsel, T., and Most, E. (1990a) Neural Network Based Multi Sensor Heart Sound Analysis. Computers in Cardiology, 23.-24. Sept. 1990, Chicago, Proc. pp. 303-306.

[4] Barschdorff, D., Ester, S., Dorsel, T., and Most, E. (1990b) Phonographische Diagnosehilfe bei Herzfehlern unter Verwendung neuronaler Netze - A New Phonographic Technique for Congenital and Acquired Heart Disease Using Neural Networks. Biomedizinische Technik 35, pp.271 - 279.

[5] Barschdorff, D., Ester, S., Dorsel, T., and Most, E. (1992a) Neue Ansätze in der Herzauskultation durch ein Intelligentes Stethoskop - New Approaches in Heart Auscultation using an "intelligent" Stethoscope. CorVas 1 (1992), pp. 23 - 30.

[6] Barschdorff, D., and Ester, S. (1992b) Artificial Neural Net Based PCG Analysis of Congenital and Acquired Heart Diseases, American College of Cardiology 41st Annual Scientific Session, Dallas Texas, 12-16 April, 1992, JACC Vol. 19, No.3, 1992, p. 5A

[7] Barschdorff, D. (1992c) Neuronale Netzwerke in der biomedizinischen Signalverarbeitung und Diagnose (Symposium: Wissensbasierte Systeme in der Laboratoriumsmedizin, (Expertensysteme-Neuronale Netzwerke). Innsbruck, 22.-23. April 1992)

[8] Barschdorff, D. (1992d) Neuronale Netze in der SIDS-Forschung. (Internationales Symposium "Prävention des SIDS", Recklinghausen, 4. u. 5. September 1992), Proc. in press.

[9] Funahashi K. (1989) On the Approximate Realization of Continuous Mappings by Neural Networks, Neural Networks, Vol. 2, pp. 183-192.

[10] Holldack K., and Wolf, D. (1974) Atlas und kurzgefaßtes Lehrbuch der Phonokardiographie und verwandter Untersuchungsmethoden. 4. Aufl., Stuttgart, Georg Thieme Verlag

[11] Joo, T.H., McClelland, J.H., Foale, R.A., Myers, G.S., and Lees, R.S. (1983) Pole-Zero Modeling and Classification of Phonocardiograms. IEEE Trans. Biomed. Engineer., Vol. BME-30, No. 2, pp. 110-117.

[12] Ninova, P., Dascalow, I., and Dimitrova, M.I. (1983) Automated Phonocardiographic screening for Heart Disease in Children. Cardiology, pp. 5-13.

[13] Krayenbühl, H.P., and Hegglin R. (1965) Zur Beurteilung der Myokardfunktion mittels einfach meßbarer Herzparameter (Systolenlänge, Frequenz, Druck, Schlagvolumen), Deutsches Archiv für klinische Medizin 211, pp. 177-196.

[14] Rummelhart, D.E., and McClelland, J.L. (1986) Parallel Distributed Processing. Vol. 1&2, MIT Press, Cambridge Mass.

[15] Schimmler, W. (1965) Untersuchung zu Elastizitätsproblemen der Aorta (Statistische Korrelation der Pulswellengeschwindigkeit zu Alter, Geschlecht und Blutdruck). Archiv für Kreislaufforschung, Band 47, Heft 3-4

[16] Weissler A.M., Peeler R.G., and Roehl W.H. (1961a) Relationships between left vintricular ejection time, stroke volume, and heart rate in normal individuals and patients with cardiovascular disease. Am. Heart J., Vol 62, 367

[17] Weissler A.M., Harris L.C., and White G.D. (1963) Left ventricular ejection time index in man. Journal of applied Physiology, Vol 12, No 5

[18] Weissler A.M., Harris W.S., and Schoenfeld C.D. (1968) Systolic Time Intervals in Heart Failure in Man, Circulation, Vol XXXVII

[19] Weissler A.M., Harris W.S., and Schoenfeld C.D. (1961b) Bedside Technics for Evaluation of Ventricular Function in Man. Am. J. Cardiol., Vol 23, pp. 577-583.

[20] Zeh, E., Quante F., Becker, D., and Haag, R. (1986) Vom Phonokardiogramm zur Phonoanalyse, Z Kardiol, Band 76, Heft 6, pp. 357-363

HYBRID SYSTEM FOR DIAGNOSIS AND TREATMENT OF HEART DISEASE

DONNA L. HUDSON†, MAURICE E. COHEN†,††, PRAKASH C. DEEDWANIA†,†††
†*University of California, San Francisco,* ††*California State University, Fresno,*
†††*Veterans Affairs Medical Center, Fresno, 93703, USA*

1. Introduction

The development of clinical decision support systems has been an active area of research for the past twenty-five years [1]. A brief history of this research is instructive in that most of the approaches have ebbed and waned in popularity a number of times, leading to current systems which may include multiple methods.

The first decision support systems in medicine relied on pattern recognition, or more correctly, pattern classification [2]. The aim of these systems was to use data along with learning algorithms to determine which parameters were useful in making a decision. The goal was two-fold: to use the results to correctly classify new cases, and to identify parameters, perhaps heretofore unknown, which were important in the decision making process. A number of these systems were quite effective [3,4]. This approach fell out of favor partially due to a seminal article [5] which criticized these systems because they were incapable of explaining their conclusions. Shortly thereafter MYCIN appeared, which was the first knowledge-based expert system in medicine [6]. The attention received by MYCIN probably has been as far-reaching as any program ever developed because for the first time a practical medical system utilized symbolic processing. Interestingly enough, MYCIN has never been used in clinical practice, in spite of its ability to prescribe antibiotic therapy. After a number of knowledge-based systems had been developed, it became popular to distinguish between shallow and deep reasoning systems, with deep reasoning systems utilizing actual known causative effects in the human body [7]. Unfortunately, at this point in time, such deep reasoning models are unknown for many medical applications. It also appears that most diagnoses are not made through causal reasoning [8].

The next wave to sweep decision support systems, and likewise medical decision support systems, was the neural network approach [9]. Like the early pattern recognition systems, neural network models use learning algorithms. The difference lies in the patterning of the neural network models after biological nervous systems, incorporating thresholding and, at least in theory, parallel processing [10]. In fact, neural networks are a revival of early work in the 1950's which fell out of favor because of limitations of the initial algorithms and the impossibility of implementing realistic systems on the then-existing hardware [11]. Both hardware and software advances have made this approach both feasible and attractive [12]. In the last decade neural network systems have abounded in many areas of medicine [13,14].

As the information for knowledge-based systems is derived from experts and the information for pattern recognition and neural network systems is derived from data, it seems reasonable to combine the two to take full advantage of all available information [15]. In this chapter, a hybrid system is described which comprises a knowledge-based and a neural network component, both of which contain some unique features developed by the authors over the past fifteen years [16,17]. In addition, the combined system can handle a variety of data types including crisp, fuzzy, temporal, and chaotic [18].

This hybrid approach is illustrated in a decision support aid for cardiology, including several facets of heart disease: myocardial infarction, coronary artery disease, and congestive heart failure. The following section analyzes the different data types which are found in typical medical applications. The knowledge-based component and the neural network component are discussed in turn, along with the means by which they handle various data types. The combined system is then explained. Finally, the application of this hybrid system to heart disease is illustrated.

2. Data Types

2.1. Crisp Versus Fuzzy Data

First we will consider continuous fuzzy data. An example of continuous data is a test result or instrument reading such as body temperature or potassium level. A potassium level of 4.2 may have been obtained. However, all instrument readings and test results are subject to some degree of uncertainty, so in fact it may be more accurate to represent the potassium level to be in the interval (4.1,4.3). In other words, it can be considered to be a fuzzy number. In the crisp case, this interpretation would degenerate into (4.2,4.2), or just the number itself. An example of a fuzzy number representing a test result is shown in Figure 1. Fuzzy numbers are generally considered to be either triangular or trapezoidal. These data can be represented in the neural network by means of intervals, whose use is explained in the following section. A second construct which is useful is the idea of a membership function. A membership function assigns a quantifier to a numerical value based on a pre-defined function. An example is given in Figure 2.

2.2. Temporal Data

Temporal data can be divided into the following categories:

1. Δ Data: Change in value from previous recording (example: blood pressure);
2. Normalized Δ Data: Change in value relative to time interval (example: weight loss or gain per week);
3. Duration Data: Duration of time for which finding persisted (example: fatigue).
4. Sequence Data: Particular sequence of events (example: pain occurring before sweating occurring before nausea).

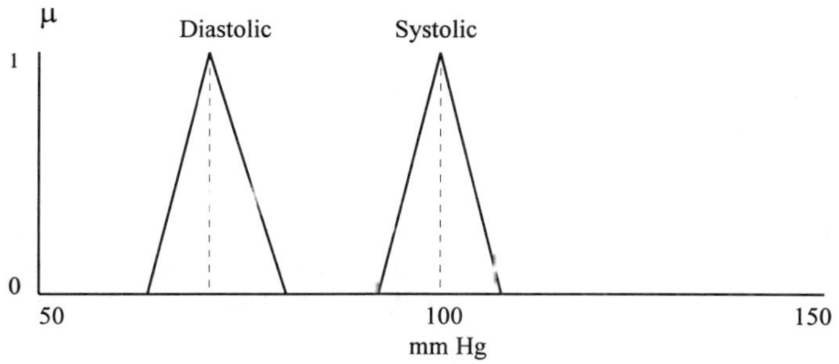

Figure 1: Fuzzy Number for Continuous Variables

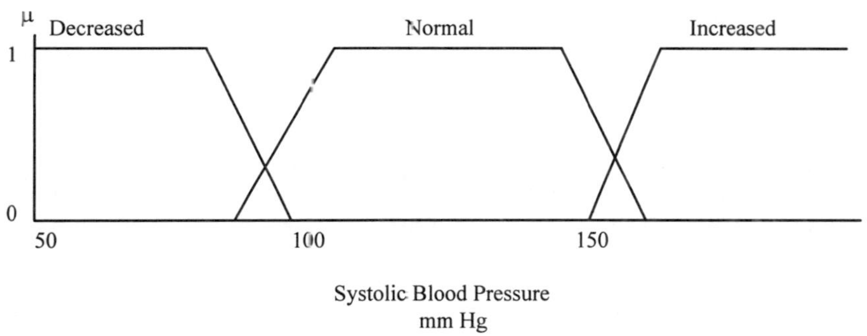

Figure 2: Membership Functions

2.3. Chaotic Data

The basic common thread in chaos theory is the recursive evaluation of seemingly simple functions which produce unexpectedly complex results. An iterative function does not suddenly become chaotic, but rather goes from the stage of convergence to a single value to a bifurcation, or convergence to two values. Additional bifurcations occur, and finally chaos results.

For the Poincaré equation (also known as the logistic equation):

$$a_n = A\, a_{n-1}(1 - a_{n-1}) \tag{1}$$

where A is a constant whose value changes the behavior of the function. The recursion is dependent on the selection of a_0, which must be chosen between 0 and 1. For increasing values of A, the equation progresses from single value convergence to chaos. Within the chaotic area, regions of stability unexpectedly appear. It will be shown in this paper that these regions of stability are only a matter of perception when discrete values of n are considered. They do not exist if continuous values are taken. For integer values of n, this function exhibits chaotic properties for $A > 3.57$. These properties include apparent lack of periodicity and sensitivity to initial conditions.

Many processes in medicine appear to exhibit chaotic properties. These analyses have become increasingly useful, especially in cardiology [19,20]. Chaotic analysis is still in its infancy, with new techniques needed to determine the degree to which a data set appears to be chaotic. Such an approach is described below.

2.3.1. Continuous Versus Discrete Equations

In the traditional approach to chaotic modeling, a recurrence relation is established which is evaluated at integer values, generally with each integer corresponding to a fixed time interval. These values are then plotted and connected with straight lines. However, actual non-integer values of these recurrence relations are unknown. We have developed an approach which permits an approximate solution of the logistic equation not only for integer values but for all real values of n and for any value of A in the important range $2 \leq A \leq 4$.

These results show that the chaotic behavior of this function is not apparent when viewed as a continuous, and not as a discrete, model, except in the narrow mathematical definition. This work emphasizes the danger of approximating any continuous process by a discrete model when the underlying principles are not understood [21].

2.3.2. Difference Equations and Graphs

Chaotic equations are sometimes used to generate graphs which are known as Poincaré plots. For example, using the logistic equation (1), a Poincaré plot is obtained by plotting a_{n+1} vs. a_n. The resulting plot is a measure of the degree of chaos in the system. We produced similar graphs using the continuous solution. Figure 3 shows two discrete Poincaré plots, at A=3.5 and A=4.0, while Figure 4 shows the continuous Poincaré plot for the same two values [22]. Note that the character of these plots is totally different.

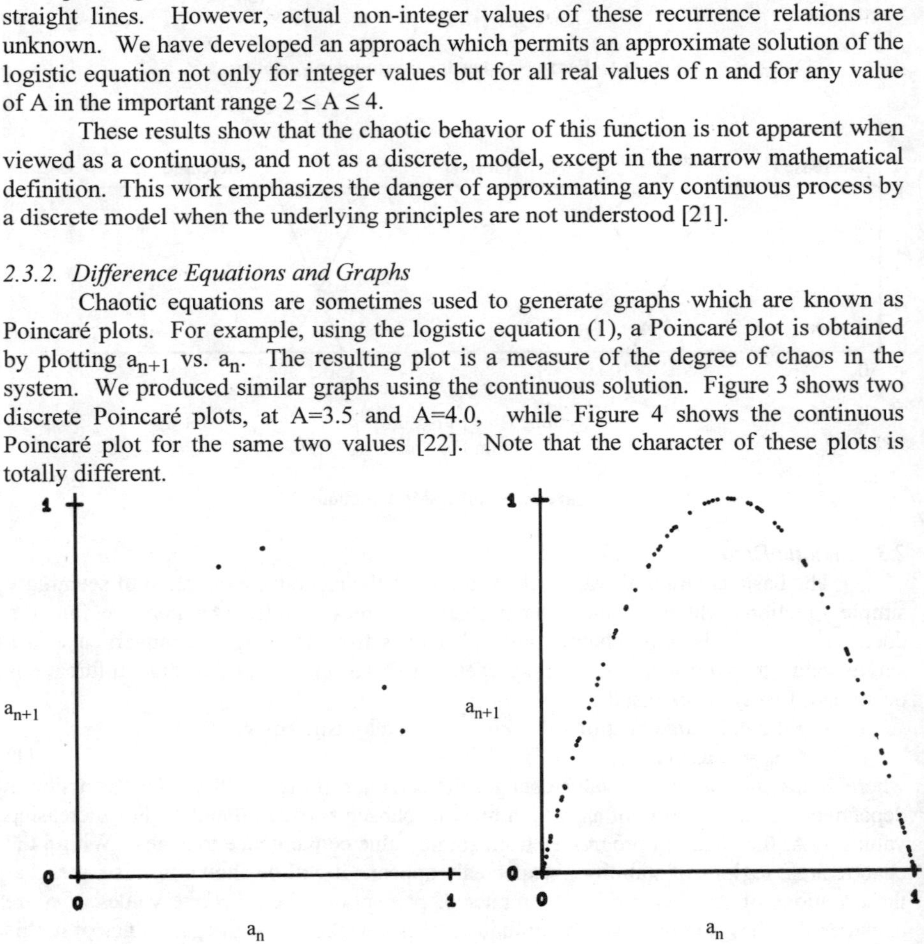

Figure 3: Discrete Poincaré Plots, A=3.5 and A=4.0

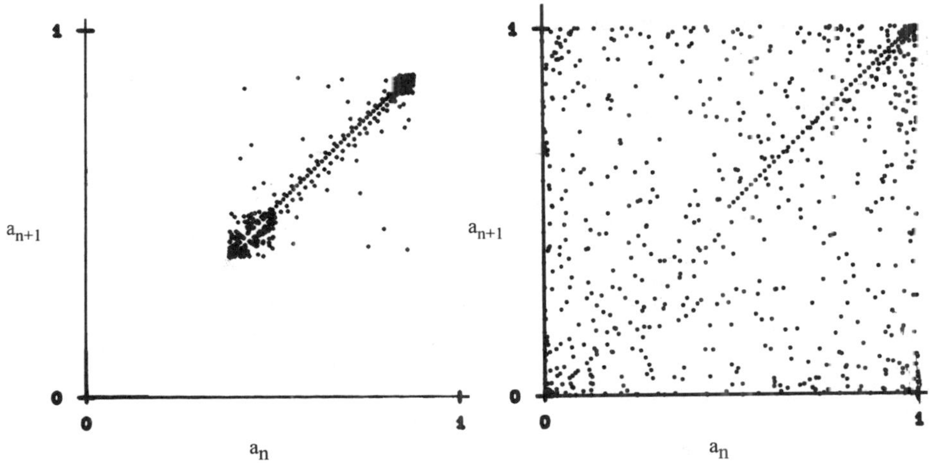

Figure 4: Continuous Poincaré Plots, A=3.5 and A=4.0

2.3.3. Second Order Difference Equations

Another useful graph for practical applications is the second order difference: $(a_{n+2}-a_{n+1})$ vs. $(a_{n+1}-a_n)$. This results in plots centered around the origin and is useful in modeling biological systems, such as hemodynamics and heart rate variations. The difference approach appears to give a more robust picture of the problem and fits well within our theoretical results of the continuous logistic equation [23]. Examples for low and high n values are shown in Figure 5.

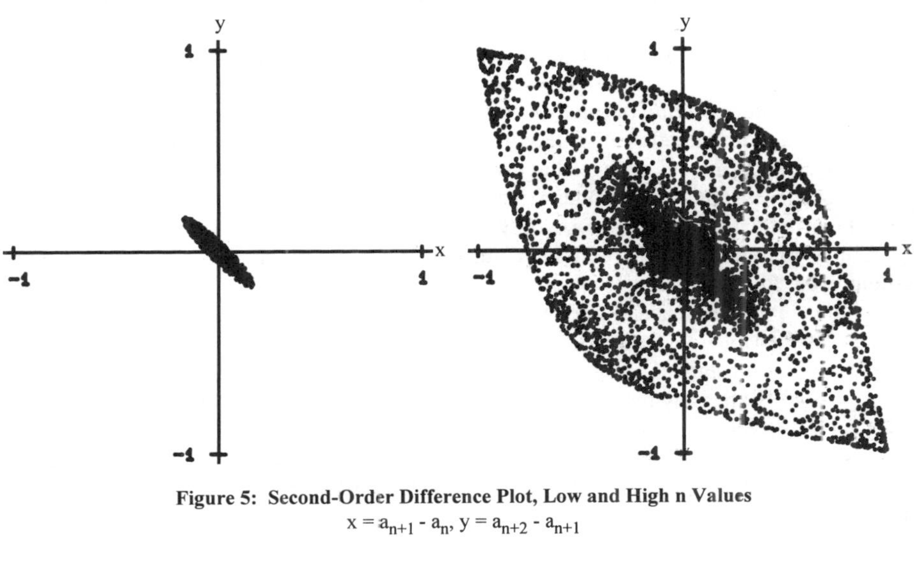

Figure 5: Second-Order Difference Plot, Low and High n Values

$x = a_{n+1} - a_n$, $y = a_{n+2} - a_{n+1}$

3. Knowledge-Based Component

Different components of the expert system are activated depending on the aspects of uncertainty which are present. They fall into three categories [24]:

- Crisp implementation;
- Partial substantiation of antecedents;
- Weighted antecedents and partial substantiation of rules.

Each will be discussed in turn.

3.1. Crisp Implementation

The crisp implementation allows rule antecedents in three forms: conjunctions (AND), disjunctions (OR), and a specified number in a list (COUNT) [25]. These constructs are summarized in Figure 6. Note that COUNT is followed by an integer which indicates how many in the list must be substantiated. The inclusion of these three logical constructs permits the types of reasoning most often identified in the human thought process. In fact, the AND and OR are special cases of the COUNT, with AND equivalent to COUNT m, where m is the number of antecedents, and OR equivalent to COUNT 1.

When using this form of the expert system, the presence of all symptoms and results of all tests are considered to be all or nothing, with no degrees of severity indicated. Thus all operations are implemented in straightforward binary logic. The only uncertainty included is the presence of certainty factors associated with each rule which indicate the certainty that the substantiation of the rule points to the presence of the relevant condition.

In reality, it is seldom the case that it is acceptable to ignore degrees of presence of symptoms, as important nuances in the data are lost. This is in fact more important for borderline cases, the exact cases for which it is important that the expert system function properly. The next section discusses partial substantiation of antecedents.

3.2. Partial Substantiation of Antecedents

Partial substantiation of antecedents can be accomplished in a number of ways. The most straightforward changes the user interaction with the system so that, instead of yes/no responses, the user responds with a degree of presence (a number between 0 and 10) which indicates a degree of severity. In this case, it is necessary to provide some guidelines to guard against individual differences in interpretation of severity. For example, the following may be used.

0	No evidence of presence
1-3	Moderate amount
4-6	Substantial amount
7-9	Extremely high amount
10	Maximum possible amount

This is still an area of controversy, and no completely satisfactory solution has been found. However, for subjective evaluations of symptoms such as pain, no better solution has presented itself.

Another possibility is that the user enters a value, for example a test result, and then pre-defined membership functions are invoked to determine a degree of presence. This is feasible for readings such as cholesterol or blood pressure.

In any case, once partial presence of symptoms is allowed, the binary logic inference engine will no longer suffice. Each of the three conditions in Figure 6 must be re-implemented.

For the conjunctive case

$$V_1 \text{ is } A_1 \text{ AND } V_2 \text{ is } A_2 \text{ AND} \ldots V_n \text{ is } A_n \tag{2}$$

then

$$P_{v_1,\ldots,v_n}(x_1,\ldots,x_n) = \min_{i=1,\ldots n} [A_i(x_i)] \tag{3}$$

Similarly for disjunctions

$$P_{v_1,\ldots,v_n}(x_1,\ldots,x_n) = \max_{i=1,\ldots n} [A_i(x_i)] \tag{4}$$

For the case where neither a conjunction or disjunction is appropriate (e.g. COUNT), linguistic quantifiers are used [26,27]. Let

$D(x_1,\ldots,x_n)=\{A_1(x_1),\ldots,A_n(x_n)\}$, and let

$D_i(x_1,\ldots,x_n)$ be the ith largest element in the set $D(x_1,\ldots,x_n)$.

Then for any quantifier Q

$$H(x_1,\ldots,x_n) = \max [Q(i) \wedge D_i(x_1,\ldots,x_n)]. \tag{5}$$

This definition suffices for the special cases AND and OR also. For AND,

$$Q(i) = 0, i=1,\ldots,n-1 \tag{6}$$
$$Q(n) = 1$$

IF **SC_1**
THEN Diagnosis A

IF **SC_2**
THEN Diagnosis B

IF **SC_3**
THEN Diagnosis

where

SC_1	**AND**	**SC_2**	**OR**	**SC_3**	**COUNT i**
	Antecedent 1		Antecedent 1		Antecedent 1
	Antecedent 2		Antecedent 2		Antecedent 2
	.		.		.
	.		.		.
	.		.		.
	Antecedent n		Antecedent m		Antecedent p

Figure 6: Rule Structure

3.3. Weighted Antecedents and Partial Substantiation of Rules

The rule structure below illustrates the combination of weighted antecedents along with the partial substantiation of each antecedent. The a_i's must be determined by some means, which is discussed later. The d_i's are determined by information entered from the user, perhaps in conjunction with pre-defined membership functions.

	Antecedent	**Weighting Factor**	**Degree of Substantiation**
IF	Antecedent 1	a_1	d_1
	Antecedent 2	a_2	d_2
.			
.			
.			
	Antecedent n	a_n	d_n
THEN	Conclusion (If S > Threshold)		

In order to determine S, the following is used. Let Q be a kind 1 linguistic quantifier (such as all, most, some), replacing the statement "QV's are A" with

$$Q_1(Q_2V\text{'s}) \text{ are A.} \tag{7}$$

The quantifier Q in this case replaces traditional binary logic operations, such as AND, OR, or more generally, m out of n conditions required for substantiation. The truth of the proposition is then determined by assuming there exists some subset C of V such that 1) the number of elements in C satisfies Q; or 2) each element in C satisfies the property A. The degree S to which P is satisfied by C is given by

$$S = \max_{C \,\varepsilon\, A} \{V_p(c)\} \tag{8}$$

where

$$V_p(c) = \max[(Q \sum_{i=1}^{n} c_i \wedge a_i) \wedge \min_{i=1,\ldots,n} (d_i^{\,c_i \wedge a_i})] \tag{9}$$

where ^ indicates minimum, a_i and d_i are the weighting factor and degree of substantiation, respectively, of the ith antecedent, and n is the number of antecedents.

3.4. Handling of Temporal Data

Temporal data are difficult to handle in knowledge-based systems. In general, temporal information is treated in special rules. For example, an antecedent of one rule in the chest pain rule base is "Duration of pain". The consequent of the rule is dependent upon this temporal information. Usually the incorporation of temporal reasoning is accomplished by the addition of specific rules to the knowledge base which may be purely temporal or may combine temporal and other data items.

4. Neural Network Component

4.1. Learning Algorithm

Variables are incorporated into a neural network model which utilizes a learning algorithm developed by the authors [28]. It features a non-statistical approach based on supervised learning. Weights are adjusted using orthogonal functions.

The learning algorithm utilizes supervised learning techniques. The basis of the technique is generalized vector spaces which permits the development of multidimensional nonlinear decision surfaces. This learning algorithm has a number of advantages over more traditional statistically-based back propagation networks: dependent features are easily handled, missing information can be accommodated, and convergence of the system is assured. In many applications, a number of the input nodes will represent dependent information. Although statistically-based systems can accommodate dependent features, great care must be taken in handling them. The model described here is also quite robust in handling missing information. Guaranteed convergence is especially important. Work in the last decade with recursive systems has shown not only that such systems can propagate error, but under some circumstances, the systems will produce chaotic behavior. It can be shown theoretically that the method used here will not result in divergence or chaos. The basic learning algorithm is [29]:

Read in values for input nodes;
Compute value P_1.
Until no changes
Compute P_i
IF $P_i > 0$ and class 1, no change
IF $P_i < 0$ and class 2, no change
IF $P_i > 0$ and class 2, or $P_i < 0$ and class 1, then Adjust P_i

Output decision hypersurface equation with weighting factors, $D(\mathbf{x}) = P_i(\mathbf{x})$.

The method used is a modification of the potential function approach to pattern recognition. The potential function is defined by

$$P(\mathbf{x},\mathbf{x}_k) = \sum_{i=1}^{\infty} k_i \, w_i(\mathbf{x}) \, w_i(\mathbf{x}_k) \tag{10}$$

for k = 1,2,3..., where $w_i(x)$, i=1,2 are orthonormal functions and k_i are non-zero real numbers. P_1 is computed by substituting the values from the first feature vector for case 1, $\mathbf{x}_1$. Subsequent values for P_k are then computed by

$$P_k = P_{k-1} + r_k \, P(\mathbf{x},\mathbf{x}_k) \tag{11}$$

where

$$r_k = \begin{cases} 1 & \text{If } P_i < 0 \text{ and class 1} \\ -1 & \text{If } P_i > 0 \text{ and class 2} \\ 0 & \text{If } P_i > 0 \text{ and class 1 or } P_i < 0 \text{ and class 2} \end{cases}$$

The orthonormal functions can in fact be replaced by orthogonal functions, since multiplication by a normalizing factor does not affect the final relative outcome. These functions are chosen from the set of multidimensional orthogonal functions developed by Cohen. These functions are represented by the general class [30]:

$$C_n(x_1,\dots,x_m)=\frac{m!}{n!(m-n)!}+\sum_{k=1}^{n}\frac{(-1)^k(m-k)!}{(n-k)!(m-n)!}\sum_{i_k=k}^{m}\;\sum_{i_{k-1}=k-1}^{i_k-1}\cdots\sum_{i_2=2}^{i_3-1}\;\sum_{i_1=1}^{i_2-1}\cdot$$

$$\sum_{p=1}^{k}\frac{x_{i_p}^{a(n,i_p)}\,[a(n,i_p)+v_{i_p}]}{v_{i_p}} \tag{12}$$

where m is the dimensionality of the data, a_i, i=1,...,k are parameters which may be arbitrarily selected, A is the normalization constant, and v_i, i=1,...,m are assigned values corresponding to the components of the first feature vector.

The general form of the decision function is

$$D_i(\mathbf{x})=\sum_{i=1}^{n} w_i x_i+\sum_{i=1}^{n}\sum_{\substack{j=1\\ i\neq j}}^{n} w_{i,j}\,x_i x_j \tag{13}$$

where n is the number of input nodes. This is the simplest nonlinear case; higher order equations can also be generated.

4.2. Handling of Special Data Types

4.2.1. Temporal Data

These data types can be handled in a straight-forward manner, according to the following schemes [31]. Let $n(t_i)$ be the value of the nth variable at time t_i, and let

$$\Delta n = n(t_i) - n(t_{i-1}). \tag{14}$$

$$\Delta t = (t_i - t_{i-1}) \tag{15}$$

Assign a new node in the network for Δ data such that

$$p_n = \Delta n. \tag{16}$$

The original network is then expanded by the number of nodes required to accommodate the items for which the change is important. For normalized Δ data follow the same procedure as before, except let

$$q_n = \Delta n/\Delta t. \tag{17}$$

Duration data can also be handled simply, by establishing

$$r_n = \Delta t \tag{18}$$

The most difficult type of temporal data to handle is sequence data in that a new variable cannot be created to deal with this entity. A major modification must be made to the neural network structure for accommodating this type of reasoning. These data are handled by embedding a procedure at each of the sequence nodes. To analyze for the presence of a sequence, let s_i, i=1,...,k be the ith symptom out of k and let t_i be the ith time interval. Define the matrix

$$S = [a_{ij}] \text{ where}$$

$$a_{ij} = \begin{cases} 1 & \text{if the } s_i \text{ occurred at time } t_j \\ 0 & \text{otherwise.} \end{cases} \tag{19}$$

Then tr [S] = k if the proper time sequence occurred, where tr [S] is the trace of the matrix S. There are two options for determining the value of node u:

$$u = \begin{cases} 1 & \text{if tr [S]} = k \\ 0 & \text{otherwise} \end{cases} \quad (20)$$

or

$$u = \{\text{tr [S]}\}/k \quad (21)$$

These choices will be discussed later with respect to fuzzy data.

4.2.2. Interval Data

In order to handle interval data as input, the following is proposed. For a data set with n variables, define a vector

$$\mathbf{x} = [(x_1,y_1), (x_2,y_2),...,(x_n,y_n)] \quad (22)$$

where (x_i,y_i) represents the interval range for the ith variable. The values for (x_i,y_i) will be determined by the input data in the training set for the learning algorithm. The objective is to obtain a decision surface which will separate data at any point in the interval. This can be accomplished if the extreme values are accommodated. In order to do, this all possible combinations of interval endpoints must be considered. For a data set with n variables, 2^n combinations will be produced. A new set of 2^n vectors is then defined:

$$\mathbf{z_k} = [z_1,z_2,...,z_n] \qquad k = 1,...,2^n \quad (23)$$

where $z_i \, \varepsilon \, (x_i,y_i) \ni$ all possible combinations of x_i,y_j are generated for i,j = 1,...,n. The learning algorithm is run for each of the 2^n cases. The weights attached to the decision surface which produces the poorest classification is chosen in order to form a robust model [32].

4.2.3. Crisp Versus Fuzzy Temporal Data

For the first three temporal data types, there are two parameters which may assume fuzzy rather than crisp values: the time dependent finding $n(t_i)$ and the time interval itself t_i. The $n(t_i)$'s can be of four types: binary, categoric, integer, or continuous. In fact, for these types of temporal data, the values themselves are not important, only the differences in the values. (If the value itself is important, it is included as a separate node in the network.) Thus the generalization of the difference operation is required. The most straight-forward generalization appears to be extended subtraction for fuzzy sets defined in [33]. According to the algorithm established by Dubois and Prade, this operation can be applied to continuous variables, with a simpler, direct computation possible for the discrete case. If the data itself is binary or categoric, these variables can first be fuzzified, if appropriate. In the case of normalized data, the extended division, also discussed in [33], can be applied. It can be shown that if M and N are fuzzy numbers, then

$$M \ominus N = M \oplus (-N) \quad (24)$$

will also be a fuzzy number, where $M \oplus N$ is extended addition, and

$$M \oslash N = M \otimes (N^{-1}) \quad (25)$$

likewise is a fuzzy number, where $M \otimes N$ is extended multiplication.

For the sequence data, the occurrence of a sequence in the correct order is a crisp result. However, the degree to which the sequence occurred in the correct order can be considered. Instead of setting node u_n as in equation (20), u_n is defined using equation (21). This definition provides a degree to which the sequence occurred in the required order.

For example, consider the k x k matrix S:

$$\begin{bmatrix} 1 & 0 & 0 & 0 & \dots & 0 \\ 0 & 0 & 1 & 0 & \dots & 0 \\ 0 & 1 & 0 & 0 & \dots & 0 \\ 0 & 0 & 1 & 1 & \dots & 0 \\ & \cdot & & & & \\ & & \cdot & & & \\ & & & \cdot & & \\ 0 & 0 & 0 & 0 & \dots & 1 \end{bmatrix} \tag{26}$$

Then $u_n = (k-2)/k$, the degree to which the required sequence was met. Each row in this matrix represents a point in time, and each column represents a symptom. $s_{ij} = 1$ if at time i symptom j is present.

4.4. Chaotic Data

Chaotic data can be incorporated into the neural network if defined in numerical terms. A number of methods exist for quantifying the degree of chaos in the system, including the fractal dimension and the Lyaponov exponent. A better method for experimental data appears to be the measure of central tendency of the second-order difference plots discussed above. This is computed by selecting a circular region around the origin of radius r, counting the number of points which fall within the radius, and dividing by the total number of points. Let t = total number of points, and r = radius of central area. Then

$$n = \left[\sum_{i=1}^{t-2} \delta(d_i) \right] / (t-2) \tag{27}$$

where $\delta(d_i) = \begin{cases} 1 & \text{if } [(a_{i+2}-a_{i+1})^2+(a_{i+1}-a_i)^2]^{.5} < r \\ 0 & \text{otherwise} \end{cases}$

The node value n will thus be a number between 0 and 1, inclusive, and can be added to the network like any other node.

5. Combined System

5.1. Weighting of Antecedents

The techniques described above are combined in a number of ways which address some of the shortcomings of each system in isolation.

First, the neural network structure can be run independently for each rule to determine the appropriate weighting of antecedents. In the simplest approximation, a hyperplane is obtained from equation (13), generating an equation of the form

$$D_i(\mathbf{x}) = \sum_{i=1}^{n} w_i x_i \tag{28}$$

The weight a_i for the ith antecedent is then determined by

$$a_i = \frac{w_i}{\sum_{i=1}^{n} w_i} \tag{29}$$

Note that these weights are normalized to sum to 1.

5.2. Determination of Thresholds

In addition, the neural network can be used to determine appropriate threshold levels for each rule [34]. The maximum and minimum values for the decision surface $D(\mathbf{x})$ must be determined. Let $A_i = \{m_1,...,m_k\}$, the set of all values which x_i can assume, where $m_i > 0$ for all i. Then to obtain the maximum value $D_{max}(\mathbf{x})$:

$$\text{If } w_i > 0, \text{ let } x_i' = \max [A_i] \tag{30}$$

If $w_i < 0$, let $x_i' = 0$ for all $i=1,...,n$. Then

$$D_{max}(\mathbf{x}) = \sum_{i=1}^{m} w_i x_i' + \sum_{i=1}^{m} \sum_{\substack{j=1 \\ i \neq j}}^{m} w_{i,j} x_i' x_j' \tag{31}$$

Similarly, $D_{min}(\mathbf{x})$ is obtained by the following:

$$\text{If } w_i > 0, \text{ let } x_i' = 0 \tag{32}$$

If $w_i < 0$, let $x_i' = \max[A_i]$ and apply equation (31).

All decisions are then normalized by

$$D_n(\mathbf{x}) = \begin{cases} D(\mathbf{x})/D_{max}(\mathbf{x}) & \text{if } D(\mathbf{x}) > 0 \quad \text{(class 1)} \\ D(\mathbf{x})/|D_{min}(\mathbf{x})| & \text{if } D(\mathbf{x}) < 0 \quad \text{(class 2)} \\ 0 & \text{if } D(\mathbf{x}) = 0 \quad \text{(indeterminate)} \end{cases} \tag{33}$$

The result is a value between -1 and 1, inclusive, which gives a degree of membership in that category. The values are then shifted to give an answer between 0 and 1, inclusive by

$$V(\mathbf{x}) = [1 + D_n(\mathbf{x})]/2 \tag{34}$$

5.3. Neural Network with Symbolic Layer

The nonlinear decision function produces a normalized numerical value between 0 and 1, inclusive. A separate decision function $D_i(\mathbf{x})$ is attached to each of the output nodes. A threshold value $T_i(\mathbf{x})$ (or values) is also attached to each level three node. If the value of the decision function exceeds the corresponding threshold value, a certain symbol is produced; if it does not, a different symbol is produced. This process can be extended by having any number of threshold values produce as many symbols as desired. An additional layer is added to the network which combines the symbols generated by adjacent nodes according to a well-structured grammar. A grammar provides the rules by which a symbol can be combined. The following notation is used. A grammar G is defined by (V_n, V_t, P, S), where V_n are the variables, V_t are the terminals, P are productions, and S is the start symbol. A simple grammar would be

$$V_n=\{S\}$$
$$V_t=\{0,1\} \quad (35)$$
$$P=\{S \rightarrow 0S1, S \rightarrow 01\}.$$

The result of this grammar is to produce the sequence 0^n1^n.

5.4. Example of Combined System

Consider a medical application in which it is necessary to choose among three conditions. It is possible that none, one, or a combination of these conditions are present. A neural network is set up to learn on data of known classification, determining which variables are pertinent to making the decision and the appropriate weighting factors for each of these variables [35]. The decision algorithm is represented by a multi-layered network as shown in Figure 7. The bottom level is the input level. This is followed by a number of additional levels, with each level accounting for fractional contributions. In Figure 7, two such levels are shown. The next level is the decision level. In traditional neural networks this would be the final level. In the combined system described here, the output from this level is used to produce an additional level, denoted the action level. In the case of medical decision making, level n-1 would determine which condition or conditions are present, and level n would determine what treatment or follow-up testing should be done based on these results. Table I shows a sample grammar. A possible interpretation is the following. Each node has an potential excitatory action (represented by a) or inhibitory action (represented by b). This is determined by threshold values: If $D_i(\mathbf{x}) > T_i$, then "a" else "b". In the grammar, each node is numbered N_i. A response of "a" at node i indicates that condition C_i is present. To simplify the grammar, a sequential evaluation of nodes is assumed. If random evaluation is done, additional entries in the grammar are required.

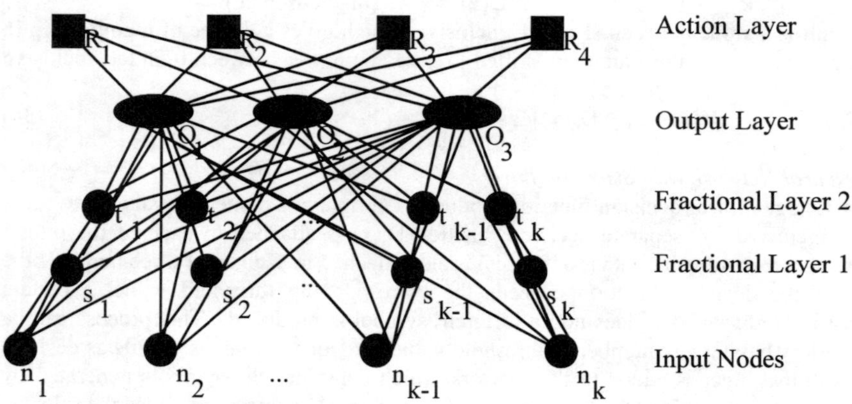

Figure 7: Neural Network Diagram

Table I: Sample Grammar

V_n= {S,A,B,C,D,T}	V_t= {a,b,r_1,r_2,r_3,r_4}		
P:	$S \to N_1$	$N_1 \to aN_2$	$aaaT \to r_1$
		$N_1 \to bN_2$	$bbbT \to r_4$
		$N_2 \to aN_3$	$bbaT \to r_3$
		$N_2 \to bN_3$	$baaT \to r_3$
		$N_3 \to aT$	$abbT \to r_2$
		$N_3 \to bT$	$aabT \to r_2$
			$abaT \to r_2$
			$babT \to r_2$

For the example, four possible actions are assumed:

r_1: No action
r_2: Re-do test
r_3: Do additional tests
r_4: Begin treatment

6. Diagnosis and Treatment of Heart Disease

6.1. Categories of Heart Disease

To illustrate these methods, a problem from medical decision making, analysis of chest pain in the emergency room, will be used. Medical systems represent an application in which numerous types of complex data are involved. These techniques are applicable to other areas which require complex reasoning.

When a patient presents to the emergency room with chest pain, it is vital to make a rapid decision regarding whether the patient should be hospitalized, and if so, if he or she should be assigned to a coronary care unit. Relevant information for this decision comes from number of sources, including description of symptoms, observable symptoms, patient history, ECG results, x-ray results, and blood analysis. The objective is to combine these data into one model which is capable of producing a rapid and accurate decision. The variables illustrated below have been selected to illustrate the different data types which have been described in the previous section.

6.2. Knowledge-Based Information

Typical rules and standard conditions (SC's) are illustrated in Figure 8. Note that a number of types of information are represented in these rules. Data types include integer, categoric, continuous, and binary. Variable types may be fuzzy or crisp, and temporal data are also included. The information in these rules was derived through expert input over a ten-year period. Expert-derived rules are always subject to change as medical knowledge improves, thus it is necessary to continually update the rule base.

Rule 010	IF		Blood Pressure < 100/60
			AND **SC_1**
	THEN		Patient should be admitted to CCU
Rule 020	IF		**SC_{10}**
	THEN		Patient should be admitted
Rule 030	IF		**SC_{15}**
			AND Associated with onset
	THEN		Patient should be observed
	SC_1	(OR)	Abnormal mental status
			Cold, clammy skin
			Gray, cyanotic skin
			Weak peripheral pulses
			Urinary output < 30 cc/hr
	SC_{10}	(AND)	Pain excruciating
			Pain unremitting
	SC_{15}	(COUNT 2)	Sweating
			Nausea
			Dizziness

Figure 8: Rules and SC's for Chest Pain Analysis

6.3. Data-Based Information

Some information may not be available through expert consultation. This is particularly true for new areas in which data are in the collection process, or in areas for which experts disagree about the relative importance of contributing factors. Some examples of items which appear to be crisp data in this system are listed below, along with the data type. In the following section, the interpretation of these same items as fuzzy data is presented.

6.3.1. Crisp Data

Some data items which appear to be crisp are listed here, along with their data types [31]:

- x_1: Duration of chest pain (Duration data)
- x_2: Change in diastolic blood pressure (Δ data)
- x_3: Number of PVC's per minute (normalized Δ data)
- x_4: Pain occurring before sweating occurring before nausea (sequence data)
- x_5: Abnormal ECG (Binary data)
- x_6: Type of Arrhythmia (Categoric data)
- x_7: Blood gas values (Continuous data)

6.3.2. Fuzzy Data

It is possible that some of the above variables can in fact be fuzzy variables. For x_1, the duration of chest pain may be approximate; instead of reporting 2 hours duration, a more likely response is "about 2 hours." This value can be represented as a fuzzy number, as illustrated above. For x_2, the change in blood pressure can be interpreted as fuzzy due to the approximate nature of the blood pressure reading. In this case, both readings would be approximate, and the difference would be computed using fuzzy subtraction as illustrated in equation (24). As x_3 is an actual count, it is inherently crisp. For x_4 the algorithm for partial presence of a sequence would be invoked (equation (21)). Although x_5 appears to be a straight-forward binary variable, in fact more information is imparted by indicating the degree of abnormality. Instead of entering a 0 or 1, a number between 0 and 10 can be entered which indicates the level of abnormality. As x_6 is strictly categoric, it could only be fuzzified if each category is considered separately, and a degree of membership is established for each category, as discussed above. In the case of x_7, the blood gas levels can be considered fuzzy numbers because of the limited accuracy of the test.

The decision of whether these variables should be included as crisp or fuzzy depends on the impact that the fuzzified version will have on the decision. This can be determined experimentally by establishing different models and comparing classification results.

6.3.3. *Chaotic Data*

Chaotic analysis is useful in many aspects of heart disease. For example, data obtained from twenty-four hour Holter monitoring of patients produces a record of electrocardiogram activity during normal day-to-day activities. Analysis of R-R intervals for the Holter data, which is the time between heart beats, yields interesting patterns. Typically, around 100,000 points are included in the twenty-four hour period. Figure 9 shows a second-order difference graph for the R-R intervals for a normal patient. By comparison, Figure 10 shows a patient with congestive heart failure. The visual difference is quite dramatic. The total number of points corresponding to Figures 9 and 10, respectively, are

$$t_{normal} = 104{,}443$$
$$t_{chf} = 109{,}374$$

Using equation (27), the corresponding central tendencies are as follows:

$$n_{normal} = 0.986$$
$$n_{chf} = 0.232$$

These numerical representations of central tendency can thus be included in the neural network model. Note that a rule could also be established in which a subjective measure of the degree of chaos is used.

6.4. *Sample System*

Figure 11 shows a consultation as it would appear to the user, invoking both the rule-based system and the neural network model where appropriate. The neural network model is imbedded in the rule-based model and is triggered by the invocation of certain rules. In addition to this direct connection, the neural network model is used to obtain weighting factors and thresholds for many of the rules in the knowledge-based program.

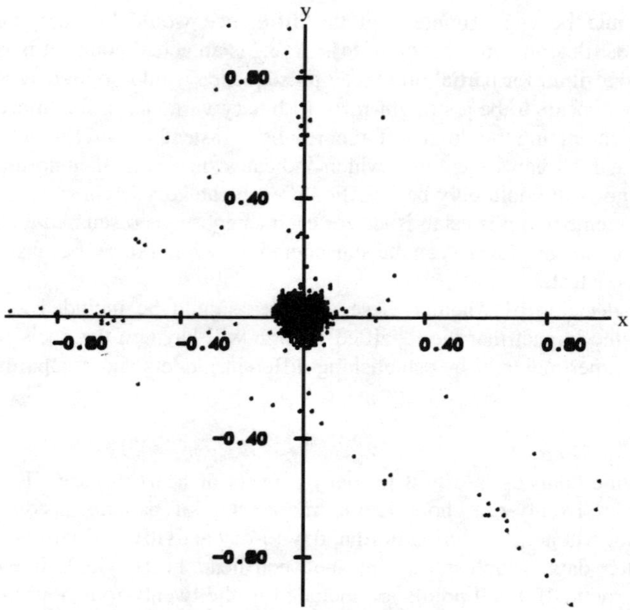

Figure 9: Second Order Difference Graph, Normal Patient, $x = hr_{t+1} - hr_t$, $y = hr_{t+2} - hr_{t+1}$

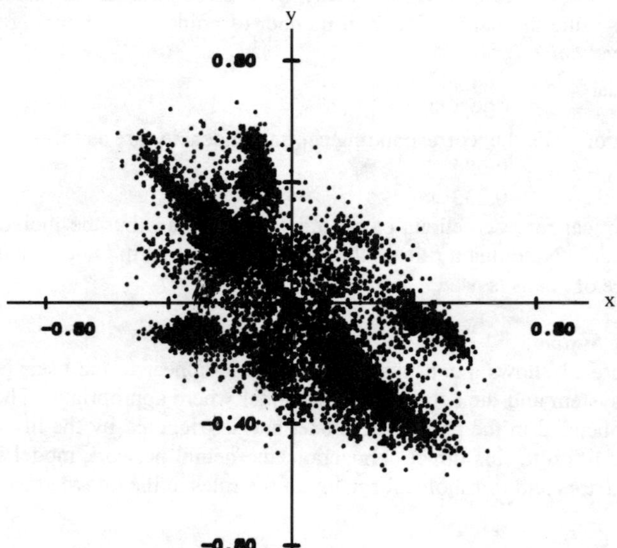

Figure 10: Second Order Difference Graph, Patient with CHF, $x = hr_{t+1} - hr_t$, $y = hr_{t+2} - hr_{t+1}$

Patient name: CH
Age: 73
Chief complaint: Recurrent chest pain
Hx of coronary problems y/n? y
Hx CAD y/n? y
Recent ETT data available y/n?: y
From ETT *(Neural Network)*

  Max ST depression in mm: 3.0
  HR at beginning of ETT: 94
  HR at end of ETT: 100
  BP at beginning of ETT: 133
  BP at end of ETT: 131

Hx of CHF y/n? y
Computer file of Holter data available y/n? y
Enter file name: CHholter *(Chaotic Analysis)*
List current symptoms, followed by a degree of severity between 0 (n) and 10 (y):

  Chest pain 7 *(Knowledge-Based System)*
  Sweating 9
  Syncope 6
  *

Dizziness? 8
Nausea? 6
Associated with onset? y

Patient should be admitted to hospital as inpatient.
ETT data indicate 2 vessel CAD
Holter data indicates significant chaos in R-R intervals related to CHF

Do you want an explanation of these conclusions? y

The following rules from the knowledge-based chest pain analysis were substantiated (in reverse order):

```
IF      Any 2 of
                Sweating
                Dizziness
                Nausea
        AND
                Associated with onset
THEN    Patient should be admitted
IF      Chest pain
THEN    Proceed to other symptom analysis
```

The neural network model for ETT concluded 2-vessel disease based on change in HR during test, change in BP during test, double produce of HR and BP, and maximum ST depression.

Chaotic analysis of R-R intervals from the 24-hr Holter tape indicates a central tendency of 57%, indicating a high level of variability.

Figure 11: Consultation

The information in italics in the consultation are not part of the system but are added to indicate the origin of the data. Note that the consultation contains a mixture of data types. However, the underlying complexity of the system is not apparent to the user. As shown, the user can obtain an explanation. When the neural network model is invoked, the variables used and their relative ranking are provided instead of a rule.

7. Conclusion

Although many clinically useful systems have been developed, they have been put to little practical use for a number of reasons. In order to become useful decision aids, these systems must provide relevant advice, be easy to use, and incorporate all available medical knowledge. The combination of expert input and information derived from accumulated data through automated learning algorithms ensures that all available information can be used in the same system.

Both knowledge-based systems and neural network models offer the advantage of providing easy updating to keep pace with changing medical knowledge. Because of the modular structure of the knowledge-based system, its rule base can be changed without any modification to the program, or inference engine, itself. Likewise, as new data are accumulated, a new neural network model can be generated simply by re-running the learning algorithm on the new data set. Thus these two approaches are not only adaptable to new medical knowledge, but in fact allow the same system to be utilized for different medical applications by replacement of the knowledge and data bases. Although in theory this is true, some systems will incorporate specific design features which may change with the application.

In the hybrid system presented here, the knowledge structure developed by the authors expands the usual production rule format to permit more complicated reasoning structures, and also allows complete departure from binary logic to permit reasoning with uncertainty.

The authors' neural network model is quite different from the back-propagation model in that results can be easily interpreted for clinical significance. Thus the results can be used to generate rules, if one prefers the knowledge-based format. The neural network model allows variables of all types to be used, including temporal and chaotic variables. The combined system provides a general framework for inclusion of medical knowledge from whatever source in whatever form.

8. References

1. R, Davis, D.B. Lenat, *Knowledge-Based Systems in Artificial Intelligence*, McGraw-Hill, New York (1982).
2. E. Patrick, F. Stelmock, L. Shen, Review of pattern recognition in medical diagnosis and consulting relative to a new system model, *IEEE Trans. on Systems, Man, and Cybernetics*, **SMC4(1)** (1974) 1-16.
3. F.T. deDombal, D. Leaper, J. Horrocks, J. Staniland, A. McCann, Human and computer-aided diagnosis of abdominal pain, *Brit. Med. J.* **1** (1974) 376-380.

4. M. Ben-Bassat, R. W. Carlson et al., Pattern-based interactive diagnosis of multiple disorders: The MEDUS system, *IEEE Trans. Pattern Analysis and Machine Intelligence* **PAMI-2** (1980) 148-160.
5. G.A. Gorry, Computer-assisted clinical decision making, *Method. Inform. Med.* **12** (1973) 45-51.
6. E.H. Shortliffe, *Computer-Based Medical Consultations, MYCIN*, Elsevier/North Holland, New York (1976).
7. P.L. Miller, P.R. Fisher, Causal models in medical artificial intelligence, in *Computer Applications in Medical Care*, IEEE Computer Society Press **11** (1987) 17-22.
8. W.R. Swartout, S.W. Smoliar, Explaining the link between causal reasoning and expert behavior, *Computer Applications in Medical Care*, IEEE Computer Society Press **11** (1987). 37-42.
9. S. Grossberg, *Neural Networks and Natural Intelligence*, MIT Press, Cambridge, MA (1988).
10. D.E. Rummelhart, J.L. McClelland and the PDP Research Group, *Parallel Distributed Processing*, vols. 1 and 2, MIT Press, Cambridge (1986).
11. N.J. Nilsson, *Learning Machines*, McGraw Hill, New York (1965).
12. B. Widrow, R. Winter, *Neural nets for adaptive filtering and adaptive pattern recognition*, Computer (March 1988) 25-39.
13. R.M.E. Sabbatini, Applications of connectionist systems in biomedicine, in K.C. Lun et al. (Eds.), *MEDINFO 92*, Elsevier Science Publishers (1992) 418-425.
14. Rocha, A. F., et al., A neural network for extracting knowledge from natural language data bases, *IEEE Trans. on Neural Networks*, **3(5)** (1992) 819-828.
15. A. Kandel, G. Langholz, *Hybrid Architectures for Intelligent Systems*, CRC Press (1992).
16. M.E. Cohen, D.L. Hudson, P.C. Deedwania, Pattern recognition analysis of coronary artery disease, in A. H. Levy, B. T. Williams, (Eds.): *American Association for Medical Systems and Informatics* (1985) 262-266.
17. D.L. Hudson, M.E. Cohen, An approach to management of uncertainty in a medical expert system, *International Journal of Intelligent Systems* **3(1)** (1988) 45-58.
18. M.E. Cohen, and D.L. Hudson, Integration of neural network techniques with approximate reasoning techniques in knowledge-based systems, in A. Kandel, G. Langholz, (Eds.): *Hybrid Architectures for Intelligent Systems*, CRC Press (1992) 72-85.
19. A.L. Goldberger, B.J. West, Fractals in physiology and medicine, *Yale Journal of Biology and Medicine* **50** (1987) 421-435.
20. A.L. Goldberger, Cardiac chaos, *Science*, **243 (2987)** (1989) 1419.
21. M.E. Cohen, D. L. Hudson, M.F. Anderson, Importance of sampling rate for analysis of hepatic blood flow data demonstrated by non-chaotic solution of Poincaré equation, in J.P. Morucci, et al. (Eds.): *Engineering in Medicine and Biology*, IEEE, Piscataway, NJ (1992) 982-983.
22. M.E. Cohen, D.L. Hudson, M.F. Anderson, A conjectured continuous approach to chaotic modeling, *Nonlinear Theory and Its Applications* (1993) 783-786.

23. M.E. Cohen, D.L. Hudson, M.F. Anderson, Blood flow data exhibit chaotic properties, *International Journal of Microcomputer Applications* **12(3)** (1993) 37-40.
24. D.L. Hudson, M.E. Cohen, P.W. Banda, M.S. Blois, Medical diagnosis and treatment plans derived from a hybrid expert system, in A. Kandel, G. Langholz (Eds.): *Hybrid Architectures for Intelligent Systems*, CRC Press (1992) 329-344.
25. D.L. Hudson, T. Estrin, EMERGE, a data-driven medical decision-making aid, *IEEE Transactions on Pattern Analysis and Machine Intelligence* **PAMI-6** (1984) 87-91.
26. R.R. Yager, Approximate reasoning as a basis for rule-based expert systems, *IEEE Transactions on Systems, Man, and Cybernetics*, vol. SMC-14, 4 (1984) 636-643.
27. D.L. Hudson, M.E. Cohen, Fuzzy logic in a medical expert system, in M. Gupta, T. Yamakawa, (Eds.): Fuzzy Computing: *Theory, Hardware Realization and Applications*, North Holland (1988) 273-284.
28. M.E. Cohen, D.L. Hudson, M.F. Anderson, A neural network learning algorithm with medical applications, in L. C. Kingsland, (Ed.): *Computer Applications in Medical Care*, , IEEE Computer Society Press, Washington **13** (1989) 307-311.
29. D.L. Hudson, M.E. Cohen, M.F. Anderson, Use of neural network techniques in a medical expert system, *International Journal of Intelligent Systems* **6(2)** (1991) 213-223.
30. M.E. Cohen, D.L. Hudson, J.J. Touya, P.C. Deedwania, A new multidimensional polynomial approach to medical pattern recognition problems, in R. Salamon, B. Blum, M. Jorgensen, (Eds.), *MEDINFO 86* (1986) 614-618.
31. D.L. Hudson, M.E. Cohen, Combination of spatial and temporal variables in a neural network model, *Proceedings, International Society for Computers and Their Applications* (1993) 69-73.
32. D.L. Hudson, M.E. Cohen, Approaches to handling of fuzzy input data in neural networks, *IEEE Conference on Fuzzy Systems* (1992) 93-100.
33. D. Dubois, H. Prade, *Fuzzy Sets and Systems: Theory and Applications*, **144** Academic Press, Orlando (1980).
34. D.L. Hudson, M.E. Cohen, Use of fractional powers to moderate neuronal contributions, *IEEE Conference on Neural Networks* (1993) 517-522.
35. D.L. Hudson, M.E. Cohen, A nonlinear neural network combined with symbolic processing, *Nonlinear Theory and Its Applications* (1993) 937-940.

INDEX

N

O

P